Advances in
Intervertebral Disc Disease in Dogs and Cats

Advances in Intervertebral Disc Disease in Dogs and Cats

Edited by

James M. Fingeroth
Orchard Park Veterinary Medical Center, USA

William B. Thomas
College of Veterinary Medicine, University of Tennessee, USA

WILEY Blackwell

Editorial Offices

1606 Golden Aspen Drive, Suites 103 and 104, Ames, Iowa 50014-8300, USA

The Atrium, Southern Gate, Chichester, West Sussex, PO19 8SQ, UK

9600 Garsington Road, Oxford, OX4 2DQ, UK

This Work is a co-publication between the American College of Veterinary Surgeons Foundation and Wiley-Blackwell.

For details of our global editorial offices, for customer services and for information about how
to apply for permission to reuse the copyright material in this book please see our website at
www.wiley.com/wiley-blackwell.

Library of Congress Cataloging-in-Publication Data

Advances in intervertebral disc disease in dogs and cats / edited by James M. Fingeroth,
William B. Thomas.
   p. ; cm.
  Includes bibliographical references and index.
  ISBN 978-0-470-95959-6 (cloth)
  1. Intervertebral disk–Diseases. 2. Dogs–Diseases. 3. Cats–Diseases. 4. Musculoskeletal system–Diseases.
I. Fingeroth, James M., editor. II. Thomas, William B., 1959– , editor.
  [DNLM: 1. Intervertebral Disc Degeneration–veterinary. 2. Cat Diseases–physiopathology. 3. Dog Diseases–
physiopathology. 4. Intervertebral Disc–physiology. 5. Intervertebral Disc Displacement–veterinary. SF 992.M86]
  SF992.M86A37 2015
  636.7'0896–dc23

                       2014029624

A catalogue record for this book is available from the British Library.

Wiley also publishes its books in a variety of electronic formats. Some content that appears in print may not be available in
electronic books.

Set in 9.5/11.5pt Palatino by SPi Publisher Services, Pondicherry, India
Printed and bound in Singapore by Markono Print Media Pte Ltd

Contents

Contributors

Filippo Adamo, DVM
Diplomate, European College of Veterinary
Neurologists
Chief, Section of Neurology/Neurosurgery
East Bay Veterinary Specialists
Walnut Creek, CA, USA

Kenneth Bartels, DVM, MS
McCartland Professor of Laser Surgery
Cohn Chair for Biophotonics
Department of Veterinary Clinical Sciences
Center for Veterinary Health Sciences
Oklahoma State University
Stillwater, OK, USA

Niklas Bergknut, DVM, PhD
Resident in Neurology
Department of Clinical Sciences of Companion
Animals
Faculty of Veterinary Medicine
Utrecht University
Utrecht
The Netherlands

James F. (Jeff) Biggart III, MS, DVM
President
Veterinary Surgical Services, Inc
Rancho Murieta, CA, USA

Brigitte A. Brisson, DMV, DVSc
Diplomate, American College of Veterinary
Surgeons
Professor of Small Animal
Surgery
Department of Clinical Studies
Ontario Veterinary College
University of Guelph
Guelph, ON
Canada

Claude Carozzo, DVM, PhD
Diplomate, European College of Veterinary
Surgeons
Ecole Nationale Vétérinaire de Lyon
Marcy l'étoile
France

Alexander de Lahunta, DVM, PhD
Diplomate, American College of Veterinary
Internal Medicine (Neurology)
Diplomate, American College of Veterinary
Pathologists (Honorary)
Emeritus James Law Professor
of Anatomy
College of Veterinary Medicine
Cornell University
Ithaca, NY, USA

Luisa De Risio, DMV, MRCVS, PhD
Diplomate, European College of Veterinary
Neurology
Head of Neurology/Neurosurgery
Animal Health Trust
Lanwades Park
Kentford, Newmarket
Suffolk
UK

**Michael Farrell, BVetMed, CertVA,
CertSAS**
Diplomate, European College of Veterinary
Surgeons
Fitzpatrick Referrals
Halfway lane
Eashing
Godalming
Surrey
UK

Amy E. Fauber, DVM, MS
Diplomate, American College of Veterinary
Surgeons
Diplomate, American College of Veterinary
Internal Medicine (Neurology)
Assistant Professor of Small Animal Surgery
and Neurology
Department of Veterinary Clinical
Sciences
Purdue University College of Veterinary
Medicine
West Lafayette, IN, USA

James M. Fingeroth, DVM
Diplomate, American College of Veterinary
Surgeons
Senior Staff Surgeon
Orchard Park Veterinary Medical
Center
Orchard Park, NY, USA

**Noel Fitzpatrick, MVB, MRCVS, D Univ CVR,
DSAS (Ortho)**
Diplomate, American College of
Veterinary Sports Medicine and
Rehabilitation
Director, Fitzpatrick Referrals
Professor of Veterinary Orthopaedics
University of Surrey
Guildford, Surrey UK

Franck Forterre, Dr Med Vet
Diplomate, European College of Veterinary
Surgeons
Professor of Neurosurgery
Small Animal Clinic
Vetsuisse Faculty of Bern
Bern
Switzerland

Patrick R. Gavin, DVM, PhD
Diplomate, American College of Veterinary
Radiology (Radiology and Radiation Oncology)
Emeritus Professor of Radiology
College of Veterinary Medicine
University of Washington
Pullman, WA
President, MR Vets
Sagle, ID, USA

Ragnvi Hagman, DVM, MSc, PhD
Associate Professor in Small Animal Surgery
Department of Clinical Sciences
Swedish University of Agricultural Sciences
Uppsala, Sweden

Michael J. Higginbotham, DVM
Diplomate, American College of Veterinary
Internal Medicine (Neurology)
Bush Veterinary Neurology Service
Richmond, VA, USA

**John F. Innes, BVSc, PhD, MRCVS, CertVR,
DSAS (Ortho)**
Professor of Small Animal Surgery
RCVS Specialist in Small Animal Surgery
(Orthopaedics)
Department of Musculoskeletal Biology
Institute of Aging and Chronic Disease
School of Veterinary Science
University of Liverpool
Leahurst Campus
Neston, UK

Sharon Kerwin, DVM, MS
Diplomate, American College of Veterinary
Surgeons
Professor of Small Animal Surgery
Department of Small Animal Clinical Sciences
College of Veterinary Medicine and Biomedical
Sciences
Texas A&M University
College Station, TX, USA

Otto I. Lanz, DVM
Diplomate, American College of Veterinary
Surgeons
Associate Professor of Surgery
Department of Small Animal Clinical Sciences
Virginia-Maryland Regional College of Veterinary
Medicine
Virginia Tech
Blacksburg, VA, USA

Steven D. Lasser, MD
Fellow, American Academy of Orthopaedic
Surgeons
Orthopaedic Spine Surgery
Interlakes Orthopaedics/Geneva (NY) General
Hospital/
Rochester (NY) General Hospital
Chief of Staff
Geneva General Hospital
Geneva, NY, USA

Gwendolyn J. Levine, DVM
Diplomate, American College of Veterinary
Pathologists (Clinical Pathology)
Department of Veterinary Pathobiology
College of Veterinary Medicine and Biomedical
Sciences
Texas A&M University
College Station, TX, USA

Jonathan M. Levine, DVM
Diplomate, American College of Veterinary
Internal Medicine (Neurology)
Associate Professor, Neurology and
Neurosurgery
Chief, Section of Surgery
Department of Small Animal Clinical Sciences
College of Veterinary Medicine
Texas A&M University
College Station, TX, USA

Joseph M. Mankin, DVM
Diplomate, American College of Veterinary
Internal Medicine (Neurology)
Clinical Assistant Professor
Department of Small Animal Clinical Sciences
College of Veterinary Medicine
Texas A&M University
College Station, TX, USA

James Melrose, Bsc (Hons), PhD
Honorary Senior Research Fellow
Department of Surgery, North Clinical School
E25-Royal North Shore Hospital
College of Medicine
The University of Sydney
Sydney, New South Wales
Australia

Natasha Olby, Vet MB, PhD, MRCVS
Diplomate, American College of Veterinary
Internal Medicine (Neurology)
Professor, Neurology and Neurosurgery
Department of Clinical Sciences
College of Veterinary Medicine
North Carolina State University
Raleigh, NC, USA

Núria Vizcaíno Revés, DVM
Small Animal Clinic
Vetsuisse Faculty of Bern
Bern
Switzerland

Lucas A. Smolders, Dr Med Vet, DVM, PhD
Vetsuisse Faculty of Zurich
Small Animal Clinic
Zurich University
Zurich
Switzerland

William B. Thomas, DVM, MS
Diplomate, American College of Veterinary
Internal Medicine (Neurology)
Professor, Neurology and Neurosurgery
Department of Small Animal Clinical
Sciences
College of Veterinary Medicine
University of Tennessee
Knoxville, TN, USA

Rick Wall, DVM
Certified Canine Rehabilitation Practitioner
American Academy of Pain Management
Certified Myofascial Trigger Point Therapist
Center for Veterinary Pain Management and
Rehabilitation
The Woodlands, TX, USA

Foreword

Hippocrates (460–370 B.C.), perhaps the most prominent physician of the distant past, is recognized as a founder of scientific medicine. The bases of the Hippocratic method were *accurate observation* and *sound reasoning*. The Hippocratic study of medicine attributed diseases to "natural causes," thereby eradicating the concept of "luck" as a creative force. This application of scientific method to medicine was revolutionary, as the thinking of the time is epitomized in the works of the philosopher Plato (fifth to fourth century B.C.) who believed that "a divine intervention contributed to the creation of the flexible spine," or the famous philosopher and physician Empedocles (fifth century B.C.), who suggested that at birth the spine was rigid, and that subsequently this osseous column was broken into pieces as a result of body movements.

Hippocrates considered knowledge of vertebral column anatomy essential to physicians: "One should first get a knowledge of the structure of the spine; for this is also requisite for many diseases." Centuries later, an eminent physician of the time, Galen (second century A.D.), promoted this principle, and criticized physicians for their ignorance of the structure of the vertebral column.

What might Hippocrates have accomplished with modern technology such as magnetic resonance imaging, computed tomography, balanced anesthesia regimens, advanced surgical instrumentation, and force plate analysis? Throughout history, great minds have been limited only by the technology of the time.

Perhaps, it is the lack of technology available at the time he made his observations that makes Hippocrates' findings so significant. Hippocrates was forced to substitute *thought* and *reasoning* for technology. He actually had to think through problems, and to reason solutions. Hippocrates had to observe what was in front of him and describe things for the first time. Because of his thorough study of spinal diseases and their management, which was the first such study in orthopedics in the history of medicine, Hippocrates should be regarded as the *father of spine surgery*.

Now let's jump forward to the present day of *evidence-based veterinary medicine*, where technology is available to address some of the questions previously addressed by means of thought and reasoning alone.

Evidence-based veterinary medicine may be defined as the conscientious, judicious, and explicit use of current best evidence in making decisions about individual patients. The practice of evidence-based veterinary medicine means integrating *individual clinical expertise* with the *best available external clinical evidence* obtained from systematic research.

- *Individual clinical expertise* describes the proficiency and judgment that individual clinicians acquire through clinical experience and clinical practice. This includes the essential aspects of the Hippocratic method—namely, accurate observation and sound reasoning.
- *Best available external clinical evidence* describes an aspect of evidence-based medicine that was denied to Hippocrates because of a lack of technology—namely, the results of clinically relevant research.

It should be noted that the best available external clinical evidence is not restricted to double-blinded, randomized, placebo-controlled, prospective trials with quantifiable and reliable outcome assessments. Nor is it restricted to meta-analyses. Results of such studies may be considered the "gold standard" for some types of evidence, particularly when addressing the efficacy of a particular therapeutic approach. However, results of such studies cannot take the place of the individual clinical expertise that is necessary to decide whether the external evidence applies to an individual patient, and if so, how it should be integrated into a clinical decision.

The chapters included in this book are written by authors who understand that evidence-based veterinary medicine is not "cookbook" veterinary medicine. The authors also understand that management of intervertebral disc (IVD) disease in an individual patient requires careful integration of both the best external evidence and the best individual clinical expertise. Without individual clinical expertise, the management of IVD disease risks becoming "tyrannized" by evidence, for even outstanding external evidence may be inappropriate for an individual patient or an individual situation. On the other hand, without the continual generation of best available external clinical evidence, management of IVD disease risks becoming outdated to the detriment of patients.

Several major developments have led to the present base of knowledge that permits the publication of this book. In this context, I would like to attempt an explanation of the reasons I am well qualified to write the Foreword to this extraordinary book.

In 1951, Dr Sten-Erik Olsson (1921–2000) published his doctoral thesis titled "On Disc Protrusion in the Dog." Sten-Erik was both a human physician and a veterinarian, and an imposing figure in every sense of the word.

At a 1986 conference on IVD disease in Lund, Sweden, Sten-Erik and I were speakers on the program along with a legend in the field of vertebral column veterinary radiology, Dr Joe Morgan. After each of my presentations, Sten-Erik would correct all the "information" I had shared, not privately, but in front of the entire conference. At one stage, he had prepared his own set of slides to project after one of my lectures to debate some of the assertions I had made! I learned more during those days than anyone else at the conference. For example, I learned that data are not the plural for anecdote and that the beginning of wisdom is to call things by their correct names. In addition, I survived a focused lesson in evidence-based veterinary medicine. This experience profoundly influenced my career.

The face page of Sten-Erik's landmark publication is something I still retain and cherish, along with Sten-Erik's message to me written after we had been debating aspects of IVD disease for several days. The significance of this publication, as Sten-Erik stated to the entire audience, was that he had published this landmark work "in the year Rick was born." This publication is a reminder of the importance of distinguishing data, information, knowledge, understanding, and wisdom, in the application of clinical expertise to an individual patient with clinical signs of IVD disease.

Sten-Erik and I remained good friends until he died in 2000. In my opinion, Sten-Erik Olsson is "the Hippocrates of canine IVD disease." It was during those valuable lessons he imparted all those years ago that I learned that individual clinical expertise and best available evidence must be applied *together* to effect the best strategies for management of IVD disease in an individual patient.

It is an honor to have been asked to write the Foreword to this book, edited by two of the most experienced and talented veterinarians in the fields of surgery, neurology, and neurosurgery. I have been privileged to have known Drs Fingeroth and Thomas for many years. Careful reading of the Preface of this book reveals much about these two clinicians, researchers, and teachers, and I highly recommend that the Preface be read before a reader proceeds to delve into the chapters within this volume. The contributions of a remarkable group of authors have been included in this most comprehensive body of information on IVD disease in dogs and cats to date. The authors have successfully combined the Hippocratic method of *accurate observation and sound reasoning* with the *best available external clinical evidence* to produce a landmark work.

Rick LeCouteur, BVSc, PhD,
Diplomate ACVIM (Neurology),
Diplomate ECVN
Professor of Neurology & Neurosurgery
University of California, Davis,
California, USA

Bibliography

Marketos SG, Skiadas P: Hippocrates: The Father of Spine Surgery. Spine 24(13):1381–1387, 1999.
Morgan JP: Sten-Erik Olsson. Vet Radiol & Ultrasound 41(6):581–583, 2000.
Sackett DL et al.: Evidence based medicine: What it is and what it isn't. BMJ 312:71–72, 1996.

Foreword

The American College of Veterinary Surgeons Foundation is excited to present *Advances in Intervertebral Disc Disease in Dogs and Cats* in the book series titled *Advances in Veterinary Surgery*. The ACVS Foundation is an independently charted philanthropic organization devoted to advancing the charitable, educational, and scientific goals of the American College of Veterinary Surgeons. Founded in 1965, the ACVS sets the standards for the specialty of veterinary surgery. The ACVS, which is approved by the American Veterinary Medical Association, administers the board certification process for diplomates in veterinary surgery and advances veterinary surgery and education. One of the principal goals of the ACVS Foundation is to foster the advancement of the art and science of veterinary surgery. The Foundation achieves these goals by supporting investigations in the diagnosis and treatment of surgical diseases; increasing educational opportunities for surgeons, surgical residents, and veterinary practitioners; improving surgical training of residents and veterinary students; and bettering animal patients' care, treatment, and welfare. This collaboration with Wiley-Blackwell will benefit all who are interested in veterinary surgery by presenting the latest evidence-based information on a particular surgical topic.

Advances in Intervertebral Disc Disease in Dogs and Cats is edited by Drs James Fingeroth and William Thomas. Dr Fingeroth is a diplomate of the American College of Veterinary Surgeons, and Dr Thomas is a diplomate of the American College of Veterinary Internal Medicine (Neurology). Both are prominent in their fields of neurosurgery and neurology, particularly as it applies to intervertebral disc disease of dogs and cats. They have assembled the leaders in this field presenting the structure and function of the intervertebral disc, the pathophysiology of disc disease in dogs and cats, the clinical features of intervertebral disc disease, and the surgical management of this important condition. They conclude this series with future directions in the field. The ACVS Foundation is proud to partner with Wiley-Blackwell in this important series and is honored to present this book in the series.

Mark D. Markel
Chair, Board of Trustees
ACVS Foundation

Preface

Clinical syndromes related to the vertebral column are among the most common and consternating problems addressed by general practitioners, emergency clinicians, diagnostic imagers, neurologists, and surgeons. Of the various causes for neck and back pain, pain referred to a limb, gait disturbance, and sphincter disturbance, intervertebral disc disease (IVDD) in its several guises is certainly the most prevalent etiology in dogs and is occasionally identified in cats. And even when the cause for such signs is something other than IVDD, there is often a *presumption* of IVDD by many clinicians who too often assume that IVDD underlies all such spinal syndromes. Yet, despite the commonness of clinical disorders related to the intervertebral disc, and decades of clinical experience in diagnosing and treating these disorders, there remains among all of the aforementioned groups of veterinarians (and their staffs and clientele) a substantial and sometimes astounding array of differing thought processes with respect to the criteria for appropriate diagnostic testing, the type and timing of interventions for treatment, and the prognostication for outcome. Moreover, while IVDD has been addressed in its various component parts in scattershot fashion in journals and previous texts, there has never been a single comprehensive source focused solely on all the aspects related to the intervertebral disc and its

diseases. While there may not be one universally agreed-upon consensus that can be derived from the extant knowledge base on how to diagnose and treat IVDD, there should be an effort to at least get everyone "on the same page," and identify those things we know as facts, those things we speculate are true but perhaps lack sufficient evidence for, and those areas that, even as they remain controversial, ensure that we establish a common framework for arguing our theories.

To this end, the book herein is an attempt to identify areas of established fact as well as areas of established controversy, with an effort to cogently describe what we know, what we don't know, and what we speculate is true in all the areas related to intervertebral disc disease. As with any textbook, we expect subsequent discoveries and developments to confirm some of the material presented, refute some material, and perhaps render some of it obsolete. But, even in the face of such natural expansion of knowledge, we anticipate that this book will remain a solid foundation from which present and future readers will still be able to find, in a single source, a compilation of subject areas, topics, and expression of opinion that will continue to be germane to the understanding and treatment of IVDD.

As experienced clinicians working in academia and referral centers, we have been exposed to the wide array of thought processes, dogma, and extreme variations in knowledge that guides our veterinary students, interns, residents, general practitioners, emergency clinicians, and fellow specialists when considering the issue of "IVDD." Each of these groups of veterinary professionals is our target audience in presenting this book. For the specialists, our goal is to compile, in a single place, all the currently existing reference material that touches upon issues related to the intervertebral disc in dogs and cats. For the nonspecialists, our goal is to provide a core of material that will enhance their understanding of IVDD, help them in dispensing with dogma, and provide a sound scientific and clinical basis for decision making as they confront patients suspected of having some form of IVDD. We may not settle every area of controversy, and we expect some of what is

presented to perhaps stir up new controversy. But regardless of our ability to "settle, once and for all" any of the disagreements that exist in our understanding or management of IVDD, we hope this book at least establishes a common playing field, where each of these controversies are acknowledged and discussed, and where each of the reader groups mentioned can more fully understand the basis for any disagreements or controversies that persist. If we are successful, we anticipate this book becoming a valuable reference to the clinician on the front lines, perhaps drawing readers to a more centralized and common understanding of IVDD and its management, and ultimately improving the quality of care offered to our patients.

JMF
WBT

Acknowledgments

Perhaps only those who have preceded me in cajoling colleagues into contributing to a multiauthor text can truly appreciate the efforts required to translate an initial concept into a publishable tome. I for one did not imagine what a painstaking and ultimately drawn-out process this would be. But it is precisely because of the knowledge, expertise, collegiality, patience, and friendship of those contributors and my coeditor that we are now able to offer what we hope will be a cogent treatise on the subject of intervertebral disc disease. To all those who have written within, my heartfelt thanks.

When it comes to patience and forbearance, no one deserves more acknowledgment than the two people at Wiley-Blackwell who have shepherded this book from its inception to the volume that now rests in your hands. Thank you to Erica Judisch and Susan Engelken!

This book is part of a series sponsored by the ACVS Foundation. To the Foundation trustees I express my deep appreciation for approving this project initially, and then waiting patiently for it to be completed. It is my sincere hope that the final product has matched their expectations, and will sit proudly next to the other excellent texts in the series *Advances in Veterinary Surgery*.

I can make no claim to being a great neurosurgeon or scholar. My ability to conceive this project, to draw upon the expertise of others, and to synthesize those things that I have encountered and learned over the past 30-plus years of my veterinary education, I owe to the mentors, residents, interns, and patients I have worked with over that time. It has been both humbling and my great pleasure to have been educated by and exposed to some truly legendary figures in the fields of veterinary neurology and surgery. And it is some of the intense disagreement between and differing viewpoints held by those mentors that has helped me both avoid a lot of strict dogma, and force me to formulate my own opinions based on the evidence. It is that attitude that has guided me in the formulation of this book.

My late father always thought I would one day write a book. I don't know if this is what he conceived, but it does remind me of the importance of and support from my family as I have traveled through my education and life. And family of course can be no more valuable than the ones who share our day-to-day lives, especially when it comes to the hours sacrificed at the computer, or listening to one's venting about the various problems and obstacles that turn up during the writing and editing of a book. So, how can I say "thank you" strongly enough to my wife, Robbie, for her indulgence as I hammered away at this text these past few years? But anyway, thank you!

Finally, any one of us in this profession of veterinary medicine could have earned more money and had more prestige had we become physicians, and done almost exactly what we do now, but with human patients. We are here, most of us, because of our abiding love for animals and interest in using our scientific talents to bettering their lives. It is therefore to my patients, and to the animals in my life who have been my own "fur kids," that I really dedicate this book, and who deserve acknowledgment as the inspiration for what I and all of us do.

James M. Fingeroth

I would like to thank the many contributors who unselfishly shared their expertise and experience and Erica Judisch and Susan Engelken at Wiley-Blackwell for their dedicated editorial assistance in the preparation of this book.

I am indebted to the neurology residents I have worked with at the University of Tennessee—Avril Arendse, Christina Wolf, Joe Mankin, Amy Hodshon, Curtis Probst, Lindsay Williams, Jennifer Michaels and German Venegas—who have taught me more than I could ever have taught them. I could not get through a day in the hospital without the help of Karen McLucas.

Most importantly, thanks to Sherri, Emelie, and Jenna for their love and support.

William Thomas

Section I

Intervertebral Disc Structure and Function

The causes and consequences of intervertebral disc (IVD) degeneration and clinical disease are best understood in the context of the normal anatomy, physiology, and biomechanics of the IVD itself and its relationship with spinal function. In the following chapters, these fundamental principles are elucidated. And because IVD disease (IVDD) afflicts both domestic animals and humans, we include a chapter that compares and contrasts IVDD in dogs and people. The last has esoteric value, but also can be clinically useful in that many clients have or know someone who has "back problems" or a "slipped disc," and may make erroneous assumptions and extrapolations when trying to understand IVDD that has been diagnosed in their pet.

Embryology, Innervation, Morphology, Structure, and Function of the Canine Intervertebral Disc

John F. Innes and James Melrose

Introduction

The intervertebral disc (IVD) is composed of a disparate collection of connective tissues of differing structure and function, and it is the dynamic interplay of these components in the composite IVD which endows it with its unique ability to withstand tensional stresses, to act as a viscoelastic hydrodynamic weight-bearing cushion, and to provide spinal flexibility [1]. While the cross-sectional area and angulation of IVDs vary with spinal level, all share common structural features. The outer region of the IVD, the annulus fibrosus (AF), is a collagen-rich tissue, while the central region of the IVD, the nucleus pulposus (NP), is rich in proteoglycans. The intervening region between the AF and NP is called the transitional zone (TZ). The areas of the IVD that interface with the adjacent vertebral bodies are called the cartilaginous end plates (CEPs); these are hyaline-like cartilaginous tissues containing cells of a rounded chondrocyte-like morphology.

Embryology of the IVD

During gastrulation, three somatic germ cell layers are initially laid down in the developing embryo: outer ectodermal, middle mesodermal, and inner endodermal layers [2–4]. A midline longitudinal rod-shaped column of the mesoderm, the notochord, subsequently develops from cell aggregates located between the ectoderm and endoderm and establishes cranial/caudal and ventral/dorsal axes in the developing embryo [2]. Ectoderm dorsal to the notochord gives rise to the neuroectoderm from which the neural tube develops. Adjacent mesodermal tissue develops into discrete tissue units, termed as the somites [5]. The somites consist of three tissue types: (1) the dermatome which gives rise to the dermis, (2) the myotome which gives rise to the axial musculature, and (3) the sclerotome from which vertebral structures arise. Cells of the sclerotome migrate medially and ventrally to form a continuous tube of mesenchymal cells (the perichordal sheath)

Advances in Intervertebral Disc Disease in Dogs and Cats, First Edition. Edited by James M. Fingeroth and William B. Thomas.
© 2015 ACVS Foundation. Published 2015 by John Wiley & Sons, Inc.

which surround the notochord. Increased proliferation of cells at regular lengths along the perichordal tube creates areas of low and high cell density from which the vertebrae and AF, TZ, and spinal ligaments develop [5]. Formation of the vertebral bodies results in segmentation of the notochord. Each notochordal segment persists in the central region of the developing IVD to give rise to the NP [3]. Thus, during embryonic disc development, cells of the AF are derived from the sclerotome, whereas the NP originates from the notochord [3]. In nonchondrodystrophoid breeds, notochordal cells persist into adulthood, whereas in chondrodystrophoid breeds they disappear within 2 years of birth. This correlates with an earlier onset of IVD degeneration in chondrodystrophoid breeds.

Innervation of the IVD

There are major neuroanatomical differences between the human and canine spines in terms of how far the spinal cord extends along the vertebral canal. In humans, the spinal cord extends as far as the second lumbar vertebra with nerves exiting the spinal cord descending inside the remaining lumbar and sacral vertebral segments to exit through their respective foramina. The spinal cord in dogs ends at approximately L6 with nerves that serve the IVDs descending through the last lumbar, sacral and coccygeal vertebral segments. The canine cervical IVDs are served by 8 pairs of nerves, the thoracic IVDs have 13 pairs, the lumbar IVDs have 7 pairs, and the coccygeal region contains 2 nerves per IVD.

The human lumbar IVD is innervated by several nerves. The sinuvertebral nerve (meningeal rami) innervates the posterior (i.e., dorsal) aspect of the disc and the posterior (dorsal) longitudinal ligament. Branches from the rami communicantes innervate the lateral aspects of the disc and the anterior (ventral) longitudinal ligament [6]. A structure similar to the sinuvertebral nerve is not apparent in the canine thoracolumbar spine and in contrast to the human IVD, sensory nerves are sparse in the outermost annular lamellae. However, the dorsal longitudinal ligament is innervated profusely [7]. The nerves in the outer AF communicate with caudal and cranial spinal levels two positions removed from the actual site of annular innervation,

which explains the referred pain reported at sites distant from damaged annular nerves.

Obvious postural differences in man and dogs and effects on IVD loading contribute to differences in the resolution of forces along the spine and the incidence and distribution of spinal neurological deficits of clinical relevance [8, 9]. The upright stance of humans results in axial spinal forces being transferred down the spinal column to the lumbar region and it is this region that has the highest incidence of IVD degeneration. Posterior lumbar IVD prolapse in man can lead to significant generation of sciatic pain and impairment in mobility; however, paralysis is rarely encountered. In the canine spine, the juncture of the immobile thoracic and mobile lumbar spine is the region that has the highest incidence of disc herniation. Furthermore, since the spinal cord extends to this level in dogs, compression of the spinal cord by extruded disc material can have a significant neurological impact [10–12]. IVD degenerative diseases are generally more common in the chondrodystrophoid breeds than nonchondrodystrophoid breeds and more prevalent in older than younger dogs [13, 14] (Figure 1.1). The clinical presentation of thoracolumbar disc herniation in dogs can be severe with profound paralysis of their pelvic limbs from the resulting spinal cord damage [15]. The thoracolumbar vertebral canal is almost entirely filled by the spinal cord, and there is very little extradural space, which explains why herniations in canine thoracolumbar IVDs are so debilitating [16].

IVD morphology, structure, and function

The immature nonchondrodystrophoid canine IVD has an extremely gelatinous NP that with age becomes progressively more fibrous and less hydrated with the decline in proteoglycan levels (Figure 1.1 A). IVDs of chondrodystrophoid canine breeds have a relatively fibrous NP (Figure 1.1 B). The NP is surrounded by well-defined collagenous annular lamellae (Figure 1.1 B). Calcification of the NP occurs in the chondrodystrophoid canine breeds but infrequently in nonchondrodystrophoid dogs (Figure 1.1 C).

The annular lamellae contain collagenous fibers of type I and II collagen, which comprise 40–60%

COLLAGENOUS
ANNULAR LAMELLAE

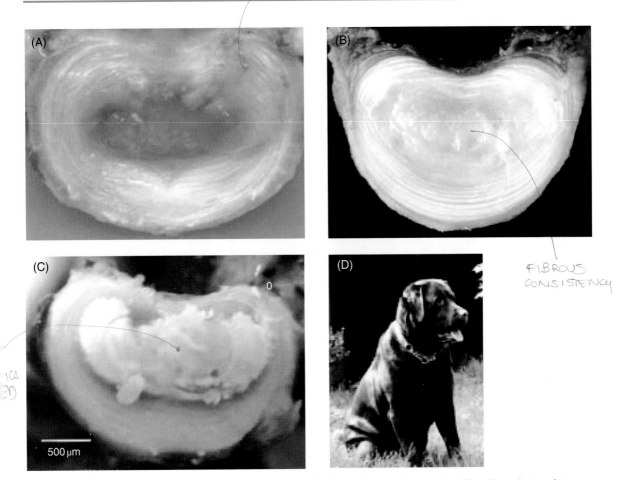

FIBROUS
CONSISTENCY

Figure 1.1   Composite figure depicting macroviews of horizontally bisected lumbar intervertebral discs demonstrating their characteristic morphology with the peripheral annular lamellae clearly evident and central nucleus pulposus. Discs typical of nonchondrodystrophic (A) and chondrodystrophic (B, C) canine breeds are shown. In plate (A), the nucleus pulposus is gelatinous, while in (B) the nucleus pulposus has a fibrous consistency typical of a chondrodystrophic breed (beagle). In plate (C), the entire nucleus pulposus has undergone calcification (Hansen type I). Plate (D) depicts an example of typical nonchondrodystrophic canine breed, labrador retriever. Labradors typically present with disc degeneration at ages of 5–12 years. Figures (A) and (C) supplied by courtesy of Dr PN. Bergknut, Faculty of Veterinary Medicine, Utrecht University.

of the dry weight of the outer annulus and 25–40% of the inner annulus. Type I and II collagens are radially distributed in opposing gradients from the disc periphery to the NP with the concentration of type I collagen greatest in the outer AF, while type II collagen predominates in the NP (Figure 1.2 A, B, D, and E). The tension-bearing properties of the AF are principally conveyed by type I collagen fiber bundles; however, the resistance to compression provided by the NP is provided by proteoglycans (aggrecan) and their associated hydration entrapped within a type II collagen network (Figure 1.2C and F). Collagen fibers are virtually inextensible and their major role is in the provision of tensile strength. Elastin fibers located in intralamellar margins interconnect adjacent lamellae and return the fully extended collagen fibers to their preloaded dimensions. The elastin content of the IVD is small (1–2%) but nevertheless essential in the provision of elastic material properties [17]. Type I collagen fiber bundles insert firmly but imperceptibly with the CEPs and underlying vertebral bone to form anchorage points for the IVD to adjacent bony structures (Figures 1.2G–I).

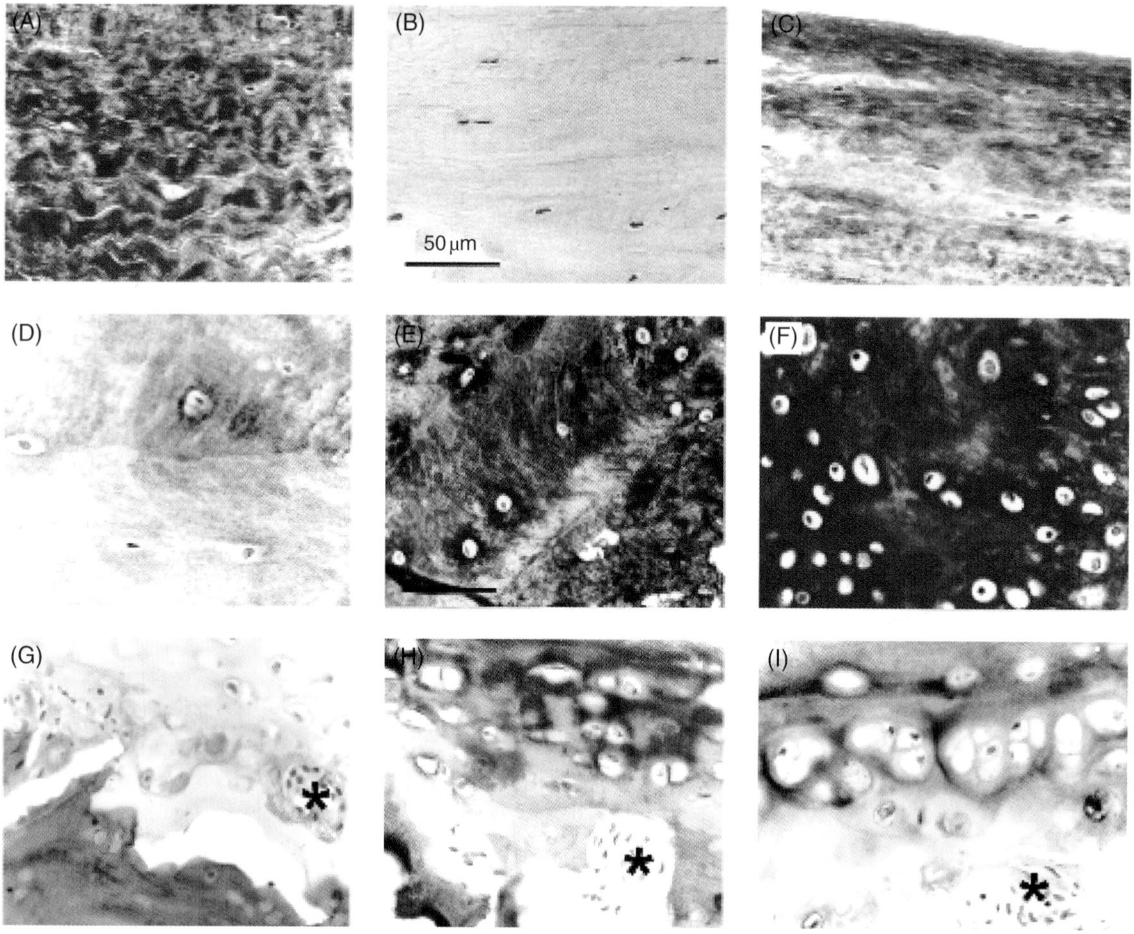

Figure 1.2   Composite figure depicting the immunolocalization of type I (A, D, G) and type II collagen (B, E, H) and the major space-filling and water-imbibing disc proteoglycan aggrecan (C, F, I) in the outer annulus fibrosus (A–C), inner annulus fibrosus/nucleus pulposus (D–B), and cartilaginous end plate (G–I). Plate (A) depicts strong localization of type I collagen displaying a crimp pattern in the outer annulus fibrosus. This is consistent with the hoop stresses generated within and tensional forces carried by this tissue. The outer annulus fibrosus is devoid of type II collagen (B) while it contains a sparse distribution of aggrecan (C). The characteristic elongated fibroblastic morphology of the annular cells is also evident (A–C). The inner annulus fibrosus/nucleus pulposus contains a little type I collagen (D) but is rich in type II collagen (E) and aggrecan (F). The cells in this region of the intervertebral disc display a characteristic rounded morphology (E–F). The cartilaginous end plate is a hyaline cartilage-like tissue that forms the interface of the intervertebral disc with the vertebral bodies (G–I). This tissue also contains cells of a rounded chondrocytic morphology surrounded by type II collagen (H) and aggrecan (I) but does not contain type I collagen (G), while the underlying vertebral bone is stained positively for type I collagen (G). The cartilaginous end plate has important roles to play in the nutrition of the disc cells with small blood vessels (*) clearly in evidence in the underlying vertebral vascular bed (G–I). The intervertebral discs shown are vertical midsaggital sections from an L1–L2 disc of a 2-year-old French bulldog, a typical chondrodystrophic canine breed.

The NP acts as a viscoelastic hydrodynamic cushion that counters compressive loading of the spine. Upon axial loading of the spine, compression of the NP results in load transference to the AF which is arranged in collagenous lamellar layers with collagen fiber bundles arranged at a 50–60° angle relative to one another in adjacent lamellae (Figure 1.3). This results in bulging of the annular lamellae with the generation of hoop stresses that dissipate axial compressive forces.

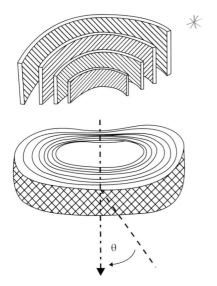

Figure 1.3 Schematic depiction of the lamellar structure of the annulus fibrosus in a partially exploded view and surrounding the central nucleus pulposus with the parallel arrays of collagen fiber bundles indicated oriented at 50–60° (q) relative to collagen fiber bundles in adjacent lamellae in the transverse plane.

References

1. Bray JP, Burbidge HM. The canine intervertebral disk: part one: structure and function. J Am Anim Hosp Assoc. 1998 Jan–Feb;34(1):55–63.
2. Sinowatz F. Musculoskeletal system. In: Hyttel P SF, Veijlstad M, editors. Essentials of domestic animal embryology 1st edition. Edinburgh, London, NY, Oxford, Philadelphia, St. Louis, Sydney, Toronto: Saunders, Elsevier; 2010. pp. 286–316.
3. Risbud MV, Schaer TP, Shapiro IM. Toward an understanding of the role of notochordal cells in the adult intervertebral disc: from discord to accord. Dev Dyn. 2010 Aug;239(8):2141–8.
4. Smits P, Lefebvre V. Sox5 and Sox6 are required for notochord extracellular matrix sheath formation, notochord cell survival and development of the nucleus pulposus of intervertebral discs. Development. 2003 Mar;130(6):1135–48.
5. MacGeady TA QP, FitzPatrick ES. Muscular and skeletal systems. In: MacGeady TA QP, FitzPatrick ES, editors. Veterinary Embryology. Oxford: Blackwell Publishing; 2006. pp. 184–204.
6. Bogduk N, Tynan W, Wilson AS. The nerve supply to the human lumbar intervertebral discs. J Anat. 1981 Jan;132(Pt 1):39–56.
7. Forsythe WB, Ghoshal NG. Innervation of the canine thoracolumbar vertebral column. Anat Rec. 1984 Jan;208(1):57–63.
8. Verheijen J, Bouw J. Canine intervertebral disc disease: a review of etiologic and predisposing factors. Vet Q. 1982;4(3):125–34.
9. Miller JA, Schmatz C, Schultz AB. Lumbar disc degeneration: correlation with age, sex, and spine level in 600 autopsy specimens. Spine (Phila Pa 1976). 1988 Feb;13(2):173–8.
10. Gage E. Incidence of clinical disc disease in the dog. J Am Anim Hosp Assoc. 1975;135:135–8.
11. Goggin JE, Li AS, Franti CE. Canine intervertebral disk disease: characterization by age, sex, breed, and anatomic site of involvement. Am J Vet Res. 1970 Sep;31(9):1687–92.
12. Hansen HJ. A pathologic-anatomical interpretation of disc degeneration in dogs. Acta Orthop Scand. 1951;20(4):280–93.
13. Bray JP, Burbidge HM. The canine intervertebral disk. Part Two: Degenerative changes—nonchondrodystrophoid versus chondrodystrophoid disks. J Am Anim Hosp Assoc. 1998 Mar–Apr; 34(2):135–44.
14. Preister W. Canine intervertebral disc disease-occurrence by age, breed, and sex among 8,117 cases Theriogenology. 1976;6:293–303.
15. Hoerlein BF. Intervertebral disc protrusions in the dog. I. Incidence and pathological lesions. Am J Vet Res. 1953 Apr;14(51):260–9.
16. Ferreira AJ, Correia JH, Jaggy A. Thoracolumbar disc disease in 71 paraplegic dogs: influence of rate of onset and duration of clinical signs on treatment results. J Small Anim Pract. 2002 Apr;43(4):158–63.
17. Johnson EF, Caldwell RW, Berryman HE, Miller A, Chetty K. Elastic fibers in the anulus fibrosus of the dog intervertebral disc. Acta Anat (Basel). 1984;118(4):238–42.

2 Biomechanics of the Intervertebral Disc and Why Do Discs Displace?

Lucas A. Smolders and Franck Forterre

Biomechanical function of the healthy intervertebral disc

From a biomechanical viewpoint, the intervertebral disc (IVD) can be regarded as a water-filled cushion that mediates and transmits compressive forces between vertebral bodies and provides mobility as well as stability to the spinal segment [1–4]. The IVD functions in relation to the ligamentous apparatus of the spine, which consists of the interspinal, interarcuate, dorsal longitudinal, and ventral longitudinal ligaments and the annulus fibrosus of the IVD. The healthy IVD exerts a high swelling pressure, which accounts for the separation of contiguous vertebrae. The separation of adjacent vertebrae creates constant tension on the spinal ligaments, preventing uncontrolled displacements that would cause stress peaks of the vertebrae. Therefore, the IVD creates the necessary tension for optimal functionality and stability of the ligamentous apparatus of the spine [4].

The healthy IVD is composed of three distinct components: the nucleus pulposus (NP), annulus fibrosus (AF), and cartilaginous end plates (EPs). Each component exhibits specialized physical–mechanical properties and specific biomechanical functions. The collaboration of these individual structures results in optimal biomechanical function of the IVD.

The healthy NP is composed of approximately 80% water. This high water content results in a high intradiscal swelling pressure that allows the NP to serve as a hydraulic cushion transmitting compressive forces while providing spinal mobility and stability [1–3, 5–9]. The NP is surrounded ventrally, dorsally, and laterally by the AF, with the ventral part of the AF being 2–3 times thicker than the dorsal part [10–12]. The fibers of the AF provide reinforcement when the IVD is twisted (axial rotation), bent (flexion/extension), and/or compressed (axial compression), with the inner and outer AF mainly resisting compressive and tensile forces, respectively [5, 6, 8]. The AF contains the NP, preserving its internal swelling pressure and protecting it against shearing [5, 6, 8, 13].

The cranial and caudal borders of the IVD are formed by the cartilaginous EPs, situated between the disc and the epiphyses of the respective cranial

Advances in Intervertebral Disc Disease in Dogs and Cats, First Edition. Edited by James M. Fingeroth and William B. Thomas.
© 2015 ACVS Foundation. Published 2015 by John Wiley & Sons, Inc.

and caudal vertebral bodies [5, 11, 14]. The EPs are partially deformable due to their high water content (50–80%) and serve to contain the NP during loading of the spine [15].

All in all, this IVD can be viewed as an inflated tire, with the NP providing intradiscal pressure and resistance to compressive loads, the AF coping with tensile forces, and the partially deformable EP containing the NP. Owing to the specialized conformation of these structurally and functionally divergent entities, the IVD concurrently provides mobility and stability to compressive, tensile, and shear stresses applied to the spine [2, 5, 6, 8].

Biomechanical failure of the IVD

Degeneration of the IVD is the fundamental process that lies at the root of most IVD displacements. Due to this degeneration, the NP loses the ability to absorb and maintain water and thereby to function as a hydraulic cushion [16–20]. Consequently, more of the compressive load bearing, which is normally resisted by the hydrated NP, is transmitted to the AF [21–23]. This results in a compensatory increase in functional size of the AF [21, 24–26]. However, the AF is not built to resist compressive forces, and the increase in functional size consists of biomechanically inferior matrix [17–19, 25]. As a result, the AF becomes stiffer and weaker leading to structural failure that impedes the ability of the AF to resist tensile forces and to contain the NP. Eventually, these degenerative changes result in outward bulging of the IVD when subjected to physiological loading [16]. In addition, structural failure of the AF can result in annular defects or tears, through which degenerated NP material can extrude and which further compromise the function of the IVD [12, 16]. In essence, the degenerated IVD functions as a flat tire, being unable to cope with physiological loading, with consequent displacement of the IVD. Since the dorsal AF is 2–3 times thinner than the ventral AF, the dorsal side is usually where the AF shows structural failure and IVD displacement. In addition to structural failure of the NP and AF with consequent disc displacement, degeneration of the NP and AF results in an uneven distribution of load onto the EP, making the EP more susceptible to damage [27]. Although the EPs are deformable when axially loaded, they are a weak link within the IVD [13].

Degeneration of the IVD can cause cracks in the EP [28–30]. The degenerated NP can displace through these EP defects, which is referred to as a Schmorl's node [31].

Although displacement of the IVD is commonly the result of IVD degeneration, displacement can also occur as a result of strenuous exercise or trauma. This type of IVD displacement involves abrupt extrusion of nondegenerated NP material through the dorsal or dorsolateral AF and is referred to as acute noncompressive nucleus pulposus extrusion [12, 32–34] (see Chapter 13).

The biomechanical alterations involved in degeneration of the IVD can occur in any dog. However, when speaking of actual herniation of the IVD, a clear distinction can be made between chondrodystrophoid (CD) and nonchondrodystrophoid (NCD) dogs. Chondrodystrophoid and NCD dogs display significant differences in the character, age of onset, prevalence, and spinal location of IVD displacement. Due to these distinct differences, it is conceivable that the etiological factors for IVD displacement are different between these two groups of dogs.

Displacement of the IVD in CD dogs

Chondrodystrophoid dog breeds are characterized by an accelerated form of IVD degeneration [12]. Consequently, the NP abruptly loses its hydraulic function, with consequent degenerative changes in the AF [12]. This predisposes to explosive herniations of the IVD, with complete rupture of the AF and dorsal longitudinal ligament, and extrusion of the NP into the vertebral canal [12]. These disc displacements are referred to as Hansen type I IVD herniations [12, 35–37].

Another remarkable feature of CD dogs is that IVD degeneration occurs throughout the entire vertebral column [12, 38, 39]. Therefore, biomechanical factors inherent to individual spinal levels seem to be of less importance to IVD degeneration in CD dogs. At first impression, a logical biomechanical factor in CD dogs may be the disproportion between the length of the spine and the length of the legs. However, there is no correlation between a relatively long spine and IVD degeneration in these dogs [12, 28]. Moreover, CD dogs with a relatively shorter spine, a larger height at the withers, and a large pelvic circumference are at higher risk for IVD herniation [29]. In CD dogs, all IVDs show signs of degeneration at an early age; therefore, a genetic component linked to the CD trait causing aberrant synthesis of the NP extracellular matrix appears to be the main etiological factor [12, 30, 38, 40]. However, causative factors for the high susceptibility of IVD herniation at certain spinal levels (cervical and thoracolumbar spine) in CD dogs are still unclear. It has been proposed that the transition from the rigid, thoracic spine to the more flexible, lumbar spine is a causative biomechanical factor for herniation of thoracolumbar IVDs in CD dogs; however, definitive evidence to support this theory is still lacking [41]. In contrast, it is well known that IVD displacement is seldom seen in the midthoracic spine (T1–T9). This may be because of the intercapital ligaments present ventral to the dorsal longitudinal ligament at each level from T1–T2 to T9–T10 [12, 42, 43]. These ligaments may prevent dorsal and dorsolateral displacement of the IVD at these levels [12, 36].

Displacement of the IVD in NCD dogs

In NCD dogs, degeneration of the IVD occurs more gradually [17, 18]. Degeneration of the AF can occur independently of NP degeneration, and mainly consists of partial ruptures of the AF fibers [12]. Due to the more gradual character of IVD degeneration in NCD dogs, lesions in the IVD are less dramatic, generally characterized by partial herniation of the NP through a partial rupture of the AF, and protrusion of the IVD and dorsal longitudinal ligament. This type of disc displacement is referred to as Hansen type II IVD herniation [12].

In NCD dogs, IVDs at specific spinal levels, such as C5–C7 and L7–S1, have the highest rate of degeneration and displacement [12, 44–47]. Therefore, it seems that in NCD dogs biomechanical factors related to individual spinal levels play a key role in degeneration and consequent displacement of the IVD.

In the cervical spine of large-breed NCD dogs, the caudal cervical spine is at the highest risk for developing IVD degeneration and displacement [44, 45, 48]. This may be related to the conformation of the facet joints of the caudal cervical spine. Due to their shape and conformation, the facet joints of the caudal cervical spine allow considerably more axial rotation and can induce significantly more spinal

instability compared to more cranial spinal segments [49, 50]. Therefore, the workloads and stresses on the IVDs of the caudal cervical spine may be relatively high, thereby promoting IVD degeneration and displacement at these locations [51].

The L7–S1 disc of NCD large-breed dogs is also frequently affected by IVD displacement [46, 52–54]. This may be related to the conformation and mobility of the L7–S1 junction in these breeds. The conformation of the IVD and facet joints of the L7–S1 spinal segment permits considerable mobility in flexion/extension, axial rotation, and ventrodorsal translation [51, 55–58]. Also, the L7–S1 junction in large-breed dogs is subject to proportionally higher loads due to an imbalance between body weight and the dimensions of the lumbosacral contact area (IVD and facet joints) as compared to smaller dogs [57]. These factors indicate that the L7–S1 IVD of large-breed dogs is subject to relatively high workloads and stress (wear and tear), predisposing the disc to degeneration and structural failure, with consequent displacement of the IVD.

In addition to these factors for NCD dogs in general, specific biomechanical factors apply to the German shepherd dog, which is highly predisposed to degeneration and displacement of the L7–S1 IVD [53]. In this breed, the orientation of the L7–S1 facet joint causes a disproportionally high workload in the L7–S1 IVD [46, 47, 51]. Also, lumbosacral transitional vertebrae are relatively common in the German shepherd dog. This developmental abnormality is associated with abnormal mobility and distribution of force on the lumbosacral IVD [59–61]. Last, the German shepherd dog is predisposed to sacral osteochondrosis, which involves degeneration and fragmentation of the sacral end plate [62–64]. Besides aberrant nutritional supply to the IVD, the abnormal shape of the sacral end plate may cause aberrant mechanical loading of the IVD [62–64]. These specific factors in the German shepherd dog may cause aberrant loading of the IVD with consequent IVD degeneration and displacement.

References

1. Adams MA, Hutton WC. Mechanics of the Intervertebral Disc. In: Ghosh P, editor. The Biology of the Intervertebral Disc. 2. 1 ed. Boca Raton, FL: CRC Press, Inc.; 1988. pp. 39–73.

2. White AA, 3rd, Panjabi MM. Clinical Biomechanics of the Spine. Philadelphia, PA: J.B. Lippincott Company; 1978. pp. 1–56.

3. Smit TH. The use of a quadruped as an in vivo model for the study of the spine—biomechanical considerations. Eur Spine J. 2002 Apr;11(2):137–44.

4. Putz RL, Muller-Gerbl M. The vertebral column—a phylogenetic failure? A theory explaining the function and vulnerability of the human spine. Clin Anat. 1996;9(3):205–12.

5. Hukins DWL. Disc Structure and Function. In: Ghosh P, editor. The Biology of the Intervertebral Disc. 1. 1 ed. Boca Raton, FL: CRC Press, Inc.; 1988. pp. 1–38.

6. Roughley PJ. Biology of intervertebral disc aging and degeneration: involvement of the extracellular matrix. Spine (Phila Pa 1976). 2004 Dec 1;29(23):2691–9.

7. Hendry NG. The hydration of the nucleus pulposus and its relation to intervertebral disc derangement. J Bone Joint Surg Br. 1958 Feb;40-B(1):132–44.

8. Setton LA, Chen J. Mechanobiology of the intervertebral disc and relevance to disc degeneration. J Bone Joint Surg Am. 2006 Apr;88 Suppl 2:52–7.

9. Urban JP, Maroudas A. Swelling of the intervertebral disc in vitro. Connect Tissue Res. 1981;9(1):1–10.

10. Cassidy JJ, Hiltner A, Baer E. Hierarchical structure of the intervertebral disc. Connect Tissue Res. 1989; 23(1):75–88.

11. Samuelson DA. Cartilage and Bone. In: Samuelson DA, editor. Textbook of Veterinary Histology. St. Louis, MO: Saunders Elsevier; 2007. pp. 100–29.

12. Hansen HJ. A pathologic-anatomical study on disc degeneration in dog, with special reference to the so-called enchondrosis intervertebralis. Acta Orthop Scand Suppl. 1952;11:1–117.

13. Brinckmann P, Frobin W, Hierholzer E, Horst M. Deformation of the vertebral end-plate under axial loading of the spine. Spine (Phila Pa 1976). 1983 Nov–Dec;8(8):851–6.

14. Eurell JA, van Sickle DC. Connective and Supportive Tissues. In: Eurell JA, Frappier BL, editors. Dellmann's Textbook of Veterinary Histology. 6 ed. Ames, IA: Blackwell Publishing; 2006. pp. 31–60.

15. Roberts S, Menage J, Urban JP. Biochemical and structural properties of the cartilage end-plate and its relation to the intervertebral disc. Spine (Phila Pa 1976). 1989 Feb;14(2):166–74.

16. Adams MA, Roughley PJ. What is intervertebral disc degeneration, and what causes it? Spine (Phila Pa 1976). 2006 Aug 15;31(18):2151–61.

17. Ghosh P, Taylor TK, Braund KG. The variation of the glycosaminoglycans of the canine intervertebral disc with ageing. I. Chondrodystrophoid breed. Gerontology. 1977;23(2):87–98.

18. Ghosh P, Taylor TK, Braund KG. Variation of the glycosaminoglycans of the intervertebral disc with ageing. II. Non-chondrodystrophoid breed. Gerontology. 1977;23(2):99–109.

19. Ghosh P, Taylor TK, Braund KG, Larsen LH. The collagenous and non-collagenous protein of the canine intervertebral disc and their variation with age, spinal level and breed. Gerontology. 1976;22(3): 124–34.

20. Gillett NA, Gerlach R, Cassidy JJ, Brown SA. Age-related changes in the beagle spine. Acta Orthop Scand. 1988 Oct;59(5):503–7.

21. McNally DS, Adams MA. Internal intervertebral disc mechanics as revealed by stress profilometry. Spine (Phila Pa 1976). 1992 Jan;17(1):66–73.

22. McNally DS, Shackleford IM, Goodship AE, Mulholland RC. In vivo stress measurement can predict pain on discography. Spine (Phila Pa 1976). 1996 Nov 15;21(22):2580–7.

23. Adams MA, McMillan DW, Green TP, Dolan P. Sustained loading generates stress concentrations in lumbar intervertebral discs. Spine (Phila Pa 1976). 1996 Feb 15;21(4):434–8.

24. Adams MA, McNally DS, Dolan P. 'Stress' distributions inside intervertebral discs. The effects of age and degeneration. J Bone Joint Surg Br. 1996 Nov;78(6):965–72.

25. Cole TC, Ghosh P, Taylor TK. Variations of the proteoglycans of the canine intervertebral disc with ageing. Biochim Biophys Acta. 1986 Feb 19;880(2–3): 209–19.

26. Johnson JA, da Costa RC, Allen MJ. Micromorphometry and cellular characteristics of the canine cervical intervertebral discs. J Vet Intern Med. 2010 Nov–Dec;24(6):1343–9.

27. Grant JP, Oxland TR, Dvorak MF, Fisher CG. The effects of bone density and disc degeneration on the structural property distributions in the lower lumbar vertebral endplates. J Orthop Res. 2002 Sep;20(5): 1115–20.

28. Jensen VF, Christensen KA. Inheritance of disc calcification in the dachshund. J Vet Med A Physiol Pathol Clin Med. 2000 Aug;47(6):331–40.

29. Levine JM, Levine GJ, Kerwin SC, Hettlich BF, Fosgate GT. Association between various physical factors and acute thoracolumbar intervertebral disk extrusion or protrusion in Dachshunds. J Am Vet Med Assoc. 2006 Aug 1;229(3):370–5.

30. Ghosh P, Taylor TK, Braund KG, Larsen LH. A comparative chemical and histochemical study of the chondrodystrophoid and nonchondrodystrophoid canine intervertebral disc. Vet Pathol. 1976; 13(6):414–27.

31. Schmorl CG. Die pathologische Anatomie der Wirbelsäule. Verhandlungen der Deutschen orthopädischen Gesellschaft 1926;21:3–41.

32. De Risio L, Adams V, Dennis R, McConnell FJ. Association of clinical and magnetic resonance imaging findings with outcome in dogs with presumptive acute noncompressive nucleus pulposus extrusion: 42 cases (2000–2007). J Am Vet Med Assoc. 2009 Feb 15;234(4):495–504.

33. Griffiths IR. A syndrome produced by dorso-lateral "explosions" of the cervical intervertebral discs. Vet Rec. 1970 Dec 12;87(24):737–41.

34. Chang Y, Dennis R, Platt SR, Penderis J. Magnetic resonance imaging of traumatic intervertebral disc extrusion in dogs. Vet Rec. 2007 Jun 9;160(23):795–9.

35. Hansen HJ. A pathologic-anatomical interpretation of disc degeneration in dogs. Acta Orthop Scand. 1951;20(4):280–93.

36. Olsson SE, Hansen HJ. Cervical disc protrusions in the dog. J Am Vet Med Assoc. 1952 Nov;121(908):361–70.

37. Olsson SE. On disc protrusion in dog (enchondrosis intervertebralis); study with special reference to roentgen diagnosis and to the value of disc fenestration. Acta Orthop Scand Suppl. 1951;8:1–95.

38. Braund KG, Ghosh P, Taylor TK, Larsen LH. Morphological studies of the canine intervertebral disc. The assignment of the beagle to the achondroplastic classification. Res Vet Sci. 1975 Sep;19(2):167–72.

39. Hoerlein BF. Intervertebral disc protrusions in the dog. I. Incidence and pathological lesions. Am J Vet Res. 1953 Apr;14(51):260–9.

40. Ghosh P, Taylor TK, Yarroll JM. Genetic factors in the maturation of the canine intervertebral disc. Res Vet Sci. 1975 Nov;19(3):304–11.

41. Braund KG, Taylor TK, Ghosh P, Sherwood AA. Spinal mobility in the dog. A study in chondrodystrophoid and non-chondrodystrophoid animals. Res Vet Sci. 1977 Jan;22(1):78–82.

42. Dyce KM, Sack WO, Wensing CJG. The Neck, Back, and Vertebral Column of the Dog and Cat. In: Dyce KM, Sack WO, Wensing CJG, editors. Textbook of Veterinary Anatomy. 4 ed. Philadelphia/London/New York/St. Louis/Sydney/Toronto: Saunders Elsevier; 2010. pp. 407–19.

43. Evans HE, Christensen GC. Joints and Ligaments. In: Evans HE, Christensen GC, editors. Miller's Anatomy of the Dog. 2 ed. Philadelphia/London/Toronto: W.B. Saunders Company; 1979. pp. 225–68.

44. da Costa RC, Parent JM, Partlow G, Dobson H, Holmberg DL, Lamarre J. Morphologic and morphometric magnetic resonance imaging features of Doberman Pinschers with and without clinical signs of cervical spondylomyelopathy. Am J Vet Res. 2006 Sep;67(9):1601–12.

45. De Decker S, Gielen IM, Duchateau L, Van Soens I, Bavegems V, Bosmans T, et al. Low-field magnetic resonance imaging findings of the caudal portion of the cervical region in clinically normal Doberman Pinschers and Foxhounds. Am J Vet Res. 2010 Apr;71(4):428–34.

46. Rossi F, Seiler G, Busato A, Wacker C, Lang J. Magnetic resonance imaging of articular process joint geometry and intervertebral disk degeneration in the caudal lumbar spine (L5-S1) of dogs with clinical signs of cauda equina compression. Vet Radiol Ultrasound. 2004 Sep–Oct;45(5):381–7.

47. Seiler GS, Häni H, Busato AR, Lang J. Facet joint geometry and intervertebral disc degeneration in the L5-S1 region of the vertebral column in German Shepherd Dogs. Am J Vet Res. 2002;63(1):86–90.

48. da Costa RC. Cervical spondylomyelopathy (Wobbler syndrome) in dogs. Vet Clin North Am Small Anim Pract. 2010 Sep;40(5):881–913.

49. Breit S, Kunzel W. Shape and orientation of articular facets of cervical vertebrae (C3-C7) in dogs denoting axial rotational ability: an osteological study. Eur J Morphol. 2002 Feb;40(1):43–51.

50. Johnson JA, da Costa RC, Allen MJ, editors. Kinematics of the cranial and caudal cervical spine in large breed dogs. American College of Veterinary Internal Medicine Forum Proceedings; 2010; Lakewood (CO).

51. Farfan HF, Cossette JW, Robertson GH, Wells RV, Kraus H. The effects of torsion on the lumbar intervertebral joints: the role of torsion in the production of disc degeneration. J Bone Joint Surg Am. 1970 Apr;52(3):468–97.

52. De Risio L, Sharp NJ, Olby NJ, Munana KR, Thomas WB. Predictors of outcome after dorsal decompressive laminectomy for degenerative lumbosacral stenosis in dogs: 69 cases (1987–1997). J Am Vet Med Assoc. 2001 Sep 1;219(5):624–8.

53. Meij BP, Bergknut N. Degenerative lumbosacral stenosis in dogs. Vet Clin North Am Small Anim Pract. 2010 Sep;40(5):983–1009.

54. Suwankong N, Meij BP, Voorhout G, de Boer AH, Hazewinkel HA. Review and retrospective analysis of degenerative lumbosacral stenosis in 156 dogs treated by dorsal laminectomy. Vet Comp Orthop Traumatol. 2008;21(3):285–93.

55. Benninger MI, Seiler GS, Robinson LE, Ferguson SJ, Bonel HM, Busato AR, et al. Three-dimensional motion pattern of the caudal lumbar and lumbosacral portions of the vertebral column of dogs. Am J Vet Res. 2004 May;65(5):544–51.

56. Benninger MI, Seiler GS, Robinson LE, Ferguson SJ, Bonel HM, Busato AR, et al. Effects of anatomic conformation on three-dimensional motion of the caudal lumbar and lumbosacral portions of the vertebral column of dogs. Am J Vet Res. 2006 Jan;67(1):43–50.

57. Breit S, Kunzel W. Breed specific osteological features of the canine lumbosacral junction. Ann Anat. 2001 Mar;183(2):151–7.

58. Hediger KU, Ferguson SJ, Gedet P, Busato A, Forterre F, Isler S, et al. Biomechanical analysis of torsion and shear forces in lumbar and lumbosacral spine segments of nonchondrodystrophic dogs. Vet Surg. 2009 Oct;38(7):874–80.

59. Fluckiger MA, Damur-Djuric N, Hassig M, Morgan JP, Steffen F. A lumbosacral transitional vertebra in the dog predisposes to cauda equina syndrome. Vet Radiol Ultrasound. 2006 Jan–Feb;47(1):39–44.

60. Geissbühler AD. Kinetische Studien am lumbosakralen Uebergang von Berner Sennenhunden und Deutschen Schäferhunden. Bern: Universität Bern; 1999.

61. Morgan JP, Bahr A, Franti CE, Bailey CS. Lumbosacral transitional vertebrae as a predisposing cause of

cauda equina syndrome in German shepherd dogs: 161 cases (1987–1990). J Am Vet Med Assoc. 1993 Jun 1;202(11):1877–82.

62. Hanna FY. Lumbosacral osteochondrosis: radiological features and surgical management in 34 dogs. J Small Anim Pract. 2001 Jun;42(6):272–8.

63. Mathis KR, Havlicek M, Beck JB, Eaton-Wells RD, Park FM. Sacral osteochondrosis in two German Shepherd Dogs. Aust Vet J. 2009 Jun;87(6):249–52.

64. Lang J, Hani H, Schawalder P. A sacral lesion resembling osteochondrosis in the German Shepherd Dog. Vet Radiol Ultrasound. 1992;33:69–76.

3 Comparisons between Biped (Human) and Quadruped (Canine/Feline) Intervertebral Disc Disease

Niklas Bergknut, Franck Forterre, Jonathan M. Levine, Steven D. Lasser, and James M. Fingeroth

There are many similarities between the canine and human spines and their vertebral components. The vertebral units comprising two adjacent vertebrae—an intervertebral disc and facet joints—are comparable in both species. The human spine averages 33 vertebrae, whereas the canine spine generally averages 50 [1]. Humans generally have 12 thoracic and 5 lumbar vertebrae, whereas dogs generally have 13 thoracic and 7 lumbar vertebrae.

Intervertebral disc (IVD) degeneration and herniation are considered the main causes of acute and chronic low back pain in humans [2–6], with a lifetime prevalence of over 70% in the global population [7]. Also, dogs commonly suffer from back pain caused by degenerated IVDs subsequently herniating; it is in fact the most common cause of neurological deficits in dogs [8] and is one of the most common causes for euthanasia in dogs less than 10 years of age [9]. Moreover, the clinical presentation, macroscopic and microscopic appearance, diagnostics, and treatment of IVD degeneration and herniation are similar in humans and dogs [6, 10–12].

Decompressive surgery and spinal fusion are common treatments for IVD disease (IVDD) in both humans and dogs, with fusion less often used in the latter species.

The many similarities between canine and human spines and their diseases have led to dogs being frequently used for translational studies of surgical procedures and biomechanical studies of the spine [13–18]; and recently, the dog has been proposed as a translational model for acute spinal cord injury (SCI) [19] as well as for IVD degeneration [20].

Anatomy and gross pathology

The occurrence of asymptomatic degenerated IVDs is common in both dogs and humans [21, 22]; and in general, similar pathological changes have been reported in degenerated IVDs from humans and dogs [23]. A notable difference between human and canine vertebrae is the absence of growth plates in growing human vertebrae and the thicker cartilaginous end plates in humans.

Advances in Intervertebral Disc Disease in Dogs and Cats, First Edition. Edited by James M. Fingeroth and William B. Thomas.
© 2015 ACVS Foundation. Published 2015 by John Wiley & Sons, Inc.

Whereas in dogs most vertebral growth takes place in the growth plates, in humans, vertebral growth takes place in the junction between the vertebrae and the end plates, which may explain the thicker end plates found in humans [20, 24].

The overall appearance of both healthy and degenerating IVDs from humans and dogs has been found to be similar. All five stages of degeneration described in human IVDs by Thompson et al. have also been described in dogs [23]. The healthy IVDs of both species comprise (1) a fibrocartilaginous annulus fibrosus (AF) consisting of well-organized lamellar layers, (2) a soft gelatinous nucleus pulposus (NP), and (3) cartilaginous end plates lining the vertebral end plates. In the healthy IVDs, these structures are clearly distinguishable from each other; but once degeneration starts, the borders between these three structures are progressively more difficult to discern. Disorganization of the tissue structure, mainly with the AF showing increasing numbers of clefts and cracks, becomes visible with increasing degree of degeneration. In the later stages of degeneration of discs in both humans and dogs, a marked loss of IVD space can be noted, with new bone formation (spondylosis deformans) apparent, especially, on the ventral/anterior aspect of the intervertebral segments [20].

Although canine IVDs are generally smaller than human IVDs, the ratio of NP area/IVD area is reported to be similar in the two species. However, the ratios of IVD height/width, NP/IVD width, and end plate thickness/IVD height are reported to significantly differ between healthy human and healthy canine IVDs [20]. As in humans, the height of the canine lumbosacral IVD is reported to be greater than that of the lumbar IVDs (Table 3.1) [20].

Contrary to the well-innervated human IVDs [28], the innervation of the canine IVD tissue itself is sparse: nerve endings have only been found in the outer lamellae of the AF and not in the NP, the transitional zone, or the inner AF [29–31]. However, soft tissue structures surrounding the canine IVDs, such as the dorsal longitudinal ligament, are profusely innervated [29, 30].

Table 3.1   Measurements and dimensions of the midsagittal surface of canine and human lumbar intervertebral discs (IVDs) as determined by gross and histopathological examinations

Measurement	Dog		Human		P-value
	Mean±SD	Range	Mean±SD	Range	
Gross pathology					
IVD height (mm)	3.5±0.6	2.4–4.7	10[a]	6–14[a]	N/A
IVD width (mm)	15.9±2.0	11.0–18.9	35[a]	27–45[a]	N/A
Ratio of IVD height/width	0.22±0.03	0.14–0.28	0.29±0.05	0.23–0.34	<0.01*
Ratio of NP/IVD width	0.30±0.05	0.21–0.41	0.38±0.05	0.31–0.44	<0.01*
Ratio of NP/IVD area	0.25±0.05	0.17–0.34	0.28±0.02	0.24–0.31	0.18
Histology					
EP thickness (mm)	0.22±0.06	0.1–0.42	1.58±0.35	1.25–2.51	<0.01*
EP thickness/IVD height (%)	6	3–11	13	9–19	<0.01*
Number of cell layers in EP	5	3–8	21	18–23	<0.01*
Cortical thickness (mm)	0.90±0.36	0.27–1.78	0.66±0.33	0.25–1.59	0.06

Published with permission from Bergknut et al. [20].
The P-values reflect significant differences between the values obtained in dogs and humans.
EP, end plate; N/A, not available; NP, nucleus pulposus; SD, standard deviation.
[a]Measurements obtained from the literature [25–27].
*Statistically significant difference between dogs and humans at $P < 0.01$.

Biomechanics

The canine spinal column is so constructed as to make the vertebrae able to resist powerful compressive forces. According to Wolff's law, the trabecular structure of the cortical bone adapts to strengthen the bone to cope with compressive forces. By following this principle, the quadruped spine appears to be loaded mainly by axial compression in a way that is similar to the bipedal human spine [32]. Dogs and other quadrupeds have higher vertebral bone densities than humans, indicating that axial compression stress is greater in dogs than in humans [33]. The other mechanical loads are transformed by the surrounding musculature into axial compression, and eventually facet joint loads.

The size of the vertebral canal is much larger in humans than in dogs. However, in both humans and dogs, the areas with the largest vertebral canal diameter (lumbar and cervical regions) are also the most mobile ones [1]. The human vertebral canal is more triangular in its vertical dimension, whereas a more oval shape in the horizontal dimension is observed in dogs. The spinal cord fills about 80% of the vertebral canal in dogs.

The vertebral facet joints have two functions: the first is to enable but also to limit the segmental range of motion, and the second is to absorb the energy that results from the ventrally directed shearing forces [34]. The joints are therefore somewhat differently oriented at different levels of the spinal column. Comparing the orientation of the human articular processes with that in dogs, it becomes obvious that these processes show a high degree of adaptation to the movement patterns of each species [35]. In humans, articular surfaces have an angle of more than 60° to the frontal plane, while in quadrupeds, it is less than 30° [36]. Further, the cancellous bone of the most lateral extended parts of the cranial articular processes possesses a characteristic architecture that can be recognized as an adaptation to bending [37]. Together with ligaments, the facet joints determine the direction and degree of displacement of the vertebrae one to another. Because of their intrinsic fiber orientation, the AF, the dorsal longitudinal, interspinal, and supraspinous ligaments contribute to kinematic control, while the ventral longitudinal ligament has a very important static function [38]. Further, the lumbar ligaments,

together with their vertebral joints, behave like a gear system without a constant center of rotation. As an adaptive consequence, the thickness of the ventral and dorsal parts of the AF is distributed unequally, and rotation is limited by the facet joints in conjunction with the thicker ventral part of the AF. The facet joints thus play an important stabilizing role in jumping and running [32, 35].

The canine IVDs represent about 20% of the length of the spine, while in humans, the discs represent 25% [1]. It was generally recognized that the two main functions of the IVD are the absorption of shock to the spine and the provision of flexibility to the spinal column [39]. The consistent arrangement of the trabecular bone at right angles to the dorsal/posterior and ventral/anterior surfaces of the vertebral body makes it obvious that these surfaces, under normal conditions, take on an undeviating and equally distributed axial pressure. The IVD acts not as much as a shock absorber *per se* but as a kind of water-filled cushion that mediates the equal distribution of pressure [35, 40]. If its hydrostatic function is impaired as a result of the loss of water, this cushioning effect is lost as well. A second disc function is related to the associated ligamentous apparatus. The aforementioned gear mechanism only works optimally when as many as possible of the ligaments and fiber bundles are under pretension. The swelling pressure of the nucleus pulposus helps maintain the separation of the contiguous vertebrae and thus creates the necessary tension for the ligamentous apparatus to work effectively [35].

The most important clinical/anatomical difference between both species is the relationship between the length of the vertebral column and the spinal cord. Usually in dogs, the spinal cord terminates between the two last lumbar vertebrae (L6–L7), while in humans, it terminates between the first two lumbar vertebrae (L1–L2). Therefore, the usual disc herniation sites in the terminal lumbar area (L3–L4, L4–L5, L5–S1) in humans result in only nerve roots of the cauda equina being affected, while the usual thoracolumbar or lumbar localization of disc herniations in dogs will directly compress the spinal cord.

The spine, whether in quadrupeds or bipeds, can be regarded mechanically as a series of freely hinged vertebrae needing further support from surrounding tensile structures to control posture. During the different forms of locomotion, axial torsion, flexion–extension, and lateral bending moments are important loads that act on the spine. Tensile structures such as muscles and ligaments must be active to compensate for the applied moments, leaving the spine under considerable axial compression [32].

Histology and histopathology

In the healthy IVDs from both dogs and humans, there is a clear distinction between the cell populations and the organization of the cells in the AF and NP. In the NP of healthy IVDs in dogs under 1 year of age, and in children, notochordal cells are the predominant cell type. These large, vacuolar cells clump together in large clusters in a similar unorganized fashion in both species. Notochordal cells are also common in the NP of adult nonchondrodystrophoid dogs but not in the IVDs of adult humans or chondrodystrophoid dogs, where chondrocyte-like cells are most common [30, 41]. The cells in the healthy AF of both dogs and humans are smaller fibrocyte-like cells, located in between well-organized lamellar layers of collagen fibers.

All common features of IVD degeneration, such as chondroid cell clusters, disorganization of the AF, and the appearance of clefts and cracks, are reported to occur similarly in degenerating IVDs from both dogs and humans [20]. Using the Thompson grading scheme for describing IVD degeneration, increasing signs of degeneration are reported in humans and dogs alike, with increasing disorganization of the lamellae in the AF, increasing cell cluster size in the NP, and increasing numbers of clefts and cracks in the IVD overall.

There are also some notable histological differences between IVDs in humans and dogs, such as the end plates being relatively thicker (compared with the total IVD height) and having more chondrocyte layers in humans than in dogs. Conversely, the subchondral bony cortices are reported to be thicker relative to total IVD height and end plate thickness in dogs than in humans (Table 3.1).

Biochemical

There are a few essential components in the extracellular matrix of the IVD giving the IVD its physiological function, as explained in the Biomechanics section. These extracellular components are vastly different between the AF and NP but are very similar in humans and dogs. The AF is mainly made up of collagen type I strands held together by elastic fibers forming fibrils. The fibrils are bundled together in lamellar layers which are coated by proteoglycans, thereby enabling the lamellae to easily slide over each other [39]. The lamellar layers are meticulously organized, oriented at different angles to each other to withstand stress in multiple directions.

The most important extracellular component of the NP in both the species is the negatively charged proteoglycans that are trapped in a unorganized network of collagen type II fibers [42]. The proteoglycan molecules are made up of a core protein with covalently bound glycosaminoglycan (GAG) side chains (mostly, chondroitin sulfate or keratin sulfate) [42–44]. The GAG side chains are highly negatively charged, thereby repelling each other and causing the often described "bottlebrush" appearance of these molecules. Proteoglycans also aggregate together by binding to hyaluronic acid, forming even larger molecules such as aggrecan [45, 46]. The negatively charged proteoglycans osmotically attract water into the NP (making the healthy NP over 80% water), creating the high intradiscal pressure of the healthy NP [14, 43, 44, 46, 47].

The GAG content in canine IVDs is reported to be negatively correlated with increasing Thompson grades [20], which is also the case in degenerating human IVDs [48, 49]. The GAG content of IVDs from chondrodystrophoid dogs is lower than that of IVDs from nonchondrodystrophoid dogs of similar age [43, 44], which is consistent with IVD degeneration occurring at a lower age in chondrodystrophoid than in nonchondrodystrophoid dogs.

There is a complex mechanism, not yet fully understood, underlying the process of remodeling and breakdown of the extracellular matrix in the degenerating IVD. This process is largely regulated by enzymes such as the matrix metalloproteinases (MMPs). Although the underlying mechanisms of IVD degeneration are better described in humans than in dogs, it is likely that the degenerative pathways are similar in the two species [20, 50–55]. MMP-2 is the enzyme responsible for breakdown of collagen type II, and its activity in canine IVDs in different stages of degeneration is similar to that in humans [20].

Diagnostic imaging

Intervertebral disc degeneration/disease gives rise to similar clinical signs in humans and dogs, with neck or back pain and neurological deficits as the most common features when there is herniation. Because the human disc is more heavily innervated than the canine disc (sensory branches from the sinuvertebral nerve), people are sometimes affected with symptoms of discomfort associated with disc degeneration without actual herniation (so-called discogenic pain). This phenomenon appears to be much rarer in dogs and seems to be of little clinical significance, although some veterinarians postulate that some dogs with spondylosis deformans have signs of discomfort that cannot otherwise be explained (see Chapters 8 and 14).

The way we diagnose IVDD/H is similar between the two species, with the use of radiography, computed tomography (CT), and magnetic resonance imaging (MRI). Radiographic signs of IVDD are only present in the later stages of degeneration; and they include, regardless of the species, reduced intervertebral space and sclerosis of the vertebral end plates with or without spondylosis deformans. In more severe cases, spondylolisthesis can be seen both in dogs and in humans. The difference here, however, is that spondylolisthesis in humans occur as ventral (anterior) subluxation of the L4 or L5 vertebra; but in dogs, it is appreciated as a ventral subluxation of the sacrum in relation to L7. In humans, this terminal lumbar spondylolisthesis is also often accompanied by spondylolysis (detachment of the articular facets), while this latter phenomenon is not usually described in dogs.

MRI appearance of IVD herniation (IVDH) and IVD degeneration in different stages is similar in humans and dogs. The human MRI grading system for lumbar IVD degeneration [56] has recently been validated for the grading of IVD degeneration in dogs [57]. IVD degeneration is best graded on T2-weighted MRI where the NP in the healthy IVD is homogeneously hyperintense (white) and, with increasing degree of degeneration, the intensity of the NP is gradually reduced and might completely disappear into "black discs," representing end-stage degeneration. In humans, degeneration of the IVD on T2-weighted MRI is negatively correlated with the GAG content [58], and this appears to be the same in dogs [20].

Acute spinal cord injury

Canine thoracolumbar IVDH is a commonly occurring, spontaneous disease in dogs that is similar to acute SCI in humans. Despite its high incidence, few preclinical trials have utilized dogs with IVDH as a model for human SCI [59–63]. Human SCI is rarely the result of IVDH, since most herniations occur laterally and in areas where only nerve roots and not spinal cord are present in the vertebral canal.

Gross and histopathologic lesions seen in canine IVDH resemble those recognized in humans with traumatic myelopathies. Solid (grossly normal spinal cord with lesions only visible on histopathology), contusion/cavity (normal spinal cord surface with gross evidence of intraparenchymal hemorrhage and necrosis with evolution to cysts), and massive compression (gross anatomic disruption and necrosis) lesions represent 79% of human SCIs [64]. These patterns appear analogous to lesions identified in canine IVDH-associated SCI [65–67]. Axonal injury and associated demyelination are commonly identified in humans with SCI and dogs with IVDH [64, 66–68]. Neuronal necrosis likewise occurs in both species [64, 66–68]. Although the timing of inflammation following canine IVDH-associated SCI is not well described, the general pattern of early neutrophil infiltration followed by gitter cell predominance is analogous to what has been described in human SCI [64, 66, 69]. Cystic lesions at sites of necrosis and neovascularization have been identified in both species in the weeks and months after SCI [64, 66]. Importantly, the mechanisms and pathology underlying canine IVDH-associated SCI are similar to those in human traumatic myelopathies. The primary injury mechanisms involve both compression and contusion, and lesion severity is variable, which mimics the situation in clinically affected humans [30, 65, 66, 70].

There are some anatomical and physiological differences between the dog and human spinal cord, which have clinical relevance. For example, the corticospinal tracts are more important in ambulatory function in humans compared to dogs [71]. The relatively small canine corticospinal tract may explain why spinal shock is more transient in dogs with IVDH compared to humans with SCI [66].

Surgical treatment

The progression of disc degeneration in adult humans is considered a normal age-related phenomenon. Loss of T2 signal on MRI is defined as disc degeneration (disc desiccation) by radiologists but is asymptomatic in the vast majority of people. Inflammatory mediators can stimulate nociceptive pain generators and cause discogenic pain in response to injury, with or without disc herniation (see Chapter 14 regarding discogenic pain in humans vs. dogs). Fissures in damaged annular fibers can also, but inconsistently, provoke pain. Humans have a much more complex response to axial back pain than canines. Pain behavior can range from minimal discomfort with no disability to extreme narcotic dependency and total disability despite similar disc pathology. Secondary pain also confounds medical treatment in humans. Unfortunately, excessive spinal fusion surgery for discogenic disease has become epidemic in the United States. Symptomatic human discogenic disease has a high correlation with tobacco use. The effect of nicotine on the microcirculation of the IVD is surprisingly pervasive.

Approximately 75% of human herniated nucleus pulposus (HNP in the human literature) occurs at L4–L5 and L5–S1, as opposed to the higher levels in canines. Interestingly, the majority of human HNPs resolve spontaneously with fragment reabsorption. Most human lumbar HNPs occur to the right or left of the midline posterior longitudinal ligament (PLL). The PLL reinforces the central portion of the posterior annulus, resulting in fewer direct central HNPs compared with canine HNP, which can often be more centralized. The lateralization of HNP in humans results in fewer instances of cauda equina syndrome than in dogs with L6–L7 and L7–S1 disc herniations, where there is sometimes more centralized displacement (see Chapter 32).

In humans, a standard open lumbar discectomy with examination of the involved nerve root is the most common surgical procedure performed for patients having symptoms of back and leg discomfort. It can usually be accomplished readily with minimal disruption of the posterior elements, as the thecal sac (dural tube) can be manipulated with little effect on the cauda equina, and the spinal cord in humans ends well superior to the usual sites of HNP at L4–L5 and L5–S1. The procedure is usually performed under general or local anesthesia, with patients in the prone or knee–chest position. During surgery, loupe magnification or a microscope is frequently used because of the keyhole approach used and the depth of the operative site. A midline incision reflecting the paraspinous muscles allows the interlaminar space to be entered. In some cases, the medial border of the superior facet might be removed to provide a clear view of the involved nerve root. Using a small annular incision, the fragment of disc can be removed. The canal is finally inspected and the foramen probed for residual disc or bony pathology. The nerve root is decompressed, leaving it freely mobile. More aggressive surgeries affecting the vertebra (hemilaminectomy, laminectomy) or the intervertebral disc (lateral corpectomy, complete fenestration) just like we perform them on canine patients would require vertebral stabilization and are not indicated for treatment of IVDH in humans, except in those rare situations where there is thoracic disc herniation that requires surgical intervention. When a thoracic costotransversectomy is performed to reach the disc herniation without spinal cord retraction, a concomitant spinal fusion is always performed.

References

1. Hoerlein BF. Comparative disk disease: man and dog [for surgery]. J Am Anim Hosp Assoc. 1979;15:535–45.
2. Cappello R, Bird JL, Pfeiffer D, Bayliss MT, Dudhia J. Notochordal cell produce and assemble extracellular matrix in a distinct manner, which may be responsible for the maintenance of healthy nucleus pulposus. Spine. 2006 Apr 15;31(8):873–82; discussion 83.
3. Mooney V. Presidential address. International Society for the Study of the Lumbar Spine. Dallas, 1986. Where is the pain coming from? Spine (Phila Pa 1976). 1987 Oct;12(8):754–9.
4. Vanharanta H, Guyer RD, Ohnmeiss DD, Stith WJ, Sachs BL, Aprill C, et al. Disc deterioration in low-back syndromes. A prospective, multi-center CT/ discography study. Spine. 1988 Dec;13(12):1349–51.
5. Luoma K, Riihimaki H, Luukkonen R, Raininko R, Viikari-Juntura E, Lamminen A. Low back pain in relation to lumbar disc degeneration. Spine. 2000 Feb 15;25(4):487–92.
6. Webb A. Potential sources of neck and back pain in clinical conditions of dogs and cats: a review. Vet J. 2003 May;165(3):193–213.
7. Andersson GB. Epidemiological features of chronic low-back pain. Lancet. 1999 Aug 14;354(9178):581–5.

8. Bray JP, Burbidge HM. The canine intervertebral disk. Part Two: Degenerative changes—nonchondrodystrophoid versus chondrodystrophoid disks. J Am Anim Hosp Assoc. 1998 Mar–Apr; 34(2):135–44.

9. Agria Insurance. Five year statistical report. Stockholm: Agria Insurance, 2000, 33–38.

10. Lotz JC. Animal models of intervertebral disc degeneration: lessons learned. Spine. 2004 Dec 1;29(23): 2742–50.

11. Hansen HJ. A pathologic-anatomical interpretation of disc degeneration in dogs. Acta Orthop Scand. 1951;20(4):280–93.

12. Viñuela-Fernández I, Jones E, Welsh E, Fleetwood-Walker S. Pain mechanisms and their implication for the management of pain in farm and companion animals. Vet J. 2007 Sep;174(2):227–39.

13. Cole T, Burkhardt D, Ghosh P, Ryan M, Taylor T. Effects of spinal fusion on the proteoglycans of the canine intervertebral disc. J Orthop Res. 1985;3(3): 277–91.

14. Holm S, Nachemson A. Variations in the nutrition of the canine intervertebral disc induced by motion. Spine. 1983 Nov–Dec;8(8):866–74.

15. Cole TC, Ghosh P, Hannan NJ, Taylor TK, Bellenger CR. The response of the canine intervertebral disc to immobilization produced by spinal arthrodesis is dependent on constitutional factors. J Orthop Res. 1987;5(3):337–47.

16. Smith K, Hunt T, Asher M, Anderson H, Carson W, Robinson R. The effect of a stiff spinal implant on the bone-mineral content of the lumbar spine in dogs. J Bone Joint Surg. 1991 Jan;73(1):115–23.

17. Zimmerman MC, Vuono-Hawkins M, Parsons JR, Carter FM, Gutteling E, Lee CK, et al. The mechanical properties of the canine lumbar disc and motion segment. Spine. 1992 Feb;17(2):213–20.

18. Bushell GR, Ghosh DP, Taylor TK, Sutherland JM, Braund KG. The effect of spinal fusion on the collagen and proteoglycans of the canine intervertebral disc. J Surg Res. 1978 Jul;25(1):61–9.

19. Levine JM, Levine GJ, Porter BF, Topp K, Noble-Haeusslein LJ. Naturally occurring disk herniation in dogs: an opportunity for pre-clinical spinal cord injury research. J Neurotrauma. 2011 Apr;28(4): 675–88.

20. Bergknut N, Rutges JP, Kranenburg HJ, Smolders LA, Hagman R, Smidt HJ, et al. The dog as an animal model for intervertebral disc degeneration? Spine 2012;37:351–8.

21. Boden SD, Davis DO, Dina TS, Patronas NJ, Wiesel SW. Abnormal magnetic-resonance scans of the lumbar spine in asymptomatic subjects. A prospective investigation. J Bone Joint Surg Am. 1990 Mar;72(3):403–8.

22. Stigen O. Calcification of intervertebral discs in the dachshund. A radiographic study of 327 young dogs. Acta Vet Scand. 1991;32(2):197–203.

23. Bergknut N, Grinwis G, Pickee E, Auriemma E, Lagerstedt AS, Hagman R, et al. Reliability of macroscopic grading of intervertebral disk degeneration in dogs by use of the Thompson system and comparison with low-field magnetic resonance imaging findings. Am J Vet Res. 2011 Jul;72(7):899–904.

24. Taylor JR. Growth of human intervertebral discs and vertebral bodies. J Anat. 1975 Sep;120(Pt 1):49–68.

25. Amonoo-Kuofi HS. Morphometric changes in the heights and anteroposterior diameters of the lumbar intervertebral discs with age. J Anat. 1991 Apr;175: 159–68.

26. Aharinejad S, Bertagnoli R, Wicke K, Firbas W, Schneider B. Morphometric analysis of vertebrae and intervertebral discs as a basis of disc replacement. Am J Anat. 1990 Sep;189(1):69–76.

27. Eijkelkamp MF. On the development of an artificial intervertebral disc. Groningen: University of Groningen; 2002.

28. Bogduk N, Tynan W, Wilson AS. The nerve supply to the human lumbar intervertebral discs. J Anat. 1981 Jan;132(Pt 1):39–56.

29. Forsythe WB, Ghoshal NG. Innervation of the canine thoracolumbar vertebral column. Anat Rec. 1984 Jan;208(1):57–63.

30. Hansen HJ. A pathologic-anatomical study on disc degeneration in dog, with special reference to the so-called enchondrosis intervertebralis. Acta Orthop Scand Suppl. 1952;11:1–117.

31. Willenegger S, Friess AE, Lang J, Stoffel MH. Immunohistochemical demonstration of lumbar intervertebral disc innervation in the dog. Anat Histol Embryol. 2005 Apr;34(2):123–8.

32. Smit TH. The use of a quadruped as an in vivo model for the study of the spine—biomechanical considerations. Eur Spine J. 2002 Apr;11(2):137–44.

33. Hauerstock D, Reindl R, Steffen T, editors. Telemetric measurement of compressive loads in the sheep lumbar spine. Transactions (vol 26) of the 47th Annual Meeting of the Orthopaedic Research Society; 2001.

34. Putz R. The functional morphology of the superior articular processes of the lumbar vertebrae. J Anat. 1985 Dec;143:181–7.

35. Putz RL, Muller-Gerbl M. The vertebral column—a phylogenetic failure? A theory explaining the function and vulnerability of the human spine. Clin Anat (New York, NY). 1996;9(3):205–12.

36. Cotterill PC, Kostuik JP, D'Angelo G, Fernie GR, Maki BE. An anatomical comparison of the human and bovine thoracolumbar spine. J Orthop Res. 1986;4(3):298–303.

37. Muller-Gerbl M, Putz R, Kenn R. Demonstration of subchondral bone density patterns by three-dimensional CT osteoabsorptiometry as a noninvasive method for in vivo assessment of individual long-term stresses in joints. J Bone Miner Res. 1992 Dec;7 Suppl 2:S411–8.

38. Putz R. The detailed functional anatomy of the ligaments of the vertebral column. Ann Anat. 1992 Feb;174(1):40–7.

39. Johnson EF, Caldwell RW, Berryman HE, Miller A, Chetty K. Elastic fibers in the anulus fibrosus of the dog intervertebral disc. Acta Anat (Basel). 1984;118(4):238–42.

40. Gracovetsky S. The Spinal Engine. New York: Springer; 1988.

41. Hunter CJ, Matyas JR, Duncan NA. The notochordal cell in the nucleus pulposus: a review in the context of tissue engineering. Tissue Eng. 2003 Aug;9(4): 667–77.

42. Ghosh P, Taylor T, Braund K, Larsen L. The collagenous and non-collagenous protein of the canine intervertebral disc and their variation with age, spinal level and breed. Gerontology. 1976;22(3): 124–34.

43. Ghosh P, Taylor TK, Braund KG. Variation of the glycosaminoglycans of the intervertebral disc with ageing. II. Non-chondrodystrophoid breed. Gerontology. 1977;23(2):99–109.

44. Ghosh P, Taylor TK, Braund KG. The variation of the glycosaminoglycans of the canine intervertebral disc with ageing. I. Chondrodystrophoid breed. Gerontology. 1977;23(2):87–98.

45. Cole TC, Ghosh P, Taylor TK. Variations of the proteoglycans of the canine intervertebral disc with ageing. Biochim Biophys Acta. 1986 Feb 19;880(2–3): 209–19.

46. Cole TC, Burkhardt D, Frost L, Ghosh P. The proteoglycans of the canine intervertebral disc. Biochim Biophys Acta. 1985 Apr 17;839(2):127–38.

47. Holm S, Maroudas A, Urban JP, Selstam G, Nachemson A. Nutrition of the intervertebral disc: solute transport and metabolism. Connect Tissue Res. 1981;8(2):101–19.

48. Antoniou J, Steffen T, Nelson F, Winterbottom N, Hollander AP, Poole RA, et al. The human lumbar intervertebral disc: evidence for changes in the biosynthesis and denaturation of the extracellular matrix with growth, maturation, ageing, and degeneration. J Clin Invest. 1996 Aug 15;98(4):996–1003.

49. Lyons G, Eisenstein SM, Sweet MB. Biochemical changes in intervertebral disc degeneration. Biochim Biophys Acta. 1981 Apr 3;673(4):443–53.

50. Melrose J, Taylor TK, Ghosh P. Variation in intervertebral disc serine proteinase inhibitory proteins with ageing in a chondrodystrophoid (beagle) and a non-chondrodystrophoid (greyhound) canine breed. Gerontology. 1996;42(6):322–9.

51. Roughley PJ. Biology of intervertebral disc aging and degeneration: involvement of the extracellular matrix. Spine. 2004 Dec 1;29(23):2691–9.

52. Rutges J, Kummer J, Oner F, Verbout A, Castelein R, Roestenburg H, et al. Increased MMP-2 activity during intervertebral disc degeneration is correlated to MMP-14 levels. J Pathol. 2008 Mar;214(4):523–30.

53. Neidlinger-Wilke C, Wurtz K, Urban JP, Borm W, Arand M, Ignatius A, et al. Regulation of gene expression in intervertebral disc cells by low and high hydrostatic pressure. Eur Spine J. 2006 Aug;15 Suppl 3:S372–8.

54. Melrose J, Taylor TK, Ghosh P. The serine proteinase inhibitory proteins of the chondrodystrophoid (beagle) and non-chondrodystrophoid (greyhound) canine intervertebral disc. Electrophoresis. 1997 Jun;18(7):1059–63.

55. Erwin WM, Inman RD. Notochord cells regulate intervertebral disc chondrocyte proteoglycan production and cell proliferation. Spine (Phila, PA, 1976). 2006 May 1;31(10):1094–9.

56. Pfirrmann CW, Metzdorf A, Zanetti M, Hodler J, Boos N. Magnetic resonance classification of lumbar intervertebral disc degeneration. Spine. 2001 Sep 1;26(17):1873–8.

57. Bergknut N, Auriemma E, Wijsman S, Voorhout G, et al. Evaluation of intervertebral disk degeneration in chondrodystrophic and nonchondrodystrophic dogs by use of Pfirrmann grading of images obtained with low-field magnetic resonance imaging. Am J Vet Res. 2011 Jul;72(7):893–8.

58. Pearce RH, Thompson JP, Bebault GM, Flak B. Magnetic resonance imaging reflects the chemical changes of aging degeneration in the human intervertebral disk. J Rheumatol Suppl. 1991 Feb;27:42–3.

59. Baltzer WI, McMichael MA, Hosgood GL, Kerwin SC, Levine JM, Steiner JM, et al. Randomized, blinded, placebo-controlled clinical trial of N-acetylcysteine in dogs with spinal cord trauma from acute intervertebral disc disease. Spine (Phila, PA, 1976). 2008 Jun 1;33(13):1397–402.

60. Blight AR, Toombs JP, Bauer MS, Widmer WR. The effects of 4-aminopyridine on neurological deficits in chronic cases of traumatic spinal cord injury in dogs: a phase I clinical trial. J Neurotrauma. 1991 Summer;8(2):103–19.

61. Borgens RB, Toombs JP, Breur G, Widmer WR, Waters D, Harbath AM, et al. An imposed oscillating electrical field improves the recovery of function in neurologically complete paraplegic dogs. J Neurotrauma. 1999 Jul;16(7):639–57.

62. Jeffery ND, Lakatos A, Franklin RJ. Autologous olfactory glial cell transplantation is reliable and safe in naturally occurring canine spinal cord injury. J Neurotrauma. 2005 Nov;22(11):1282–93.

63. Laverty PH, Leskovar A, Breur GJ, Coates JR, Bergman RL, Widmer WR, et al. A preliminary study of intravenous surfactants in paraplegic dogs: polymer therapy in canine clinical SCI. J Neurotrauma. 2004 Dec;21(12):1767–77.

64. Norenberg MD, Smith J, Marcillo A. The pathology of human spinal cord injury: defining the problems. J Neurotrauma. 2004 Apr;21(4):429–40.

65. Griffiths IR. Some aspects of the pathology and pathogenesis of the myelopathy caused by disc protrusions in the dog. J Neurol Neurosurg Psychiatr. 1972 Jun;35(3):403–13.

66. Smith PM, Jeffery ND. Histological and ultrastructural analysis of white matter damage after naturally-occurring spinal cord injury. Brain Pathol (Zurich, Switzerland). 2006 Apr;16(2):99–109.

67. Wright F, Palmer AC. Morphological changes caused by pressure on the spinal cord. Pathol Vet. 1969;6(4): 355–68.

68. Kakulas BA. A review of the neuropathology of human spinal cord injury with emphasis on special features. J Spinal Cord Med. 1999 Summer;22(2): 119–24.

69. Hoerlein BF. Intervertebral disc protrusions in the dog. I. Incidence and pathological lesions. Am J Vet Res. 1953 Apr;14(51):260–9.

70. Tator CH. Review of treatment trials in human spinal cord injury: issues, difficulties, and recommendations. Neurosurgery. 2006 Nov;59(5):957–82; discussion 82–7.

71. Hukuda S, Jameson HD, Wilson CB. Experimental cervical myelopathy. 3. The canine corticospinal tract. Anatomy and function. Surg Neurol. 1973 Mar;1(2):107–14.

Section II

Disc Disease: Degenerative and other Pathology

Addressed later in the text is the issue of traumatic displacement of a previously healthy disc. However, few clinical cases of traumatic disc extrusion are seen by veterinarians in comparison with the numbers of patients who have clinical signs referable to intervertebral disc degeneration and its consequences. In this section, we start by focusing on the often confusing terminology associated with IVDD and associated disc displacement, and present the recommended nomenclature for use in professional discussions and publications. Then we address the processes of spontaneous disc degeneration in dogs and cats, and how such degeneration may lead to clinical signs. Finally, we address an important differential diagnosis for disc-herniation related myelopathy (disc-related fibrocartilaginous embolism/spinal cord infarction) and explore the relationship between disc disease and cervical spondylomyelopathies (so-called Wobbler syndromes).

4 Historical and Current Nomenclature Associated with Intervertebral Disc Pathology

Jonathan M. Levine and James M. Fingeroth

Introduction

The catch-all term "intervertebral disc disease" (IVDD) is familiar to all veterinary clinicians, but lacks any specificity of definition. It does not convey whether the "disease" is clinical or subclinical, and it neither addresses the seriousness of the problem nor offers any useful prognostic information or suggestions for proper intervention. Within the rubric of "IVDD" are other terms such as "prolapse," "rupture," "herniation," and "bulge" that are often used synonymously or with great overlap.

Devising and using appropriate nomenclature for abnormalities associated with the intervertebral disc has been an uncommonly addressed topic in veterinary medicine. In human medicine, this subject was largely avoided until efforts were made in the late 1990s by the American Society of Spine Radiology (ASSR) to develop a standardized glossary of terms that could be applied to imaging studies of the human lumbar intervertebral disc [1–3]. There were several reasons that basic scientists and physicians attempted to improve the nomenclature used to describe intervertebral disc pathology [4]. First, by standardizing reporting terms, heterogeneity in disease description is reduced. This has an immediate, positive effect on the quality of clinical and research data. Second, compelling clinicians to use the same terms for similar diseases facilitates communication with colleagues, paraprofessionals, and clients. Finally, by improving data quality and communication, standardized terminology is likely to enhance care delivery.

Several guiding principles should be used to develop appropriate nomenclature [5]. Importantly, terminology should be based on previously approved anatomical descriptors, such as those in the *Nomina Anatomica Veterinaria*. If at all possible, terms should have a basis in pathomechanisms and should not be eponymous. Medical vocabulary should allow clinicians to distinguish similar diseases that may have divergent outcomes or treatments. Finally, in veterinary medicine, adhering to systems commonly used by physicians and basic scientists is likely to be advantageous. Shared nomenclature, similar to what has

Advances in Intervertebral Disc Disease in Dogs and Cats, First Edition. Edited by James M. Fingeroth and William B. Thomas.
© 2015 ACVS Foundation. Published 2015 by John Wiley & Sons, Inc.

been attempted by the World Health Organization (WHO) Classification of Tumors of Domestic Animals, facilitates comparative medical studies and communication with those in other medical professions.

The goals of this chapter are to review the history of nomenclature associated with intervertebral disc pathology in dogs and to discuss current, appropriate terms based upon available veterinary and human medical literature.

A brief history of nomenclature for intervertebral disc displacement in dogs

To the authors' knowledge, the first report of canine intervertebral disc displacement occurred in 1881, when Janson described a young dachshund that was euthanized due to acute onset paraplegia [6]. Janson thought that the lesion grossly compressing the spinal cord resembled a cartilaginous tumor and termed it an enchondroma of the intervertebral disc. In 1893, Dexler described "pachymeningitis chronica ossificans" that resulted in spinal cord compression and was associated with mineralized material originating from the intervertebral disc [6]. In the early twentieth century, several investigators reported the presence of similar cartilaginous or mineralized debris in the epidural space of dogs with paraplegia. The presence of this material was referred to as "enostosis intervertebralis," "ekchondrosis intervertebralis," "calcinosis intervertebralis," and "ekchondroma." Small studies by Olsson [7] and McGrath [8] in the early 1950s used terms such as "disc protrusion" or "intervertebral disc syndrome" to describe spinal cord compression secondary to disc displacement in dogs.

Even 60 years after Hansen's seminal work on intervertebral disc degeneration and introduction of the term "herniation" (intervertebral disc herniation (IVDH)) in dogs, his influence remains well entrenched [6]. Hansen described the histology and structure of the nucleus pulposus, annulus fibrosus, and cartilaginous end plate. He attempted to define disc degeneration, although he noted, "it is practically impossible to give a certain and detached definition." Hansen subclassified degeneration as fibroid or chondroid and associated these phenotypes with signalment features. Additionally, two types of IVDH were defined,

Hansen type I and Hansen type II. As described, type I and type II IVDH are essentially synonymous with the modern terms "extrusive" and "protrusive" IVDH, respectively.

Much of the nomenclature proposed by Hansen does not meet modern, generally agreed upon criteria for appropriate medical terminology. For example, the descriptors "IVDH," "disc prolapse," and "disc protrusion" were used interchangeably by Hansen. Today, the ASSR defines disc herniation and disc protrusion as related, but distinct entities and does not recognize the term disc prolapse. Importantly, while many veterinary clinicians and students still describe canine IVDH as either type I or type II, this nomenclature is not accepted by ASSR, is not in common use outside veterinary medicine, and does not necessarily reflect underlying pathomechanisms [1].

Modern nomenclature

Intervertebral disc degeneration has been defined as structural failure of the intervertebral disc associated with abnormal or accelerated changes seen in aging [9]. Some of the pathological changes seen following disc degeneration include nuclear desiccation, fibrosis, narrowing of the intervertebral disc space, annular tearing, end plate sclerosis, and spondylosis deformans [1, 9]. In most species, both mechanical and biochemical factors are involved in the degenerative cascade. Importantly, disc degeneration may exist in the absence of displacement or in the presence or absence of clinical signs. In dogs, histologic degenerative changes are classically defined as fibroid or chondroid, though this may be a vast oversimplification. Chondroid metaplasia is identified most commonly in young chondrodystrophoid dogs. Specifically, early notochordal and chondrocyte-like cell senescence within the nucleus pulposus results in loss of proteoglycans, shifts in proteoglycan ratios, disc dehydration, and nuclear mineralization [10]. Fibroid metaplasia is frequently identified in older, large-breed dogs. The affected nucleus contains abundant fibrous tissue, has shifts in proteoglycan ratios, and is dehydrated; nuclear mineralization has also been recognized. Recently, magnetic resonance imaging (MRI) has been utilized to define and score the degree of disc degeneration in dogs based on the quality of T2 nuclear signal [11].

Intervertebral disc herniation is defined as abnormal, localized displacement of the intervertebral disc beyond the bounds of the intervertebral disc space [1]. Most often, IVDH in dogs occurs dorsally or dorsolaterally and impacts structures within the vertebral canal and/or intervertebral foramen. In dogs and humans, IVDH typically occurs following disc degeneration. In rare cases however, exogenous trauma can result in IVDH in the setting of a nondegenerate intervertebral disc [12, 13] (see Chapter 13).

According to most nomenclature schemes, disc "bulge" is technically not a form of IVDH and is likely to be of limited clinical significance [1]. It is identified when the outer rim of the annulus extends in the transverse plane beyond the edge of the intervertebral disc space over greater than 50% of the disc circumference [1, 14]. There is no shift in the location of the nucleus pulposus.

In veterinary medicine, the term intervertebral disc disease (IVDD) remains popular among clinicians. It is best thought of as a code word that may

(A)   (B)

(C)

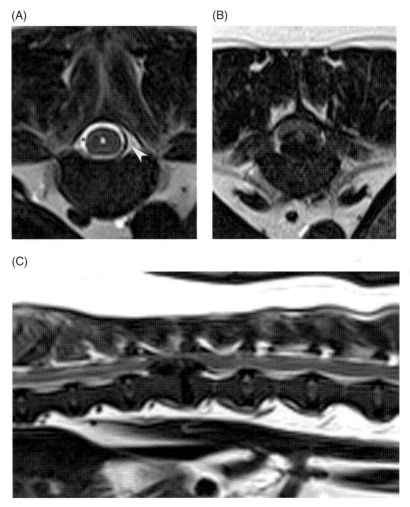

Figure 4.1   Transverse (A and B) and sagittal (C) T2-weighted MR images from a dog with intervertebral disc extrusion at the T13–L1 vertebral articulation. Image (A) was obtained at an interspace cranial to the lesion site and shows a structurally normal spinal cord, subarachnoid space (black asterisk), and epidural space (white arrow head). Image (B) was acquired at the T13–L1 articulation and demonstrates classic features of disc extrusion such as localized involvement of the annular surface and narrow attachment of herniation to the parent disc relative to dorsoventral lesion extent. Image (C) indicates that this is a migrating disc extrusion, based on the extension of herniated nucleus over adjacent vertebral bodies; there is no overt evidence of disc sequestration.

(A)   (B)

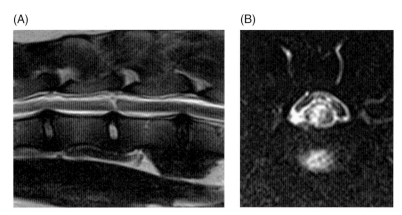

Figure 4.2   Sagittal T2-weighted (A) and transverse T2 fat saturation-weighted (B) MR images from a dog with noncompressive disc extrusion at the L1–L2 vertebral articulation. Image (A) shows a linear T2 hyperintense lesion within the spinal cord immediately overlying the intervertebral disc space. In image (B), the spinal cord T2 hyperintensity has sharp margins, does not result in mass effect, and occupies the right portion of the spinal cord. No spinal cord compression is visible, and T2 signal within the nucleus pulposus is preserved at the L1–L2 vertebral articulation, a common feature of noncompressive disc extrusion.

refer to disc degeneration, IVDH, or disc bulge [14]. As the underlying definition of IVDD is quite broad, we suggest using this term sparingly and only when more specific descriptors cannot be applied. To avoid confusion with verbiage already laden with implied meaning, we use the term disc *displacement* in lieu of IVDD to refer to either IVDH or disc bulge. In essence, disc displacement implies that some portion of the disc extends beyond the interspace. Unlike IVDD, disc displacement is well accepted in the lexicon of medical professionals and is descriptive relative to underlying pathology.

A subclassification of IVDH

IVDH in the dog is classified as disc extrusion or disc protrusion based on morphology, gross pathology, and MRI [14]. Differentiating these subtypes of IVDH may impact treatment recommendations and outcomes.

Disc extrusion occurs when a complete rent in the annulus fibrosus develops which permits displacement of the nucleus pulposus into surrounding soft tissue structures. The ASSR suggests that this can be identified via imaging when the distance of herniation beyond the interspace is greater than the base attachment against the parent disc (Figure 4.1) [1]. The terms sequestered or migrating may be used to subclassify extrusion based on anatomic relationships with the affected disc space [1].

A sequestered extrusion refers to the presence of herniated nuclear material that is no longer contiguous with the annulus. A migrating disc extrusion is one in which the herniated nuclear material extends beyond the bounds of the intervertebral disc space, and may or may not be sequestered [1]. In humans, disc extrusion is often described relative to the position of the posterior (dorsal) longitudinal ligament [1]. Subligamentous extrusions are still bounded by ligament dorsally, whereas transligamentous extrusions have herniated through the posterior longitudinal ligament. These entities have not been well described in veterinary medicine, but most extrusions in dogs appear to be transligamentous.

Relatively unique to veterinary medicine is the term "acute noncompressive nucleus pulposus extrusion" (ANNPE) which refers to a small volume IVDH event that has resulted in significant spinal cord injury (Figure 4.2) [13]. In some instances, these events may be traumatic in origin and may have occurred without the presence underlying disc degeneration. ANNPE has also been referred to as "noncompressive disc extrusion," "Hansen type III IVDH," "gunshot or bullet-like IVDH," and "high-velocity IVDH." These alternate terms may not describe the underlying pathomechanisms of this lesion adequately, since imaging studies cannot measure the velocity of IVDH and velocity is but one component that affects severity in injury models (dwell time and

(A)   (B)

(C)

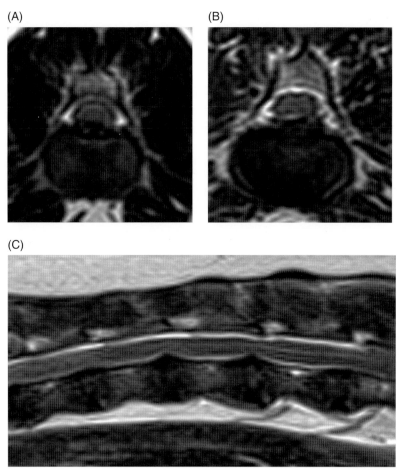

Figure 4.3   Transverse ((A), T13–L1; (B), L1–L2) and sagittal (C) T2-weighted MR images from a dog with intervertebral disc protrusion. Image (A) shows a broad-based disc protrusion that results in ventral extradural spinal cord compression with minimal loss of the dorsal epidural/subarachnoid space. Image (B) exemplifies a focal disc protrusion. Image (C) clearly shows that the distance the disc is herniated in the cranial–caudal and dorsal–ventral planes is smaller than the attachment of the herniation to the annulus in each of these planes.

impact force are also important) [15]. Nonetheless, veterinary clinicians need to be familiar with this form of IVDH, since it is commonly associated with MRI alterations to the spinal cord parenchyma and is not generally amenable to surgical treatment (see Chapters 13 and 16).

Disc protrusion is defined as rupture of the inner layers of the annulus fibrosus, partial displacement of the nucleus pulposus into the disrupted annulus, and subsequent annular hypertrophy. On imaging studies, disc protrusion is recognized when the distance of herniation (in any anatomic plane) from the disc space is less than the distance of the base attachment with the

annulus (Figure 4.3) [1]. In humans, disc protrusions can be further classified as *focal* (<25% of the disc circumference) or *broad* (between 25 and 50% of the disc circumference) [1].

Conclusions

Terminology used to describe abnormalities of the intervertebral disc in dogs dates back at least 130 years. To date, there has been limited agreement as to what descriptors are appropriate and in some instances, how terms should be defined. We propose that veterinarians should adopt terminology

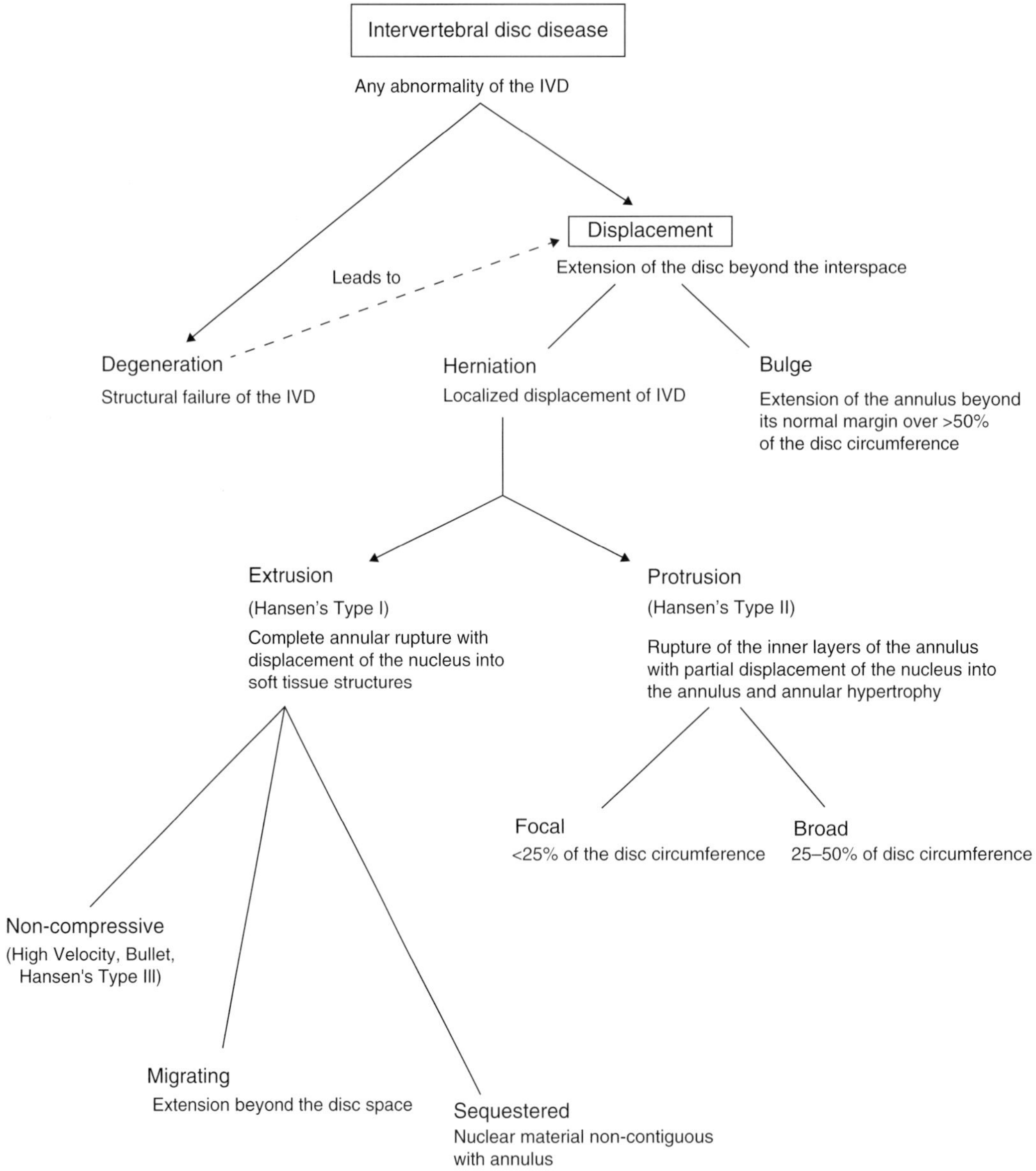

Figure 4.4   Algorithmic depiction of nomenclature (including incorporation of the commonly used Hansen terminology) for intervertebral disc degeneration and displacement.

widely accepted in the human medical, neuroimaging, and basic science fields and understand their hierarchy and proper meaning (Figure 4.4). Through doing this, we are likely to enhance communication among veterinarians and between veterinarians and other medical professionals. The use of proper terminology also facilitates understanding the clinical significance of various forms of disc displacement and how we might intervene therapeutically.

References

1. Fardon DF, Milette PC. Nomenclature and classification of lumbar disc pathology. Recommendations of the Combined task Forces of the North American Spine Society, American Society of Spine Radiology, and American Society of Neuroradiology. Spine (Phila Pa 1976). 2001 Mar 1;26(5):E93–113.
2. Milette PC, Ortiz AO. American Society of Spine Radiology: the first decade. AJNR Am J Neuroradiol. 2003 Oct;24(9):1891–2.

3. Fardon DF, Milette PC. Nomenclature and Classification of Lumbar Disc Pathology 2003. October 11, 2013. Available from: http://www.asnr.org/spine_nomenclature/glossary.shtml. Accessed on August 1, 2014.

4. Costello RF, Beall DP. Nomenclature and standard reporting terminology of intervertebral disk herniation. Magn Reson Imaging Clin N Am. 2007 May;15(2):167–74, v–vi.

5. Chalmers RJ. Health care terminology for the electronic era. Mayo Clin Proc. 2006 Jun;81(6):729–31.

6. Hansen H. A pathologic-anatomical study on disc degeneration in the dog. Acta Orthop Scand (Suppl). 1952;11:1–117.

7. Olsson SE. On disc protrusion in dog (enchondrosis intervertebralis); a study with special reference to roentgen diagnosis and to the value of disc fenestration. Acta Orthop Scand Suppl. 1951;8:1–95.

8. McGrath JT. Spinal paralysis of the dog. J Neuropathol Exp Neurol. 1951 Jan;10(1):88–9.

9. Adams MA, Roughley PJ. What is intervertebral disk degeneration, and what causes it? Spine. 2006;31:2151–61.

10. Cappello R, Bird JL, Pfeiffer D, Bayliss MT, Dudhia J. Notochordal cell produce and assemble extracellular matrix in a distinct manner, which may be responsible for the maintenance of healthy nucleus pulposus. Spine. 2006;31:873–82.

11. Bergknut N, Auriemma E, Wijsman S, Voorhout G, Hagman R, Lagerstedt AS, et al. Evaluation of intervertebral disk degeneration in chondrodystrophic and nonchondrodystrophic dogs by use of Pfirrmann grading of images obtained with low-field magnetic resonance imaging. Am J Vet Res. 2011 Jul;72(7):893–8.

12. Chang Y, Dennis R, Platt SR, Penderis J. Magnetic resonance imaging of traumatic intervertebral disc extrusion in dogs. Vet Rec. 2007 Jun 9;160(23):795–9.

13. De Risio L, Adams V, Dennis R, McConnell FJ. Association of clinical and magnetic resonance imaging findings with outcome in dogs with presumptive acute noncompressive nucleus pulposus extrusion: 42 cases (2000-2007). J Am Vet Med Assoc. 2009 Feb 15;234(4):495–504.

14. Besalti O, Pekcan Z, Sirin YS, Erbas G. Magnetic resonance imaging findings in dogs with thoracolumbar intervertebral disk disease: 69 cases (1997–2005). J Am Vet Med Assoc. 2006;228:902–8.

15. Young W. Spinal cord contusion models. Prog Brain Res. 2002;137:231–55.

5 What Do We Know about the Incidence of Disc Disease in Chondrodystrophoid Dogs?

William B. Thomas, James M. Fingeroth, and Ragnvi Hagman

Epidemiology is concerned with the frequency of disease, the course of disease, and the predilection of disease in relation to factors such as species, breed, and sex [1]. Epidemiologic data are useful for clinicians because awareness of disease frequency among different patient characteristics aids diagnosis. Knowledge of the course and severity of disease helps the veterinarian recommend treatment. Finally, identifying risk factors for a disease provides important clues to the underlying cause. This chapter reviews basic epidemiology and summarizes the current data regarding disc disease in chondrodystrophoid breed dogs.

Definitions

In epidemiology, the unit of study is a patient affected with a disease. Hence, the diagnosis of the particular disease is fundamental to all epidemiologic studies. Ideally, the criteria for diagnosis should be specified because this will affect the estimation for how common the disease is. For example, if the diagnosis of disc disease is based on clinical features of back pain, the estimate of disease frequency will be higher than if the diagnosis is based on imaging to confirm the diagnosis since not all dogs with mild clinical signs undergo further diagnostic testing.

The most basic question is, how common is the disease? The answer involves a count of the cases of the disease within a given place and time. It is common to relate the cases to the rest of the population, so that the number of cases of the disease is the numerator and all animals in the population is the denominator. If all animals in the population were examined, all the patients with the disease and without the disease could be discovered. But such a population survey is usually impractical. Instead, most veterinary studies involve patients who have come to medical attention. Much of the published information regarding disc disease arises from case series that involve cases collected from individual hospitals or databases that collect information from participating hospitals. One problem with such data is that there is little assurance that the cases or all patients in the hospital or database are representative of all animals. For example, not every animal in the population is presented for

Advances in Intervertebral Disc Disease in Dogs and Cats, First Edition. Edited by James M. Fingeroth and William B. Thomas.
© 2015 ACVS Foundation. Published 2015 by John Wiley & Sons, Inc.

veterinary care. And the patients seen at a referral practice are not necessarily a reflection of patients seen at general practices.

Prevalence

The two basic measures of disease frequency are incidence and prevalence. Prevalence is the proportion of animals that have the disease during a specified period of time. It measures the frequency of existing disease. Prevalence is affected by several factors. If the disease is severe and many animals die early in the course of disease, the prevalence is depressed. If the duration of illness is long, the prevalence increases. Since prevalence rates are influenced by so many factors unrelated to disease causation, they do not provide strong evidence of causality [2].

Incidence

Incidence is the occurrence of new cases of disease that develop in the population over a specified time period. It measures the frequency of new diseases.

Incidence rate

Data on incidence and prevalence become more useful if converted into rates. A rate is calculated by dividing the number of cases by the corresponding number of animals in the population at risk and is expressed as cases per 100 or 1000 or other number of population. Therefore, for incidence rate, each animal in the study population contributes one animal-year to the denominator for each year of observation before disease develops or the animal is lost to follow-up. The denominator is often approximated by multiplying the average size of the study population by the length of the study period. This is reasonably accurate if the size of the population is stable and the incidence rate is low.

Crude rate

When incidence rate applies to an entire population, it is referred to as crude rate, which does not take into account differences in the demographic characteristics such as breed.

Specific rate

Specific rates are used when rates are reported separately for different categories. Examples include breed-specific rate and sex-specific rate.

Mortality rate

Mortality rate or death rate is the number of deaths caused by the disease occurring within a unit of time and population. The case fatality rate refers to the proportion of affected patients who die from the disease. These rates provide a measure of the severity and course of disease.

Epidemiologic studies of disc disease in dogs

Priester studied data from 13 North American veterinary colleges participating in the Veterinary Medical Data Program from 1964 to 1974. This identified 8,117 cases of disc disease in 356,954 dogs studied, for an overall crude hospital rate of 23 new cases of canine IVDD per 1000 dogs per year. Breeds with a significantly increased risk were dachshund, Pekingese, shih tzu, Lhasa apso, and beagle. At-risk breeds had a peak incidence at 4–6 years of age, while other breeds had a peak incidence at 6–8 years [3].

Hoerlein studied 2395 cases presenting to Auburn University between 1952 and 1974 [4]. Dachshunds accounted for 65% of cases. Pekingese (8.4%), small poodles (6.3%), cocker spaniels (4.7%), and beagles (3.5%) were also commonly affected. Other breeds accounted for 12.1%. Only 1.1% of patients were 1 year of age or less. The incidence increased with age to a peak at 5 years of age and then progressively declined, with 73.1% of patients being 3–6 years old.

A study at the University of California Veterinary Medical Teaching Hospital from 1957 to 1967 showed dachshunds to have the greatest risk (12.6) relative to other breeds with Pekingese (10.3), beagles (6.4), and cocker spaniel (2.6) also being at increased relative risk [5].

A pedigree study of 536 registered dachshunds with intervertebral disc disease estimated a breed prevalence of disc disease in dachshunds of 19%. In two families, the prevalence was 62%. No obvious simple pattern of inheritance was identified [6].

Most recently, Bergknut et al. utilized insurance claims involving 677,057 dogs in Sweden, from 1995 to 2006. A major strength of this study is that the insurance database included approximately 40% of the Swedish dog population each year and these dogs are considered to be fairly representative of the entire population of dogs in the country. The lifetime prevalence for intervertebral disc disease before the age of 12 years was estimated to be 3.5%. In this study, disc disease included disc extrusions, degenerative lumbosacral stenosis, and cervical spondylomyelopathy. Overall mortality rate attributed to disc disease was approximately 1% (9.4 deaths/10,000 dog-years at risk). Miniature dachshunds had the highest risk with a lifetime prevalence of 20%, and 9 of the 10 breeds at highest risk were chondrodystrophoid. The Doberman pinscher was the only nonchondrodystrophoid breed among these 10, due to the inclusion of cervical spondylomyelopathy (see Chapter 7) [7].

The incidence of disc disease is slightly higher in males, with an incidence ranging from 53 to 67% [3, 4, 6]. Although obesity has been cited as a risk factor for disc disease, several studies have found no association between the body condition score and the development of disc disease [8, 9].

Conclusions and clinical implications

In summary, disc disease in the dog is a substantial clinical problem, with a lifetime prevalence of about 3.5% and an overall mortality rate of approximately 1%. Chondrodystrophoid breeds have the highest risk with the miniature dachshund having a lifetime prevalence of 20%. In about 25% of affected dachshunds, the disease is fatal.

The studies cited earlier, the data in other chapters in this text, and the extensive clinical experience of veterinarians clearly indicate that disc disease is common in chondrodystrophoid dogs such as dachshunds. It is also apparent that disc disease can be clinically silent in many dogs, or at least that symptoms are not clinically recognized. The incidence of signs associated with disc disease

(usually due to herniation of a disc, rather than just the degeneration of the disc) is clearly on the low side when put into perspective however, and veterinarians neither recommend against continued breeding of these dog breeds at higher risk nor prophylactic treatment of all members of a breed at risk. The challenge veterinarians face, as addressed in other chapters (see Chapters 26, 35, 36, and 37), is whether to recommend prophylactic treatment (fenestration, nucleolysis, etc.) for individual patients that have developed clinical signs associated with IVDD and disc herniation. As noted in other chapters in this text, the data are still not entirely clear. Certainly, if there was evidence that individual dogs with disc disease had a higher subsequent incidence of second or more herniations than the overall population of dogs in that breed, it would be eminently sensible to recommend routine prophylactic treatment in an effort to reduce this incidence. Similarly, if we could better identify a familial risk for IVDH (as suggested in Ball's study) [6], there could be justification for both individual and sibling prophylactic treatment in an effort to reduce the incidence of disc disease. However, if there are neither individual nor familial risk factors, and the incidence of subsequent disc herniation in any individual was no higher than for the population as a whole, then it becomes more challenging to routinely recommend prophylactic treatment for every patient with signs of disc disease. This controversy will continue to plague veterinarians until we have studies that can clearly answer the questions raised earlier in the text.

References

1. Kurtzke JF. An introduction to neuroepidemiology. Neurol Clin. 1996 1996;14(2):255–72.
2. Beaglehole R, Bonita R, Kjellstron T. Basic Epidemiology. Geneva: World Health Organization; 1993.
3. Priester WA. Canine intervertebral disk disease—Occurrence by age, breed, and sex among 8,117 cases. Theriogenology. 1976;6:293–303.
4. Hoerlein BF. Intervertebral disks. In: Hoerlein BF, editor. Canine Neurology Diagnosis and Treatment. 3rd ed. Philadelphia: WB Saunders; 1979. pp. 470–560.
5. Goggin JE, Li AS, Franti CE. Canine intervertebral disk disease: characterization by age, sex, breed, and anatomic site of involvement. Am J Vet Res. 1970 Sep;31(9):1687–92.

6. Ball MU, McGuire JA, Swaim SF, Hoerlein BF. Patterns of occurrence of disk disease among registered dachshunds. J Am Vet Med Assoc. 1982 Mar 1;180(5):519–22.

7. Bergknut N, Egenvall A, Hagman R, Gustas P, Hazewinkel HA, Meij BP, et al. Incidence of intervertebral disk degeneration-related diseases and associated mortality rates in dogs. J Am Vet Med Assoc. 2012 Jun 1;240(11):1300–9.

8. Levine JM, Levine GJ, Kerwin SC, Hettlich BF, Fosgate GT. Association between various physical factors and acute thoracolumbar intervertebral disk extrusion or protrusion in Dachshunds. J Am Vet Med Assoc. 2006 Aug 1;229(3):370–5.

9. Brown DC, Conzemius MG, Shofer FS. Body weight as a predisposing factor for humeral condylar fractures, cranial cruciate rupture and intervertebral disc disease in Cocker Spaniels. Vet Comp Orthop Traumatol. 1996;9(2):75–8.

6

Feline Intervertebral Disc Disease

Michael Farrell and Noel Fitzpatrick

Introduction

The extensive literature concerning canine and human intervertebral disc disease (IVDD) contrasts with the comparatively sparse literature detailing this condition in cats. This is probably a consequence of the relatively low prevalence of clinically significant feline IVDD. Estimates for clinical feline IVDD (i.e., signs of IVDH) prevalence vary between 0.02 and 0.12% [1, 2], whereas canine IVDD accounts for more than 2% of all diseases diagnosed in dogs [3]. Interpretation of the available literature on feline IVDD can be confusing because much of the published epidemiological data are derived from *postmortem* studies performed on clinically normal animals [4–6]. Between 1958 and 2012, there have been four histopathological studies (including a total of 355 cats) investigating the prevalence of feline spinal cord diseases [4–7]. Over the same period, 18 reports have described a total of 45 clinically affected cats with 57 IVD herniations, and 2 systematic reviews have been published summarizing the important clinical features of feline IVDD (Table 6.1). When

reviewing these data, it is important to recognize that there are significant differences between clinically unaffected and clinically affected cats in the incidence of IVDD, the common predilection sites for IVDD, and the frequency of Hansen type I *versus* type II disease (see the following text). It is also important to exercise caution when interpreting the literature concerning the relative frequency of feline IVDD compared with other causes of myelopathy. The list of differential diagnoses for cats presenting with myelopathy includes spinal fractures or luxations, infectious or inflammatory disorders, vascular disease, spinal neoplasia, and IVDD [7]. Epidemiological studies including sample populations of spinal cord segments submitted *postmortem* have the potential to bias results toward conditions carrying a poorer prognosis, which would in turn result in underestimation of the relative frequency of IVDD [7, 21]. Nevertheless, the only *antemortem* prevalence study of cats with clinical signs referable to spinal cord disease confirmed a relatively low incidence of IVDD [21]. In this study, magnetic resonance imaging (MRI) and cerebrospinal fluid (CSF) analysis findings were

Advances in Intervertebral Disc Disease in Dogs and Cats, First Edition. Edited by James M. Fingeroth and William B. Thomas.
© 2015 ACVS Foundation. Published 2015 by John Wiley & Sons, Inc.

Table 6.1 Summary of the presenting features, lesion localization, treatment, and outcome for 88 cats affected by IVDD

Reference	Signalment	Grade	Comment	IVD space	Hansen type	Treatment	Outcome	Notes
Cervical neurolocalization								
Fitzpatrick [8]	6y, FN, British shorthair	II	Chronic	C2–C3 (also C3–C4, C4–C5, C5–C6, T3–T4)	I	Non-surgically Managed	LTFU	
Lu [9]	5y, MN, DSH	III	Acute (suspected trauma)	C3–C4	HVLV	Non-surgically Managed	Fair	Residual mild hemiparesis
Heavner [10]	1.5y, M, Russian blue	III	Acute; monoparesis progressing to nonambulatory quadriparesis	C5–C6	II	Euthanasia	Euthanasia	
Maritato [11]	10y, MN, DLH	III	Acute (indoor cat)	C2–C3	I	Ventral slot	Poor	Died 3d postoperatively
Littlewood [12]	4.5y, MN, DLH	IV	Chronic; dyspneic on presentation	C5–C6	II	Euthanasia	Euthanasia	
Thoracolumbar neurolocalization								
Munana [2]	13y, FN, DLH	I	Chronic pain only	T13–L1	I	HL	LTFU	
Fitzpatrick [8]	9y, FN, DSH	I	Chronic pain; reluctant to walk	T10–T11	II	Non-surgically Managed	Good	Good improvement in 2 weeks
Munana [2]	9y, FN, DLH	I	Chronic pain only	T11–T12	II	HL	Excellent	
Fitzpatrick [8]	4.5y, FN, British shorthair	I	Chronic pain only	L4–L5	II	Non-surgically Managed	Excellent	Slow improvement over months
Fitzpatrick [8]	8y, MN, Oriental	II	Chronic	T12–T13, T13–L1	I	Non-surgically Managed	Excellent	Slow improvement to weak ambulation over 2 months
Wheeler [13]	6y, F, Siamese	II	Chronic progressive ataxia	T9–T10	I	DL	Poor	No improvement
Knipe [14]	3y, FN, Himalayan	II	Chronic; ambulatory paraparesis; urinary and fecal incontinence	T13–L1, L4–L5	I	HL	Poor	Residual urinary incontinence
Fitzpatrick [8]	12y, MN, Burmese	II	Acute	T13–L1	HVLV	HL	Poor	Significantly worse neurological status postoperatively
Fitzpatrick [8]	6.5y, MN, DSH	II	Acute trauma (fell on stairs)	L5–L6	HVLV	Non-surgically Managed	Fair	
Fitzpatrick [8]	4.5y, MN, DSH	II	Acute (unknown trauma)	T11–T12, T12–T13	I	HL	Fair	Ongoing ataxia
Fitzpatrick [8]	9y, FN, DSH	II	Acute (unknown trauma)	T13–L1	I	HL T12–L1	Fair	Ongoing ataxia

(Continued)

Table 6.1 (Cont'd)

Reference	Signalment	Grade	Comment	IVD space	Hansen type	Treatment	Outcome	Notes
Knipe [14]	6y, MN, Persian	II	Acute; ambulatory paraparesis and urinary incontinence	T12–T13	I	HL (durotomy)	Fair	Residual pelvic limb ataxia
Knipe [14]	3y, FN, DSH	II	Chronic	T13–L1	I	HL	Good	
Choi [15]	14y, MN, DSH	II	Acute	T2–T6, L2–L5	I/II	Non-surgically Managed (acupuncture)	Good	
Fitzpatrick [8]	7y, FN, DSH	II	Acute; urinary incontinent; sluggish CP	L4–L5	HVLV	Non-surgically Managed	Good	Slight residual ataxia
Fitzpatrick [8]	12y, FN, DLH	II	Acute	T12–T13	II	HL	Good	
Kathmann [16]	12y, FN, Persian	II	Acute	L4–L5	I	HL	Excellent	
Gilmore [17]	10y, FN, Siamese	II	Acute	T11–T12, T12–T13, T13–L1	I	DL	Excellent	
Munana [2]	8y, MN, DLH	II	Acute	L5–L6	I	HL	Excellent	
Bottcher [18]	7y, FN, DSH	II	Acute	T3–T4	II	Lateral corpectomy	Excellent	
Fitzpatrick [8]	14y, MN, DSH	II	Chronic; severe thoracolumbar pain	T11–T12	I	HL	Excellent	
Fitzpatrick [8]	8y, FN, DSH	II	Acute	L1–L2	I	HL	Excellent	
Fitzpatrick [8]	5 m, M, DSH	II	Chronic	T4–T5	Discospondylitis	Non-surgically Managed	Excellent	
Munana	4y, FN, Persian	III	Acute	T13–L1	I	HL	LTFU	
Fitzpatrick [8]	11 m, FN, DSH	III	Acute (unknown trauma)	T10–T11	HVLV	Non-surgically Managed	Excellent	
Knipe	9y, FN, DMH	III	Acute	T13–L1, L4–L5	I	HL	Poor	Residual urinary incontinence
Munana	10y, MN, DSH	III	Acute; flaccid tail; urinary and fecal incontinence	L5–L6	I	Non-surgically Managed	Poor	Residual urinary and fecal incontinence
Fitzpatrick [8]	6y, MN, DLH	III	Acute (unknown trauma)	L4–L5	HVLV	Non-surgically Managed	Fair	Ongoing UMN bladder
Munana	8y, MN, DSH	III	Acute paraparesis	L4–L5	I	Non-surgically Managed	Good	
Seim	2y, FN, DSH	III	Chronic (1 week)	T12–T13	I	DL	Excellent	
Fitzpatrick [8]	5.5y, FN, DSH	IV	Acute (RTA)	L5–L6	HVLV	Euthanasia	Euthanasia	
Munana	17y, MN, DSH	IV–V	Acute	L1–L2	II	Euthanasia	Euthanasia	

Reference	Signalment	Neurolocalization	Onset / Clinical signs	Disc space	Type	Treatment	Outcome	Comments
Munana	11y, FN, DSH	IV–V	Acute	L1–L2	I	HL	Poor	Residual urinary and fecal incontinence
Fitzpatrick [8]	6y, FN, DSH	IV	Acute	T13–L1	HVLV	Non-surgically Managed	Poor	Ongoing severe ataxia
Fitzpatrick [8]	9y, FN, Persian	IV	Chronic progression	L3–L4	II	HL	Fair	Ongoing mild ataxia
Fitzpatrick [8]	7y, MN, Ragdoll	IV	Acute (unknown trauma)	T13–L1	HVLV	Non-surgically Managed	Fair	
Fitzpatrick [8]	6y, MN, British shorthair	IV	Acute (unknown trauma)	L3–L4	HVLV	Non-surgically Managed	Fair	
Salisbury	12y, FN, DSH	IV	Acute	L4–L5	I	HL (durotomy)	Excellent	
Bagley	4.5y, MN, DLH	IV	Acute paraplegia and urinary incontinence	T13–L1	I	HL	Excellent	
Munana	8y, FN, DLH	IV–V	Acute	L4–L5	I	HL	Excellent	
Munana	10y, MN, DSH	IV–V	Acute	L4–L5	I	HL	Excellent	
Wheeler	6y, MN, Siamese	V	Chronic (10 days)	T13–L1	I	Fenestration	LTFU	
Fitzpatrick [8]	3y, MN, DSH	V	Acute (unknown trauma)	L1–L2	HVLV	HL	Euthanasia	Euthanasia after lack of improvement over 2.5 weeks
Knipe	7y, MN, DSH	V	Acute	L2–L3	I	HL (durotomy)	Fair	Residual mild paraparesis
Knipe	7y, MN, DMH	V	Acute	L4–L5	I	HL (durotomy)	Excellent	
Fitzpatrick [8]	10.5y, FN, DSH	V	Acute	L2–L3	I	HL	Excellent	Strongly ambulatory within 10 days

L4–S3 neurolocalization

Reference	Signalment	Neurolocalization	Onset / Clinical signs	Disc space	Type	Treatment	Outcome	Comments
Fitzpatrick [8]	6y, FN, Bengal	L4–S3 localization	Chronic; pain and paresis	L5–L6	I	Non-surgically Managed	Good	Recurrent UTI for 1 year after diagnosis
Fitzpatrick [8]	7y, MN, DSH	L4–S3 localization	Acute loss of tail sensation; dysuria; fecal incontinence; good anal tone; LS pain	L6–L7, L7–S1	I	DL L6–S1	Excellent	Manual bladder expression for 2 weeks after surgery
McConnell	5y, M, DSH	L4–S3 localization	Acute; absent anal tone and left pelvic limb nociception	L5–L6	HVLV	Euthanasia	Euthanasia	Large amount of IVD material breached dura
Sparkes	7y, MN, Siamese	L4–S3 localization	Chronic; paraparesis and absent tail nociception	L6–L7	I	HL	Good	

(Continued)

Table 6.1 (Cont'd)

Reference	Signalment	Grade	Comment	IVD space	Hansen type	Treatment	Outcome	Notes
Kathmann	6y, MN, Oriental	L4–S3 localization	Acute; paraparesis and flaccid tail	L6–L7	I	HL	Excellent	
Smith	6y, MN, DSH	L4–S3 localization	Acute; absent pelvic limb nociception (digits); dysuria	L6–L7	I	HL	Excellent	
Fitzpatrick [8]	10y, MN, DSH	L4–S3 localization	Chronic; difficulty jumping; flaccid tail; moderate LS pain	L6–L7	I	HL	Excellent	Large amount of IVD material breached dura
Fitzpatrick [8]	7y, MN, DSH	L4–S3 localization	Chronic; right pelvic limb lameness	L6–L7	I	HL	Excellent	
Fitzpatrick [8]	6y, FN, DSH	L4–S3 localization	Acute; flaccid tail; right pelvic limb paresis	L6–L7	I	HL	Excellent	
Fitzpatrick [8]	11y, FN, DSH	L4–S3 localization	Acute; right pelvic limb lameness	L7–S1	II	Non-surgically Managed	LTFU	
Fitzpatrick [8]	10y, MN, DSH	L4–S3 localization	Chronic; reluctant to jump	L7–S1	II	Non-surgically Managed	LTFU	Recurrent FLUTD
Fitzpatrick [8]	9y, MN, DLH	L4–S3 localization	Chronic; pelvic limb stiffness; lumbar transitional vertebra	L7–S1	II	Non-surgically Managed (including acupuncture)	Fair	Intermittent L/T constipation; L/T oral analgesia
Fitzpatrick [8]	11y, MN, Burmese	L4–S3 localization	Chronic; reluctant to jump	L7–S1	II	Non-surgically Managed	LTFU	
Fitzpatrick [8]	7.5y, MN, DSH	L4–S3 localization	Chronic intermittent left pelvic limb lameness	L7–S1	II	Non-surgically Managed (including acupuncture)	Good	
Fitzpatrick [8]	1.5y, MN, DSH	L4–S3 localization	Chronic; pelvic limb paresis; lumbar transitional vertebra	L7–S1	II	Non-surgically Managed	LTFU	
Fitzpatrick [8]	1y, MN, Ragdoll	L4–S3 localization	Chronic; Reluctant to jump	L7–S1	II	Non-surgically Managed	Excellent	
Fitzpatrick [8]	4.5y, MN, DSH	L4–S3 localization	Chronic; right pelvic limb lameness	L7–S1	II	Non-surgically Managed	Excellent	
Fitzpatrick [8]	10.5y, MN, DLH	L4–S3 localization	Chronic; excessive grooming over lumbar spine; concurrent surgical MPL	L7–S1	II	Non-surgically Managed	Excellent	
Fitzpatrick [8]	3y, FN, DLH	L4–S3 localization	Acute onset ataxia; constipation	L7–S1	II	Non-surgically Managed	Excellent	
Fitzpatrick [8]	10.5y, MN, DSH	L4–S3 localization	Chronic; reluctant to jump	L7–S1	II	DL	Excellent	

Author	Signalment	Localization	Clinical signs	Level	Type	Approach	Outcome	Comments
Fitzpatrick [8]	10y, MN, DLH	L4–S3 localization	Chronic; spontaneous pain; bilateral pelvic limb lameness	L7–S1	II	LSDF	LTFU	
Fitzpatrick [8]	12y, MN, DSH	L4–S3 localization	Chronic; pelvic limb paresis; reluctant to jump	L7–S1	II	LSDF	Euthanasia	Postoperative acute congestive heart failure; euthanasia
Fitzpatrick [8]	11.5y, FN, Siamese	L4–S3 localization	Acute; spontaneous pain; reluctant to jump	L7–S1	II	LSDF	Poor	Lost tail function and limited ability to jump in the L/T
Harris [19]	17y, MN, Abyssinian	L4–S3 localization	Pelvic limb paresis; reluctant to jump	L7–S1	Not recorded	DL	Fair	
Harris [19]	15y, FN, Manx	L4–S3 localization	Urinary incontinence; constipation	L7–S1	Not recorded	DL	Fair	
Fitzpatrick [8]	13y, FN, DSH	L4–S3 localization	Chronic; spontaneous pain; reluctant to jump	L7–S1	II	LSDF	Good	Slow recovery
Fitzpatrick [8]	8.5y, FN, DSH	L4–S3 localization	Chronic; reluctant to jump	L7–S1	II	LSDF	Excellent	Only STFU
Fitzpatrick [8]	9y, MN, DSH	L4–S3 localization	Chronic; bilateral pelvic limb lameness	L7–S1	II	LSDF	Excellent	
Fitzpatrick [8]	7y, MN, Maine Coon	L4–S3 localization	Spontaneous pain; reluctant to jump	L7–S1	II	LSDF	Excellent	
Fitzpatrick [8]	14y, MN, DSH	L4–S3 localization	Acute; pelvic limb paresis; flaccid tail	L7–S1	II	LSDF	Excellent	
Fitzpatrick [8]	13 m, M, Bengal	L4–S3 localization	Chronic; right pelvic limb lameness; pelvic limb paresis; lumbar transitional vertebra	L7–S1	II	LSDF	Excellent	
Jaeger [20]	8y, MN, DSH	L4–S3 localization	Acute pain and dysuria	L7–S1	II	DL	Excellent	
Harris [19]	12y, MN, DSH	L4–S3 localization	Reluctant to jump	L7–S1	Not recorded	DL	Excellent	
Harris [19]	7y, FN, DSH	L4–S3 localization	Dyschezia; lumbar transitional vertebra; low tail carriage	L7–S1	Not recorded	DL	Excellent	
Harris [19]	13y, FN, DLH	L4–S3 localization	Reluctant to jump; low tail carriage; lumbar transitional vertebra	L7–S1	Not recorded	DL	Excellent	
Harris [19]	12y, MN, DSH	L4–S3 localization	Pelvic limb paresis; reluctant to jump; low tail carriage	L7–S1	Not recorded	DL	Excellent	
Fitzpatrick [8]	10y, MN, DSH	L4–S3 localization	Chronic (3 weeks); reluctant to jump	L7–S1	Discospondylitis	NSM	Excellent	

reported in 92 cats affected by spinal cord disease. The diagnostic categories, in order of descending incidence, were neoplasia ($n = 25$), inflammatory or infectious ($n = 13$), traumatic ($n = 8$), vascular ($n = 6$), degenerative (IVDD) ($n = 5$), and anomalous ($n = 3$). The largest group in this study was the group in which no diagnosis was made ($n = 32$).

Etiology

Unlike dogs, in which there are important breed-related predispositions to IVDD, there are few known predispositions to feline IVDD. Vertebral malformations including hemivertebra and sacro-caudal dysgenesis have been reported as a cause of spinal cord compression in Manx cats [22], but there are no breed predilections to IVDD per se. The only cat breed with the chondrodystrophic type that represents a risk for similar early disc degeneration and subsequent Hansen type I herniation as seen in chondrodystrophoid dogs is the Munchkin. To date, there have not been any reports of IVDH in this breed.

Pathogenesis

In three seminal postmortem studies performed by King and Smith, dorsal IVD protrusions were noted as an incidental finding in one-quarter of a random population of adult cats that had displayed no clinical signs indicating myelopathy [4–6]. Hansen's classification for the type of IVD herniation was applied to these cats, and 79% were categorized as having fibroid disc degeneration (Hansen type II). In this population, dorsal protrusions were more common in the cervical region than in the region from T10 to S1. However, approximately half of the cervical protrusions were small Hansen type II bulges that were considered clinically irrelevant. Compared with these asymptomatic cats, the distribution and type of IVD degeneration differ markedly in clinically affected animals. Based on the information provided by single case reports or case series with inclusion of data obtained from 49 cats treated at Fitzpatrick Referrals, chondroid disc degeneration (as is usually correlated with Hansen type I herniations) was recognized in 43% of cases diagnosed between 1981 and 2012 (38/88 cats) [2, 7,

9–12, 14, 16, 17, 20, 23–30]. Only five cases of clinically significant IVD herniations were diagnosed in the cervical region [1, 10, 14, 30, 31]. Lumbar localization was most common, with L7–S1 (29 cats), L4–L5 (9 cats), L6–L7 (7 cats), and L5–L6 (6 cats) constituting the most frequently affected intervertebral discs (Table 6.1). Feline IVDD has also been reported at locations that are considered unusual in dogs, including reports of clinical herniation in the thoracic segments between T2 and T6 [11, 29]. A robust structure (the intercapital ligament) spans the floor of the vertebral canal between the paired rib heads from T1 to T10 [5, 8]. This ligament is thought to provide additional support to the disc and protection from IVD herniations in dogs but may offer less of a stabilizing function in cats in order to facilitate their superior flexibility throughout the vertebral column [15]. In contrast, canine vertebral motion is not distributed evenly, being concentrated at the thoracolumbar and lumbosacral junctions [8]. Stress concentration consequent to this regional increase in vertebral motion has been implicated in the high incidence of IVDH at these locations in dogs [13]. To date, canine studies investigating the relationship between vertebral motion and predisposition to IVDH have not been replicated in cats. Nevertheless, multiple similarities exist between canine and feline lumbosacral (LS) IVDD, which suggest that instability may be important in the pathogenesis of feline LS IVDD (see Chapter 32). These similarities include the presence of LS spondylosis deformans, IVD space collapse, end-plate sclerosis, articular facet hypertrophy, and spondylolisthesis with cranioventral tipping of S1 relative to L7 (Figure 6.1).

Histopathological studies revealed that the nucleus pulposus appears to degenerate more slowly in the cat than in the dog or man [32], and it has been speculated that tearing of the annulus fibrosus occurs in many clinically affected older cats without preexisting changes to the nucleus pulposus [33]. This implies that these discs are undergoing similar degenerative changes to that seen in humans and nonchondrodystrophoid dogs. Rayward also speculated that trauma to the IVD resulting in an acceleration of the degenerative process may account for the discrepancies between clinical features and changes reported in postmortem studies [33]. Also, some cats show clinical features suggestive of a significant

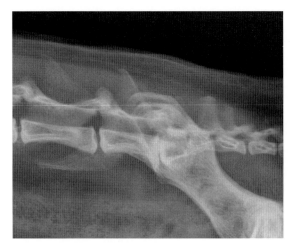

Figure 6.1 Lateral radiograph of an 11.5-year-old Siamese cat presenting acutely with spontaneous pain (vocalizing) and reluctance to jump. Note the collapsed and spondylolisthetic lumbosacral intervertebral disc space with marked end-plate sclerosis, ventral lipping of the vertebral end plates, and articular facet joint hypertrophy.

overlap between Hansen type I and II disc degenerations. Lastly, although it has only been reported once in the veterinary literature [14], we have frequently recognized explosive IVD herniation causing noncompressive spinal cord contusion in cats (Table 6.1, Figure 6.2C). This condition has been termed high-velocity low-volume (HVLV), acute noncompressive nucleus pulposus extrusion (ANNPE), or "type III" IVDD when it affects nonchondrodystrophic dogs [18] (see Chapters 4 and 13).

Clinical features, treatment, and prognosis

Data describing the signalment of 88 cats diagnosed and treated for clinical IVDD between 1981 and 2012 are listed in Table 6.1. After exclusion of the two cats affected by discospondylitis, mean age was 8 years (range, 11 months–17 years). There was a male predisposition (50 male cats (58%) and 36 female). This was particularly evident at the lumbosacral (LS) articulation (20 male (71%) and 8 female). Forty-five cats (52%) were domestic short-haired, 14 (16%) were domestic long-haired, and the remainder were pure breed (n = 25; 29%) or domestic medium-haired (n = 2).

Reported clinical signs varied according to lesion localization. Signs included:

1. Grade I myelopathy—Spinal hyperesthesia
2. Grade II myelopathy—Ataxia, ambulatory monoparesis, paraparesis, or quadriparesis
3. Grade III myelopathy—Nonambulatory paraparesis or quadriparesis
4. Grade IV—Paraplegia or quadriplegia
5. Grade V myelopathy—Paraplegia or quadriplegia with absent deep pain perception[1].

Other frequently reported clinical signs included urinary and/or fecal incontinence, low tail carriage, loss of tail tone and/or sensation, reluctance to jump and/or limping. Speed of onset and progression of clinical signs varied according to lesion localization (see the following text). Localization based on neurological examination did not always correlate with the definitive site of IVDH. Thus, in the following section (and Table 6.1), subdivision of clinical cases into cervical, thoracolumbar, and L4–S3 neurolocalization is based on neurological examination rather than the actual site of IVDH.

Cervical localization

Five cats (6%) presented with cervical neurolocalization. Presentation was acute in three cases and chronic in two. Distribution of myelopathic grade was grade I in 2/5 cats (40%), grade II in 2/5 cats (40%), and grade III in 1/5 cats (20%).

Two cats (1 grade III and 1 grade IV) were euthanized on presentation and two were managed nonsurgically. One nonsurgically managed cat had sustained suspected motor vehicle trauma causing ANNPE (traumatic IVD extrusion; see Chapter 13) (C3–C4) with grade III myelopathy [14]. This cat recovered ambulation but was affected by permanent mild hemiparesis. The other nonsurgically managed cat was lost to follow-up. The only cat managed surgically died in hospital 3 days after ventral slot surgery [10]. The small number of affected cats precludes the formulation of meaningful conclusions regarding the prognosis following nonsurgical or surgical management of feline cervical IVDD.

Thoracolumbar localization

Forty-six cats (52%) presented with thoracolumbar neurolocalization. Presentation was acute in 34

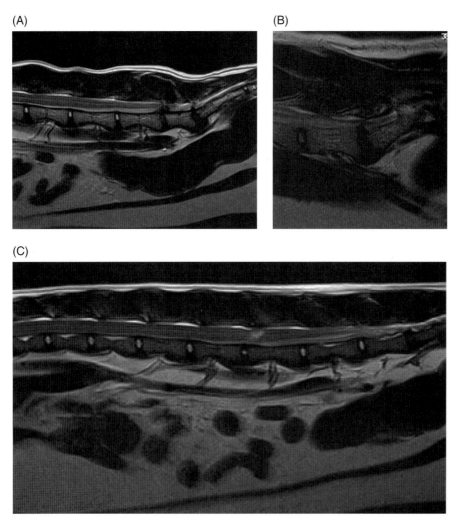

Figure 6.2   T2-weighted magnetic resonance images showing examples of the different types of intervertebral disc herniation observed in cats. (A) Hansen type I IVD herniation at L6–L7 in a 7-year-old domestic shorthair cat presenting with acute loss of tail sensation, dysuria, and fecal incontinence. The L6–L7 and L7–S1 intervertebral discs have hypointense nuclei. Extruded nucleus material is seen dorsal to the L6–L7 IVD space as a mixed intensity mass causing compression of the cauda equina. The dorsal IVD bulge at L7–S1 is typical of Hansen type II disc degeneration. (B) Hansen type II IVD herniation at L7–S1 in a 12-year-old domestic shorthair cat presenting with a chronic history of shifting pelvic limb lameness and reluctance to jump. There is hypointensity of the L7–S1 IVD nucleus pulposus with dorsal and ventral annular bulges. Bilateral abaxial IVD bulging caused bilateral neuroforaminal impingement in this cat. (C) Note the high signal intensity within the spinal cord parenchyma immediately caudal to the L4–L5 IVD space in this 6-year-old domestic longhair cat presenting with an acute grade III myelopathy after an assumed traumatic event. The spinal cord changes coupled with the reduced volume of the L4–L5 nucleus pulposus are consistent with a high-velocity low-volume (ANNPE) disc extrusion.

cats (74%) and chronic in 12 (26%). Distribution of grades for IVD lesions presenting with T3–L3 neurolocalization was grade I in 9/46 cats (19%), grade II in 19/46 cats (41%), grade III in 7/46 cats (15%), grade IV (and IV–V) in 11/46 cats (24%), and grade V in 8/46 cats (11%). Hansen type I and II disc degenerations were reported in 28/46 cats (61%) and 5/46 cats (17%), respectively (with one cat showing features common to both Hansen type I and II disc degeneration). HVLV (ANNPE) extrusions affected 10/46 cats (22%) and discospondylitis was diagnosed in only one cat.

Nonsurgical management

Of the 46 cats, 14 (30%) were managed nonsurgically. Of these 14 cats, 7 had ANNPE, 3 had Hansen type I disc degeneration, 2 had Hansen type II disc degeneration, 1 had features common to both Hansen type I and II disc degenerations, and 1 had discospondylitis. A minimum of 6 weeks of cage confinement was recommended in all cases. In our experience, the majority of physical therapy techniques applied routinely during canine rehabilitation (see Chapter 38) were more challenging to apply to cats. Nevertheless, in cats with tractable personalities, exercises intended to improve proprioception, balance, range of motion, and strength could still be performed. Moreover, hydrotherapy has the potential to facilitate an earlier return to ambulation in nonambulatory cats demonstrating slight voluntary motor function (Figure 6.3).

A single case report documented a favorable outcome after acupuncture treatment of a 14-year-old cat with grade II myelopathy attributed to multiple compressive IVD degenerations between T2 and L5 [29]. In this cat, there was a poor initial response to a course of prednisolone and the cat only started to show improvement as soon as the course of acupuncture treatments was started. The cat was able to rise, walk, and run 4 months after starting the course of 10 acupuncture treatments. In the only reported case of discospondylitis, a 5-month-old male DSH cat presented with grade II myelopathy attributed to hematogenous bacterial discospondylitis affecting the T4–T5 IVD space [30]. In this cat, complete resolution of clinical signs was recorded after a 6 weeks course of cage confinement and oral cephalexin.

Surgical management

Of the 46 cats, 30 (65%) were managed surgically. Of these 30 cats, 24 had Hansen type I IVD degeneration, 4 had Hansen type II IVD degeneration, and 1 had ANNPE. Hemilaminectomy was the most commonly applied surgical technique (25/46 cats, 54%), followed by dorsal laminectomy (3/46 cats, 6.5%). One cat was treated with fenestration alone [34]. Durotomy was performed in 4/46 cats (9%). In two cases, subdural IVD material was removed from crater defects located in the ventral aspect of the spinal cord [30, 35]. Another report documented intramedullary intervertebral disc extrusion at the L5–L6 IVD space in a cat that was euthanized immediately after completion of advanced imaging procedures [9]. In this cat, MRI

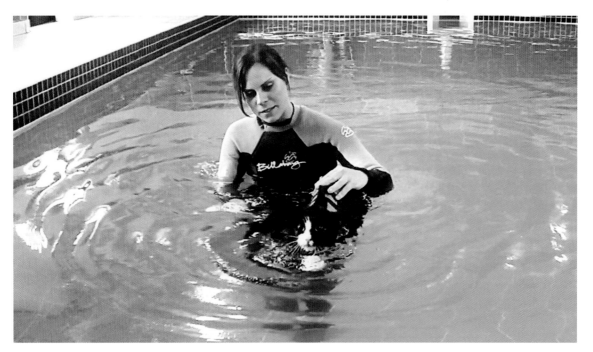

Figure 6.3   Some cats are remarkably tolerant of hydrotherapy.

revealed a linear disc trail extending from the disc space into the spinal cord. Despite the relatively higher prevalence of canine IVDH, intradural and intramedullary disc extrusions have only been reported in a few dogs [19, 36–43]. While the incidence of dura-penetrating herniations may be underreported in dogs, it nonetheless can be concluded that it is an uncommon finding. Thus, it is possible that the feline dura mater might offer less resistance than the canine dura mater to the penetration of extruded IVD material.

One case report described successful partial lateral corpectomy for the treatment of a compressive Hansen type II IVD protrusion at the T3–T4 IVD space, which had resulted in grade II myelopathy in a 7-year-old DSH cat [11]. The only reported modification of the technique as described for canine lateral corpectomy [44] was a relatively increased slot height in order to ensure unconstrained access and to enable visual control for complete decompression.

Two cats with thoracolumbar neurolocalization (one grade IV and one grade IV–V) were euthanized on presentation. Long-term follow-up data were available for 38 cats (Table 6.2). If lack of success is defined as euthanasia on presentation, or a lack of postsurgical improvement, or the long-term persistence of debilitating neurological deficits (e.g., urinary and/or fecal incontinence), 31/40 cats (77.5%) had a successful outcome (Table 6.2). After exclusion of the two cats that were euthanized on presentation, treatment was successful in 10/12 cats (83%) managed nonsurgically and 21/26 cats (81%) managed surgically. Treatment success occurred in 23/29 cats (79%) with acute presenting signs (7/9 cats (78%) after NSM and 16/20 (80%) after surgical management). In cats with chronic thoracolumbar IVDD, successful outcome occurred in 7/9 cats (78%; 2/2 (100%) after NSM and 5/7 (71%) after surgical management). There was no clear relationship between presenting myelopathic grade and outcome (Table 6.2). After exclusion of one cat managed nonsurgically for discospondylitis, 14/15 cats (93%) with excellent outcomes had been managed surgically.

L4–S3 localization

Thirty-seven cats (42%) presented with L4–S3 neurolocalization. In the 30 cats in which details of the duration of presenting signs were reported, onset was acute in 10 of the cats (33%) and chronic in 20 (67%). Lumbosacral localization was the most common (28/37 cats, 76%), followed by L6–L7 (7/37 cats, 19%) and L5–L6 (2/37 cats, 5%). One cat with Hansen type I degeneration at L6–L7 also had Hansen type II L7–S1 disc degeneration noted as an incidental MRI finding (Figure 6.2A). Nine cats with clinical L4–L5 IVD degeneration and four cats with L5–L6 IVD degeneration had neurological signs localized to the T3–L3 spinal cord segments. Presenting features varied significantly according to the affected IVD space.

L5–L6 and L6–L7 localization

Clinical signs associated with L5–L6 or L6–L7 IVD degeneration were comparatively more severe than

Table 6.2   Outcome for cats treated either nonsurgically or by decompressive surgery for thoracolumbar disc disease

Neurological grade	Treatment as % success (number of cats)	
	Non-surgically Managed	Decompression
1—no deficits	100 (2/2)	100 (1/1)
2—ambularoty paresis	100 (3/3)	70 (11/14)
3—nonambulatory paresis	67 (2/3)	50 (1/2)
4—paraplegia	67 (2/3)	83 (5/6)
5—no deep pain	0 (1/1)	100 (3/3)

2 cats euthanized on presentation, and 1 non-surgically managed cat was euthanized after a lack of improvement in the first 2.5 weeks

signs associated with L7–S1 IVD degeneration. Signs included pain, paraparesis, and loss of tone (+/–sensation) of the anus or tail. Hansen type I IVD extrusion affected 8/9 cats with L5–L6 or L6–L7 localization, and one cat was affected by ANNPE at the L5–L6 IVD space. One cat (L5–L6 ANNPE with absent anal tone and deep pain sensation) was euthanized after advanced imaging [9]. One cat that was managed nonsurgically was lost to follow-up, and the remaining seven cats were managed surgically. Of these, five cats had an excellent outcome, one had a good outcome, and one was lost to follow-up.

L7–S1 anatomical localization

Mean age of cats affected by LS IVDD was 9.3 years (range, 1–17 years). Common clinical signs included spinal hyperesthesia, reluctance to jump, reduced activity, bilateral pelvic limb ataxia, low tail carriage, limping, and difficulty when posturing to defecate. Hansen type I and II disc degeneration affected 1/28 (3.5%) and 26/28 cats (93%), respectively. One cat was affected by L7–S1 discospondylitis. In this cat, complete resolution of clinical signs was reported following a 4-week course of cage rest and potentiated amoxicillin.

Nonsurgical management

Of the 27 cats, 10 (37%) were managed nonsurgically (excluding the cat affected by discospondylitis). Treatment protocols were similar to those described in dogs. These involved body weight reduction, exercise restriction, and nonsteroidal anti-inflammatory drugs (NSAIDs). In dogs, medical management of LS IVDD using NSAIDs frequently involves treatment durations of several months. Although the long-term safety of meloxicam in cats has been demonstrated, any NSAID should be used with particular caution in this species because of the increased potential for nephrotoxicity, particularly in elderly patients [45]. In the United States, there is a proscription on the use of meloxicam beyond an initial dose.

An alternative nonsurgical approach that has been successfully applied to canine LS IVDD involves epidural infiltration of three sequential doses of methylprednisolone administered over 6 weeks [46]. Although, to date, this technique has not been reported in cats, it shows sufficient potential in dogs and humans to warrant consideration in clinically affected cats.

Surgical management

Of the 27 cats, 17 (63%) were managed surgically. Eight cats were treated using dorsal laminectomy and fenestration, and 10 cats were treated using dorsal laminectomy with dorsal stabilization via pins or screws and polymethyl methacrylate (PMMA). Lumbosacral stabilization in dogs can be achieved by placement of pins or screws through the articular processes of L7–S1 and into the body of the sacrum with dorsal fixation of the pins using a bolus of PMMA. Alternative dorsal stabilization can be achieved using pedicle screws connected by rods. In cats, these relatively large implants are inappropriate, due to the small size of the articular facets. In contrast, miniature threaded pins (IMEX Interface®, Longview, TX) are well suited to applications in cats, where their small diameter does not risk iatrogenic fracture of the smaller osseous targets (especially the articular facets). Otherwise, the principles of application are similar to those described in dogs (Figure 6.4).

In the surgically managed cats with L7–S1 IVD degeneration, 10/17 (59%) had an excellent outcome, 1/17 (6%) had a good outcome, 2/17 (12%) had a fair outcome, 2/17 (12%) had a poor outcome, and 2/17 cats (12%) were lost to follow-up.

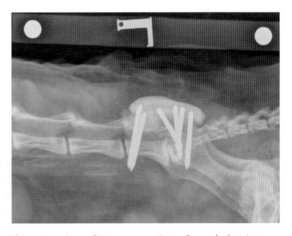

Figure 6.4 Immediate postoperative radiograph showing surgical stabilization of the lumbosacral space of the cat shown in Figure 6.1. Two miniature threaded pins (IMEX® interface, Longview, TX) have been driven into the L7 vertebral body, two pins have been driven across the L7–S1 articular facets, and two pins have been driven into the sacral alar wings from an insertion point approximately 1 cm caudal to the transfacet pins. The pins have been bonded to one another using a bolus of polymethylmethacrylate bone cement.

Conclusions

As noted elsewhere with respect to dogs, it is important to distinguish IVD *disease* from disc *herniation*. Signs of the former are often limited to clinically silent, incidental radiographic changes such as narrowed disc spaces and spondylosis. The latter appears to correlate with increasing age in cats, dogs, and humans and does not imply that disc herniation is either likely to occur or that myelopathic signs are necessarily due to disc herniation (see Chapter 8). However, the data in cats suggest that older cats with signs of lumbar or lumbosacral myelopathy/radiculopathy in particular deserve to have IVDH considered in the differential diagnosis.

Note

1. In one case series [2], specific information regarding the presence or absence of deep pain perception was absent. In the cats from this series, myelopathic grade is reported as grade IV–V.

References

1. Hoerlein BF. Intervertebral disc disease. In: Oliver JE, Hoerlein BF, Mayhew IG, editors. Veterinary Neurology. Philadelphia: WB Saunders; 1987. pp. 321–41.
2. Munana K, Olby N, Sharp AJ, Skeen TM. Intervertebral disc disease in 10 cats. J Am Anim Hosp Assoc. 2001;37:384–9.
3. Gage ED. Incidence of clinical disk disease. J Am Anim Hosp Assoc. 1975;11:135–8.
4. King AS, Smith RN, Kon VM. Protrusion of the intervertebral disc in the cat. Vet Rec. 1958;70:509–15.
5. King AS, Smith RN. Disc protrusions in the cat: Distribution of dorsal protrusions along the vertebral column. Vet Rec. 1960;72:335–7.
6. King AS, Smith RN. Disc protrusions in the cat: Age incidence of dorsal protrusions. Vet Rec. 1960;72:381–3.
7. Marioni-Henry K, Vite CH, Newton AL, Van Winkle TJ. Prevalence of diseases of the spinal cord of cats. J Vet Intern Med. 2004 Nov–Dec;18(6):851–8.
8. Evans HE. Arthrology. In: Evans HE, editor. Miller's Anatomy of the Dog. 3rd ed. Philadelphia: WB Saunders; 1993.
9. McConnell JF, Garosi LS. Intramedullary intervertebral disc extrusion in a cat. Vet Radiol Ultrasound. 2004;45:327–30.
10. Maritato KC, Colon JA, Mauterer JV. Acute non-ambulatory tetraparesis attributable to cranial cervical intervertebral disc disease in a cat. J Feline Med Surg. 2007 Dec;9(6):494–8.
11. Bottcher P, Flegel T, Bottcher IC, Grevel V, Oechtering G. Partial lateral corpectomy for ventral extradural thoracic spinal cord compression in a cat. J Feline Med Surg. 2008 Jul;10(3):291–5.
12. Sparkes AH, Skerry TM. Successful management of a prolapsed intervertebral disc in a Siamese cat. Feline Pract. 1990;18:7–9.
13. Sharp NJ, Wheeler SJ. Functional anatomy. In: Sharp NJ, Wheeler SJ, editors. Small Animal Spinal Disorders. Philadelphia: Elsevier Mosby; 2005. pp. 1–17.
14. Lu D, Lamb CR, Wesselingh K, Targett MP. Acute intervertebral disc extrusion in a cat: clinical and MRI findings. J Feline Med Surg. 2002 Mar;4(1):65–8.
15. Macpherson JM, Ye Y. The cat vertebral column: stance configuration and range of motion. Exp Brain Res. 1998 Apr;119(3):324–32.
16. Knipe MF, Vernau KM, Hornof WJ, LeCouteur RA. Intervertebral disc extrusion in six cats. J Feline Med Surg. 2001 Sep;3(3):161–8.
17. Littlewood JD, Herrtage ME, Palmer AC. Intervertebral disc protrusion in a cat. J Small Anim Pract. 1884;25:119–27.
18. De Risio L, Adams V, Dennis R, McConnell FJ. Association of clinical and magnetic resonance imaging findings with outcome in dogs with presumptive acute noncompressive nucleus pulposus extrusion: 42 cases (2000–2007). J Am Vet Med Assoc. 2009 Feb 15;234(4):495–504.
19. Liptak JM, Allan GS, Krockenberger MB, Davis PE, Malik R. Radiographic diagnosis: intramedullary extrusion of an intervertebral disk. Vet Radiol Ultrasound. 2002;43:272–4.
20. Smith PM, Jeffery ND. What is your diagnosis? A case of intervertebral disc protrusion in a cat: lymphosarcoma. J Small Anim Pract. 2006 Feb;47(2):104–6.
21. Goncalves R, Platt SR, Llabres-Diaz FJ, Rogers KH, de Stefani A, Matiasek LA, et al. Clinical and magnetic resonance imaging findings in 92 cats with clinical signs of spinal cord disease. J Feline Med Surg. 2009 Feb;11(2):53–9.
22. Newitt A, German AJ, Barr FJ. Congenital abnormalities of the feline vertebral column. Vet Radiol Ultrasound. 2008 Jan–Feb;49(1):35–41.
23. Seim HB, 3rd, Nafe LA. Spontaneous intervertebral disk extrusion with associated myelopathy in a cat. J Am Anim Hosp Assoc. 1981;17:201–4.
24. Gilmore DR. Extrusion of a feline intervertebral disk. Vet Med Small Anim Clin. 1983;78:207–9.
25. Bagley RS, Tucker RL, Harrington ML. Radiographic diagnosis: Intervertebral disk extrusion in a cat. Vet Radiol Ultrasound. 1995;36:380–2.
26. Kathmann I, Cizinauskas S, Rytz U, Lang J, Jaggy A. Spontaneous lumbar intervertebral disc protrusion in cats: literature review and case presentations. J Feline Med Surg. 2000 Dec;2(4):207–12.
27. Jaeger G, Early P, Munana K, Hardie EM. Lumbosacral disease in a cat. Vet Comp Orthop Traumatol. 2004;17:104–6.

28. Harris JE, Dhupa S. Lumbosacral intervertebral disk disease in six cats. J Am Anim Hosp Assoc. 2008 May–Jun;44(3):109–15.

29. Choi KH, Hill SA. Acupuncture treatment for feline multifocal intervertebral disc disease. J Feline Med Surg. 2009 Aug;11(8):706–10.

30. Fitzpatrick N, Farrell M. Clinical data for 49 cats treated for intervertebral disc disease between 2008 and 2012, unpublished data. 2012.

31. Heavner JE. Intervertebral disc syndrome in the cat. J Am Vet Med Assoc. 1971;159:425–7.

32. Butler WF, Smith RN. Age changes in the nucleus pulposus of the non-ruptured intervertebral disc of the cat. Res Vet Sci. 1967 Apr;8(2):151–6.

33. Rayward RM. Feline intervertebral disc disease: a review of the literature. Vet Comp Orthop Traumatol. 2002;15:137–44.

34. Wheeler SJ, Clayton Jones DG, Wright JA. Myelography in the cat. J Small Anim Pract. 1985;26: 143–52.

35. Salisbury SK, Cook JR. Recovery of neurological function following focal myelomalacia in a cat. J Am Anim Hosp Assoc. 1988;24:227–30.

36. Sanders S, Bagley RS, Gavin PR. Intramedullary spinal cord damage associated with intervertebral disk material in a dog. J Am Vet Med Assoc. 2002;221:1594–6.

37. Yarrow TG, Jeffery ND. Dura mater laceration associated with acute paraplegia in three dogs. Vet Rec. 2000 Jan 29;146(5):138–9.

38. McKee WM, Downes CJ. Rupture of the dura mater in two dogs caused by the peracute extrusion of a cervical disc. Vet Rec. 2008 Apr 12;162(15): 479–81.

39. Hay CW, Muir P. Tearing of the dura mater in three dogs. Vet Rec. 2000 Mar 4;146(10):279–82.

40. Packer RA, Frank PM, Chambers JN. Traumatic subarachnoid-pleural fistula in a dog. Vet Radiol Ultrasound. 2004 Nov–Dec;45(6):523–7.

41. Roush JK, Douglass JP, Hertzke D. Traumatic dural laceration in a racing greyhound. Vet Radiol Ultrasound. 1992;33:22–4.

42. Montavon PM, Weber U. What is your diagnosis? Swelling of spinal cord associated with dural tear between segments T13 and L1. J Am Vet Med Assoc. 1990;196:783–4.

43. Barnoon I, Chai O, Srugo I, Peeri D, Konstantin L, Brenner O, et al. Spontaneous intradural disc herniation with focal distension of the subarachnoid space in a dog. Can Vet J. 2012 Nov;53(11):1191–4.

44. Moissonnier P, Meheust P, Carozzo C. Thoracolumbar lateral corpectomy for treatment of chronic disk herniation: technique description and use in 15 dogs. Vet Surg. 2004 Nov–Dec;33(6):620–8.

45. Gunew MN, Menrath VH, Marshall RD. Long-term safety, efficacy and palatability of oral meloxicam at 0.01–0.03 mg/kg for treatment of osteoarthritic pain in cats. J Feline Med Surg. 2008 Jul;10(3): 235–41.

46. Janssens L, Beosier Y, Daems R. Lumbosacral degenerative stenosis in the dog. The results of epidural infiltration with methylprednisolone acetate: a retrospective study. Vet Comp Orthop Traumatol. 2009;22(6):486–91.

7 Is "Wobbler" Disease Related to Disc Disease?

Noel Fitzpatrick and James M. Fingeroth

Introduction

The term "wobbler" disease is a rather casual, lay-type description of signs associated with mid-to-caudal cervical spinal cord disease seen in large and giant-breed dogs. There are classically two major forms of the syndrome, one most commonly seen in young giant-breed dogs (great Danes being the most representative breed) and the other more common in older large-breed dogs (Doberman pinschers, most typically). Whether these are part of a spectrum of a single disease entity or whether they are completely different diseases that share a common location and resultant neurologic signs remains controversial. When considered as a single syndrome, the term "wobbler" disease is the most commonly used synonym for what is more properly termed cervical spondylomyelopathy (CSM) [1]. CSM is a multifactorial neurological disorder characterized by abnormal development of the cervical spinal column. Typical lesions include vertebral canal stenosis, disc protrusion, ligamentous hypertrophy, vertebral column subluxation, and articular process hypertrophy

leading to varying degrees of neurologic deficits and neck pain [1–4]. Clinical signs are associated with spinal cord and nerve root compression in addition to facet inflammation and paraspinal muscle spasm. Compressive lesions may be dynamic (improving with flexion or extension) or traction responsive (improving after application of linear distractive force), or they may be static (remaining unchanged by positional alteration) [5, 6]. Figure 7.1 depicts three different types of static compression in Doberman dogs attributable to disc protrusion and/or vertebral malformation/subluxation/"tipping" in disc-associated wobbler syndrome (DAWS). Figures 7.2 and 7.3 depict static compression in a great Dane and a basset hound affected by osseous proliferation narrowing the spinal canal and producing stenotic myelopathy or osseous-associated wobbler syndrome (OAWS). Figure 7.4 depicts the effect of flexion and extension on a Doberman affected by DAWS showing how the compressive lesion is dynamically compressing the spinal cord.

CSM is likely the most common disease of the cervical spine of large- and giant-breed dogs.

Advances in Intervertebral Disc Disease in Dogs and Cats, First Edition. Edited by James M. Fingeroth and William B. Thomas.
© 2015 ACVS Foundation. Published 2015 by John Wiley & Sons, Inc.

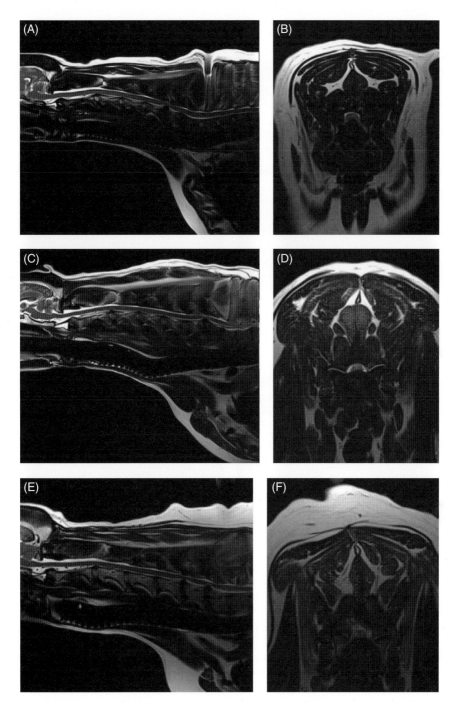

Figure 7.1 T2-weighted MRI scans in midsagittal and transverse planes from different Doberman dogs illustrating three different patterns of disc-associated wobbler syndrome (DAWS).

(A and B) A nine-year-old Doberman with intervertebral disc degeneration evident at C5–C6 and C6–C7. Central disc protrusion encroaching on the dural tube and contained spinal cord is evident on the transverse section at C5–C6.

(C and D) A five-year-old Doberman with multiple sites of cervical intervertebral disc degeneration. The C6–C7 disc has undergone protrusion in association with deformity of the cranial end plate of C7 and dorsal "tipping" of the C7 vertebral body. On the transverse section, high signal intensity is evident in the spinal cord parenchyma.

(E and F) A ten-year-old Doberman with multiple sites of cervical intervertebral disc degeneration. Disc protrusion is notable at C5–C6 and C6–C7, and a transverse section at C5–C6 shows high signal intensity within the spinal cord indicating compression-associated pathology.

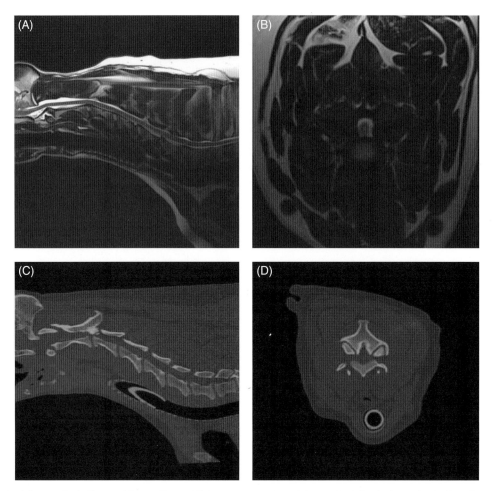

Figure 7.2 A four-and-a-half-year-old great Dane with bony compression of the cervical dural tube and spinal cord, an example of osseous-associated wobbler syndrome (OAWS) or stenotic myelopathy. (A and B) T2-weighted midsagittal plane image does not accurately define the spinal cord-compressing elements, while the transverse section at C3–C4 levels clearly demonstrates abaxial encroachment of the vertebral canal by enlarged and malformed vertebral facets. (C and D) CT scans in parasagittal image plane 2 mm lateral to midsagittal demonstrates osseous proliferation of the dorsocaudal aspect of C2 vertebral lamina. This is further manifested in the transverse plane image at this level, where narrowing of the vertebral canal is clearly apparent.

Doberman pinschers are at increased risk (incidence rate approximately 60%) and are usually presented when middle aged [7]. Other breeds, including great Danes, are also commonly affected, and this breed most commonly presents when young [2, 6, 8–10]. The C5–C6 and C6–C7 vertebral levels are most frequently affected, hence the common autonym of caudal cervical spondylomyelopathy (CCSM). Lesions affecting both of these levels simultaneously have been recognized in approximately 20% of affected dogs [11].

The question whether wobbler disease is or is not related to disc disease is probably patient dependent. Disc disease when present, often occurs concomitant with multiple other manifestations of osseous and positional anomalies of vertebrae in affected dogs, but cause or effect has been difficult to establish. This is a complex disease syndrome where different morphologic changes can cause various clinical signs. There is poor correlation between either the type or severity of the disease as diagnosed on imaging modalities and the magnitude or duration of clinical signs [12]. The disease may progress for prolonged periods and clinical debilitation can be triggered by relatively minor trauma. This is particularly true of disc-associated

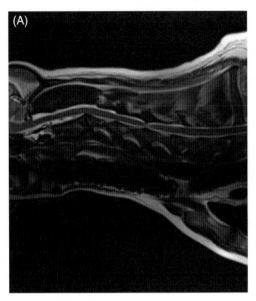 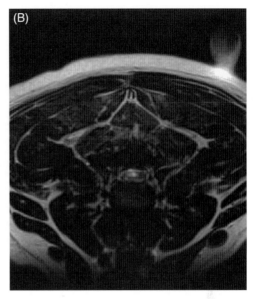

Figure 7.3   T2-weighted MRI scans in midsagittal (A) and transverse (B) planes of a 5-year-old basset hound manifesting extradural compression of the spinal cord at C3–C4 and C4–C5. Dorsal and ventral compression ("hourglass compression") is evident at C4–C5, and high signal intensity within the spinal cord parenchyma is indicative of compression-associated pathology. Spinal cord compression is caused by a combination of disc and osseous-associated elements.

CSM or DAWS, since motion can exacerbate disc protrusion resulting in acute deterioration [4, 13, 14] (Figure 7.3). Moreover, such deterioration may be difficult to address because of the chronicity of preexisting spinal cord abnormalities [4] (Figure 7.1).

Whether wobbler disease is related to disc disease has practical and prognostic relevance for a particular patient and for a population of affected dogs. When a dog is classified as being affected by DAWS based on appropriate imaging, there are significant implications regarding treatment. The fact that more than 20 different surgical techniques have been reported for treatment of CSM implies that no single technique is able to completely address all of the variable manifestations of this complex disease. With appropriate classification however, more refined protocols for intervention are possible, which might in turn improve surgical outcomes.

Etiology

The etiology of CSM is unknown. Genetic, congenital, conformational, and nutritional causes have been proposed [4]. Though canine CSM shares similarities with cervical spondylotic myelopathy of humans, etiology in human patients is likely different from dogs [15]. It has been suggested that vertebral instability may predispose to chronic degenerative disc disease in dogs, or that disc disease may itself be a primary entity and may distort the dorsal longitudinal ligament, exacerbating cord compression [1, 13, 16]. However, as discussed in the following, the whole issue of "cervical vertebral instability" (CVI) remains very controversial and undetermined. The first description of the syndrome in basset hounds suggested that the disease was likely to be sex-linked inherited [17]. A study in Borzois suggested that CSM was inherited with an autosomal recessive pattern, but no explanation was given why only females were affected [9]. In spite of the frequency of the disease in Dobermans, previous studies have failed to demonstrate the mode of inheritance implied by the high prevalence in the breed [18–21].

Computed tomography of the cervical spine of neonatal Dobermans revealed stenosis of the cranial vertebral canal and asymmetry of the vertebral bodies of the fifth, sixth, and seventh cervical vertebrae, with the seventh most affected, intimating that Dobermans may be born with congenital vertebral canal stenosis [21]. Regarding body conformation, it had been proposed that abnormal forces exerted by a large head on a long neck along with a rapid growth rate may lead to abnormal

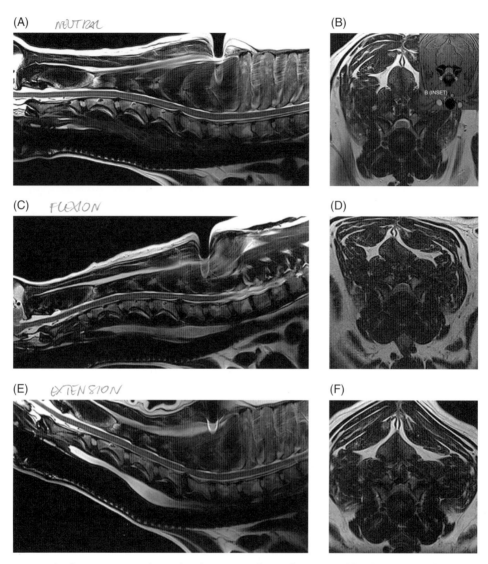

Figure 7.4   T2-weighted MRI scans in midsagittal and transverse planes of an 8-year-old Doberman dog affected by degenerative disc protrusion at C5–C6, demonstrating the effect of flexion and extension to illustrate the dynamic effect of the extradural compression.

(A and B) are neutral positioned; (C and D) show the effect of flexion, which produces more compression of the cord than neutral; (E and F) show the effect of extension, which produces even more compression than flexion.

(B (inset)) is a T2* gradient-echo transverse image of the same patient at the same level as the T2-weighted image yielding superior definition of the osseous boundaries.

stresses between vertebral bodies, inciting vertebral changes and spinal cord compression [22]. However, no correlation was found between radiographic changes associated with CSM in 138 Dobermans aged 1–13 years and head size, neck length, body length, or height at the withers [21]. Overfeeding and excessive dietary calcium were shown to increase the incidence of CSM in great Danes [23, 24], but CSM prevalence has not decreased in spite of abandonment of such feeding regimes. In a study of Dobermans affected by CSM, no association was found with dietary factors [21].

Pathogenesis

Whether CSM is related to disc disease or not, osseous malformation or soft tissue proliferation has particular relevance in terms of whether lesions compressing the spinal cord or nerve roots are static or vary with neck position [25]. This may prompt consideration of surgical interventions seeking either to preserve motion or to remove motion.

Pathogenesis of CSM includes primary developmental anomalies and secondary degenerative changes leading to vertebral canal stenosis and spinal cord compression [13]. Degenerative disc disease has been implicated in large-breed dogs such as the Doberman pinscher, where CSM is often both dynamic (influenced by position) and traction responsive (influenced by distractive force). Concurrent hypertrophy of the dorsal annulus fibrosus, hypertrophy of the dorsal longitudinal ligament, or concomitant osseous anomalies can exacerbate spinal cord compression, either symmetrically or asymmetrically, most commonly at the C5–C6 and/or C6–C7 intervertebral disc (IVD) spaces [1, 25, 26]. Thus, DAWS may represent dual pathogeneses of intervertebral disc disease and osseous malformation predisposing to changes in soft tissue morphology or facet hypertrophy. Both disease pathways likely have a combined effect producing dynamic and static spinal cord and nerve root compression. DAWS as the primary manifestation of CSM has been reported as high as 96% in Dobermans in one study [27] and 82% in large-breed dogs in another study [28].

DAWS appears to be distinct from the syndrome of CSM that occurs more commonly in giant breeds such as the great Dane, where static osseous compression attributable to dorsoventral or mediolateral vertebral canal narrowing associated with misshaped vertebral arches, articular facets, or pedicles, and secondary arthritic proliferative change of the facets with or without vertebral misalignment often constitutes the primary disease mechanism [29]. In this breed, whether osseous change is congenital or secondary to abnormal mechanics remains speculative, but it is clear that OAWS is etiopathogenically distinct from DAWS [8] (Figures 7.1 and 7.2). Extradural synovial cysts may also be present secondary to degenerative arthritic facet changes, leading to axial compression [30, 31].

Osseous changes were the primary cause of compression in 77% of the giant-breed dogs affected by CSM in one study [28]. The marked difference in both lesions and typical age of onset once again inspires the question of whether DAWS in Dobermans and OAWS in great Danes represent two different disease processes that have been improperly lumped into a single disease syndrome.

The most common sites of compression are at C5–C6 and C6–C7 in both large-breed (91%) and giant-breed (72%) dogs [28]. Multiple sites of compression have been documented in 52% of large-breed dogs and 86% of giant-breed dogs [28]. The phenomenon of OAWS in giant breeds produces severe, absolute vertebral canal stenosis [28]. Disc protrusion and ligamentous compression may also contribute to the manifestation of clinical signs, but in these dogs, disc-associated pathology is generally secondary [32] (Figure 7.2).

Stenosis, instability, and disc morphology may all contribute to the pathogenesis and the manifestation of clinical signs associated with CSM. The relative impact of each contributor is the subject of ongoing investigation and whether disc disease is a significant factor is an important focus for further research.

Stenosis

CSM-affected Dobermans have relative stenosis throughout their cervical vertebral canal compared to clinically normal Dobermans [33] (Figure 7.2). This suggests that that intrinsic conformational disturbance may predispose affected animals to clinical signs when concomitant encroachment occurs for any other reason, such as intervertebral disc protrusion [33, 34] (Figure 7.3). Corroborative evidence from human patients has documented that a small vertebral canal contributes to the development of cervical spondylotic myelopathy and the diameter of the spinal cord has been shown to correlate with clinical signs of myelopathy, duration of disease, and speed of postsurgical recovery [34–40].

It is important to acknowledge that 25–30% of clinically normal Dobermans have some degree of spinal cord compression on magnetic resonance imaging (MRI), 75% have disc degeneration, 100% have some degree of disc protrusion, and 68% have foraminal stenosis [33, 41].

However, rather than drawing into question the proposed pathogenic mechanisms of CSM, this likely represents variance in terms of how well an individual dog tolerates spinal cord or nerve root compression [14]. Also, a dog that may be clinically normal at the time of assessment may yet be at risk for the later development of signs; DAWS in Dobermans is notorious for having a late onset of signs, with many dogs not affected until past 7 years of age [14, 42]. Functional impairment due to spinal cord compression is a common manifestation of DAWS in large-breed dogs, but in our experience, large-breed dogs may also present with pain alone or with unilateral thoracic limb lameness. These may be attributable to nerve root signature secondary to foraminal impingement. As in humans, the presence in dogs of disc degeneration or foraminal stenosis *per se*, whether dynamic (intermittent claudication) or static, does not necessarily correlate with clinical signs [34, 43, 44]. But in our experience, this can produce persistent or intermittent clinical signs in some individuals. In affected humans, foraminal stenosis is a key contributor to pain associated with cervical spondylotic myelopathy, whether due to articular facet proliferation, lateralized disc herniation, or osteophyte formation [16, 45, 46].

Another factor that may account for a discrepancy between the degree of compression and clinical signs is that in giant-breed dogs where OAWS may be present from a very young age, the lesions may become symptomatic over a longer period, even with a lesser degree of compression [28]. The ratio of spinal cord diameter to vertebral canal diameter may change as the animal matures, and consequently signs may develop as the spinal cord effectively "outgrows" the surrounding vertebral canal during late juvenile development. Additionally, not only can vertebral canals be more "funnel shaped" cranially in such dogs, but intervertebral foramina are relatively larger in small breeds than in large and giant breeds [47], where the cranial aspect of the foramen is dorsoventrally flattened and the caudal region of the foramen is bilaterally narrowed (Figure 7.3). Therefore, clinical signs of stenosis are potentially triggered by a relatively smaller volume of additional soft tissue or osseous encroachment in giant breeds than in smaller breeds. This is especially so in the caudal cervical spine where the relative cross-sectional area of the spinal cord is larger [33].

Instability

Instability has been defined as a loss of spinal motion segment stiffness, such that physiologic force produces disruption of intervertebral relationships, inducing initial or subsequent damage to the spinal cord or nerve roots with incapacitating deformity or pain [15, 48, 49]. This is very distinct from and should not be considered synonymous with dynamic CSM lesions, which worsen or improve with different positions of the cervical spine [36, 50] or physiologic hypermobility, where increased segmental mobility is reversible and does not induce disc or facet pathology [49]. The canine cervical spine has more inherent mobility than the human cervical spine [51, 52], and dynamic compression may be a greater contributor to CSM than putative intrinsic instability [14, 51, 52]. In fact, restricted rather than excessive motion may produce clinical signs in some scenarios. For example, osteophyte formation subsequent to disc degeneration may contribute to increased stiffness of a vertebral motion unit and may also produce foraminal impingement and pain [53]. Nevertheless, there is evidence that both static and dynamic factors contribute to CSM regardless of the cause or direction of compressive lesions [32]. Spinal cord stretching induced by repetitive flexion and extension over a space-occupying lesion, such as a protruded intervertebral disc, would likely augment the effect of compression over time and produce strain and stress within the spinal cord, both of which are considered key mechanisms of spinal cord injury in cervical spondylotic myelopathy in humans [54–56] (Figures 7.1 and 7.3).

Whether spinal vertebral segments in affected patients are unstable or physiologically hypermobile is controversial [57], but instability has long been implicated in the pathogenesis of CSM [1, 8, 18, 58]. MRI of clinically affected and unaffected Dobermans with similar mobility patterns suggested that vertebral canal stenosis is a primary phenomenon [21] and instability is likely a secondary phenomenon in terms of manifestation of clinical signs [33], contrary to earlier interpretations [18] inferring that instability may be a primary cause of disease. Instability was purportedly responsible for 3.5% morbidity and 2.5% mortality in one study [42] and in respect to instability in CSM, it is currently speculative whether disc disease is a primary or a secondary contributor. Disc disease does not necessarily infer instability [59]; however, there is a paucity of objective criteria to define the contribution of either instability or disc disease to CSM. Subjectively, we have observed that marked end-plate deformity and relative misalignment or "tipping" of adjacent vertebrae regardless of cervical positioning occur regularly in dogs affected by CSM, although sometimes this radiographic finding can be a positional artifact and be overinterpreted (Figure 7.1C and D). Whether this is a result of congenital deformity or progressive remodeling related to or contributing to instability is unknown at this time and further research is required comparing affected and unaffected dogs to elucidate whether instability is or is not a major contributor to the disease process.

To date, there are few data regarding relative motion of cervical spinal segments in dogs. Various techniques have been used to measure kinematics of the human spine including radiography, computed tomography, electrogoniometry, radiostereometric analysis, optical motion tracking, and MRI [60–62]. In human patients with neck pain, 77% have an abnormal center of motion in at least one functional spinal unit (FSU, a pair of adjacent vertebral bodies plus the intervertebral disc) [63]. Early studies of cervical spinal motion in dogs focused on radiographic assessment only, where obfuscation of dynamic and stability issues may cloud interpretation [51, 52, 64]. The C6–C7 FSU had slightly decreased flexion/extension range of motion and increased left/right lateral bending compared to more cranial FSUs [47, 64]. Recently, a more specific *in vitro* study revealed greater mobility in the caudal cervical segments, particularly with regard to axial rotation (by 2.6 times), which is coupled with lateral bending [65]. This corroborated an earlier study finding a greater degree of rotation in the caudal cervical spine of large-breed dogs compared to smaller dogs [47]. Torsion is a more significant contributor to disc degeneration than axial compression [66], and this may in part explain why the C5–C6 and C6–C7 intervertebral discs are commonly affected in dogs with DAWS.

Stability is a product of complex interaction between the intervertebral disc, periarticular structures, and paraspinal muscles. A recent study using a porcine cervical spine model concluded that spinal stability is more significantly affected by muscle dysfunction than by disc degeneration and that muscle training could improve stability in degenerative spines [67]. Furthermore, stability or instability is time dependent in humans. In the early stages of disc degeneration (grades I–V representing increasing severity), there are greater translational motion and angular variation associated with grade II and III degeneration. Relative segmental motion decreases as ankylosis progresses with grade V disease and osteoligamentary repair mechanisms are activated [68–72]. Adaptational stabilization is apparent when disc height is reduced by 50% [73]. Finite element modeling to include the effect of the soft tissue structures found that overall and segmental stiffness of the cervical vertebral column increased with increasing severity of disc degeneration [53]. This association of stability or instability with the pathophysiology of disc disease may have important relevance for how wobbler disease is related to disc disease in dogs and may have direct consequences regarding choice of surgical intervention aiming either to preserve or to remove relative segmental motion.

Disc morphometry

Dobermans affected by CSM have larger intervertebral discs than clinically normal Dobermans and this may result in a larger volume of disc protrusion into the vertebral canal when disc disease occurs [33]. This factor coupled with relative vertebral canal stenosis and more pronounced torsion in the caudal cervical spine may help explain the significance of disc disease in the etiopathogenesis of CSM. The caudal cervical discs in nonchondrodystrophoid dogs are more rounded, and the nucleus pulposus of cervical discs occupies a greater proportion of total discal area than in chondrodystrophoid breeds [65]. These factors features may be pertinent to whether CSM is related to disc disease but the relationship of structure to function or dysfunction has not been established.

Diagnostic imaging

MRI has become the standard of care for assessment of the cervical spinal cord affected by any disease process, especially CSM. MRI permits utilization of various sequences to facilitate specific diagnosis and avoids any potential complications related to subarachnoid injection of contrast agent [1]. CT myelography is also very useful and provides excellent elucidation of osseous margins and vertebral canal soft tissue interfaces but suffers the disadvantage of not documenting intraparenchymal spinal cord pathology [28, 74, 75]. Survey radiography is obsolete, but can still be useful where finances are limited if an appropriate myelographic study is performed. It is noteworthy that 25% of clinically normal Dobermans have radiographically detected vertebral column abnormalities. This proportion is comparable to the proportion of vertebral abnormalities recorded in clinically affected Dobermans [20].

The ideal imaging modality for CSM should allow determination of the site and extent of spinal cord and nerve root encroachment, and establish whether compression derives from soft tissue or bone. Additionally, techniques that allow prediction of the nature and extent of spinal cord pathology may assist in prognostication. Lastly, the technique should allow the clinician to establish whether the lesion is dynamic, traction responsive, or both. Dynamic lesions can be identified by obtaining images during flexion and extension with conventional myelography, CT myelography, or MRI (Figures 7.4 and 7.5). Traction-responsive lesions are identified by stretching the cervical spine with a force equivalent to approximately 20% of body weight [76] (Figure 7.5 G and H).

Myelography can identify the location of the lesion in 83% of dogs but MRI imaging predicts the site, severity, and nature of spinal cord compression in 100% of affected animals [33]. Sagittal and transverse T1-weighted (T1W) and T2-weighted (T2W) images are generally employed to determine site, direction, presence and severity of spinal cord compression, discogenic disease, and degenerative or cystic articular facets [29, 33, 77] (Figures 7.1, 7.2, and 7.3).

More recently, T2* gradient-echo imaging has been used by one of us (NF) to define the osseous boundaries of compressive lesions, but caution

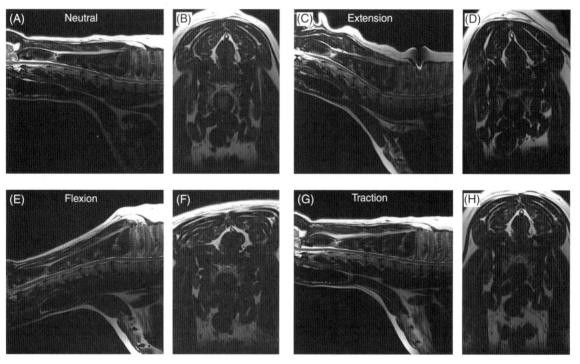

Figure 7.5 T2-weighted MRI scans in midsagittal and transverse planes from an 8-year-old Doberman dog illustrating intervertebral disc degeneration at C6–C7 associated with disc-associated wobbler syndrome (DAWS). Four positions are shown: neutral (A and B), extension (C and D), flexion (E and F), and after application of traction (G and H). These images demonstrate a dynamic and traction responsive disc lesion. Spinal cord compression by the disc is exacerbated by extension and is considerably reduced by application of traction.

must be advised regarding overinterpretation of compression as a consequence of technical factors (Figure 7.4B (inset)). Diffusion tensor imaging allows the documentation of microstructural abnormalities beyond the resolution of conventional MRI [78].

Though MRI cannot assess functional status of the spinal cord or the effect of motion *in vivo*, the transverse area and sagittal diameter of the spinal cord measured by MRI in humans correlates with clinical manifestation and duration of disease [40]. MRI also allows appreciation of severity and chronicity of lesions by characterization of intraparenchymal spinal lesions, which have been associated with abnormal histologic findings [79, 80]. Further study is warranted to establish the sensitivity and specificity of MRI cord signal changes for the prediction of prognosis or indication for surgery. MRI also helps prioritize clinical relevance of multiple lesions. Transcranial magnetic stimulation has been suggested as a diagnostic tool to differentiate clinically relevant spinal cord compression identified using MRI alone [81].

Treatment

The choice of treatment for dogs with CSM may be influenced by whether or not the pathology is related to disc disease. In humans and in dogs with signs related to radiculopathy such as spinal pain or intermittent claudication of nerve roots, medical management, manipulative therapies, physiotherapy, and acupuncture have all enjoyed anecdotal success with occasional evidence-based documentation of effect [82–87]. However, patient selection criteria have not been clearly documented and outcome measures have been poorly defined, with a broad range of disease types treated and variable outcomes reported [84, 87, 88]. One study reported no statistically significant difference in outcome between medically and surgically managed CSM patients, though 81% treated surgically improved by comparison with 54% improved in the medically treated cohort, and the authors concluded that they still recommended surgical intervention [12]. Recent reports on the use of proteolytic enzymes to address disc herniation by chemonucleolysis are discussed elsewhere in this text and have yet to be clinically validated for the management of DAWS (see Chapter 26).

Surgical intervention is usually reserved for cases where medical management or physical therapies have failed and episodes of pain, lameness, or neurologic dysfunction are recurrent or signs have been unremitting or are fulminant. Broadly, surgical treatment encompasses:

1. Decompressive techniques involving removal of dorsal structures including lamina(e) and facet(s) (dorsal laminectomy, hemilaminectomy, facetectomy, foraminotomy)
2. Decompressive techniques involving removal of ventral structures including vertebral body bone and disc (ventral slot)
3. Distraction–stabilization or just stabilization procedures with ventral and/or interbody mechanical fixation techniques with or without biologic augmentation (addition of cancellous bone or other osteogenic stimulus, such as bone morphogenetic protein)
4. Intervertebral disc replacement [89, 90] (see Chapter 40)

The controversy surrounding the type of treatment has largely arisen from suboptimal understanding or appreciation of underlying pathologic mechanisms, restricted availability of implant options, financial constraints, and surgeon bias. Optimal surgical treatment algorithms can only derive from attempts to address specific pathologic states with clearly defined disease-specific interventions and robust outcome measures.

The relative contributions of static osseous compression, disc-associated disease, and dynamic forces and whether or not instability is present may vary between breeds and clinical signs may vary between individuals. We speculate that there may be a role for enforced stabilization in multiple manifestations of CSM, but the rationale for preservation of motion with disc replacement may best be considered in patients affected by DAWS where there is no static osseous compression (OAWS) or secondary facet and ligamentous pathology. Further *in vitro* and *in vivo* studies are required for evaluation of this statement.

Ventral decompression by ventral slot or modified slot [91, 92] without stabilization [93] should be reserved for single static ventral spinal cord compression, such as intervertebral disc extrusion (see Chapter 30). This technique is not advisable for DAWS, where annular protrusion and dorsal longitudinal ligament hypertrophy prevail and cannot be effectively addressed by limited ventral approaches without stabilization [4, 94]. Cervical ventral slot in normal cadaver dogs increased neutral zone range of motion by 98% [95]. Discectomy only at C5–C6 in human cadavers resulted in increased instability of the vertebral column by as much as 70% in flexion and extension [96]. Ventral fenestration of C5–C6 has been shown to produce sagittal instability at the disc space [97] and has generally fallen out of favor for treatment of DAWS.

Extensive dorsal laminectomy, intended to address osteoproliferative changes of the articular facets or ligamentum flavum hypertrophy, carries considerable morbidity. This risk must be balanced against the rationale for stabilization with potentially less morbidity. The rate of transient postoperative neurological deterioration following dorsal laminectomy has been published to be as high as 70% [98]. Unilateral facetectomy and laminectomy techniques should be reserved for lateralized disc extrusion and unilateral osseous compression due to articular facet deformity and proliferation. In comparison with dorsal laminectomy, these techniques can be performed with minimal morbidity [99].

The chronically compressed spinal cord may become symptomatic because of dynamic forces occurring in addition to static compressive lesions (Figures 7.1, 7.2, 7.3, and 7.4). It is possible that removal of static compression without stabilization may precipitate clinically important instability, resulting in transient or permanent neurological deterioration. In contrast, surgical stabilization may produce indirect decompression by reduction of dynamic forces, resulting in gradual regression of soft tissue hypertrophy over time [100]. Both distraction and stabilization may be potentially beneficial. Distraction provides immediate nerve root and spinal cord decompression and stabilization promotes osseous union or fibro-osseous ankylosis of adjacent vertebrae. In our experience, any combination of dorsal, lateral, and ventral compression can be amenable to distraction–stabilization at multiple sites, even in the presence of vertebral malalignment with end-plate distortion.

Various indirect decompressive techniques have been reported. Distraction–stabilization techniques include intervertebral spacers such as allogenous cortical bone grafts, polymethylmethacrylate

(PMMA) cement plugs, washers, or other metallic spacers such as cages with or without screws, pins, or plates [27, 94 101–105]. Ventral bridging without spacers for stabilization has also been used by application of screws or pins with PMMA cement (internal fixators) or metallic or plastic plates [11, 106–108]. Biologic augmentation of fixation with cancellous autograft has been recommended and success rates have varied between 70 and 90% [8, 94, 105, 108]. If the vertebral canal is stenotic in multiple directions, direct decompression by tissue removal is unlikely to be completely satisfactory and may induce further instability, whereas removing the dynamic spinal cord stressors with distraction–stabilization may allow long-standing static compression to become tolerated by the patient.

Most robustly secured vertebral spacer devices facilitate satisfactory ankylosis or fusion of vertebral segments. Clinical signs will usually resolve for most forms of CSM after stabilization except where clinically significant instability remains or where osseous or soft tissue compressive lesions are inadequately addressed by the distraction–stabilization over time. It is common for any device to experience a degree of collapse into the vertebral end plates, particularly when point loaded rather than when the load is dissipated by broad-based implants [27, 94, 106]. Vertebral body spacers that induce bone ingrowth from adjacent vertebrae would obviously be advantageous, particularly if this could occur before there is significant collapse of the distracted intervertebral space. The PMMA cement plug was intended to dissipate end-plate load, but interbody fusion is only achieved if a ventral autogenous graft is applied. The cement plug may loosen over time, even if supported by metallic implants or when end-plate recesses are created for cement indentation [101]. The authors' preference is to encourage interbody fusion across the disc space and ventrally. Cortical allografts have been successful in this regard [94], as have fenestrated spacers, such as in one recent report using a titanium cage designed for tibial tuberosity advancement [109].

A novel surgical technique has been recently described for simultaneous cervical distraction and stabilization [110]. This technique uses a spacer (Fitz Intervertebral Traction Screw, FITS) and has been reported with one or two 3.5 mm string-of-pearl (SOP™) locking plates with autogenous cancellous bone graft applied ventrally to

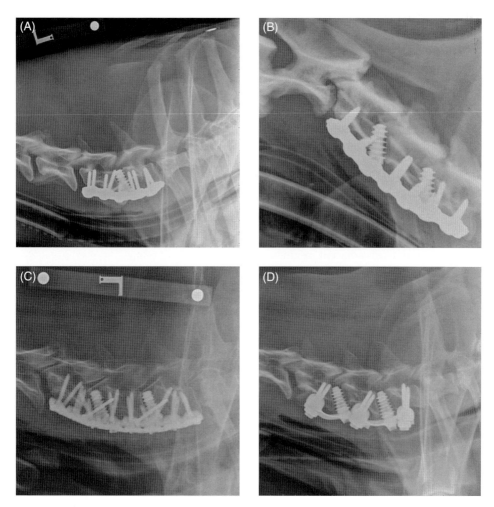

Figure 7.6   Examples of application of the Fitz Intervertebral Traction Screw (FITS) technique for cervical distraction–fusion with various linkage systems. (A) Single site fusion at C6–C7 with two 3.5 mm SOP™ plates (8-and-a-half-year-old greyhound). (B) Double site fusion at C3–C4 and C4–C5 with two 3.5 mm SOP™ plates (5-year-old basset hound). (C) Double site fusion at C5–C6 and C6–C7 with two Ventlok™ 3.5 mm plates (10-year-old Doberman). (D) Double site fusion at C5–C6 and C6–C7 with a custom CerFitz™ linkage system (8-year-old Doberman).

treat dogs affected by one- or two-segment DAWS (Figure 7.6A and B). At 6 weeks postoperatively, 15/16 (93%) operated dogs had significantly improved neurological status, with 1/16 unchanged. Long-term physical examination available for 7/16 dogs (20–36 months) revealed that 6/7 patients were normal and 1/7 patient had mild pelvic limb ataxia. Bone bridging was recorded in 10/16 (62.5%) at 6 weeks with all dogs available for long-term follow-up (7/16) achieving bone bridging. Complications included mild end-plate collapse (8/16) and single plate loosening (2/16) which were not clinically significant. More

recently, lower-profile locking plate designs have been successfully employed to address DAWS with or without facet and ligamentum flavum hypertrophy, at two or more adjacent levels (Figure 7.6C and D). Even with multiple level compressions, morbidity is limited because there is no direct manipulation of the spinal cord. The FITS device can be used in the presence of marked end-plate deformity and relative vertebral malalignment and also in dogs affected by OAWS, where distraction–stabilization compensates for the loss of vertebral canal caused by osseous compression. In selected cases, this technique has been employed by one of us (NF) to fuse up to six sites, from C2–C3 to C7–T1 in dogs severely affected by OAWS. However, as yet, there are no definitive advantages documented for any one distraction–fusion system over any other.

One potential disadvantage of stabilization or distraction–stabilization of one or more FSUs is adjacent segment disease [4, 14]. Dynamic stresses are redirected to adjacent intervertebral discs, and a "domino" effect may occur whereby these aberrant forces precipitate disc disease [4, 104]. The risk of clinically significant adjacent disc disease following any surgical intervention for treatment of DAWS is estimated to be approximately 20% [4]. Postsurgical imaging in human patients also reveals increased motion at adjacent segments [111, 112]. Disc disease at these sites may be associated with deterioration after anterior cervical fusion [113–115].

Preservation of motion at the surgery site may reduce the rate of adjacent-level cervical disc disease after anterior cervical discectomy and fusion in humans, and this has promoted the popularity of disc replacement in human patients affected by discogenic spinal cord or nerve root compression [116]. A variety of different designs with various bone anchorage, bone ingrowth, and impact or kinetic force absorption mechanisms have been designed and implanted in humans [117] (see Chapter 40). It is unknown whether long-term mobility is maintained at the operated site or whether spondylosis and pseudoankylosis occur at the surgical site. Whether or not disc replacement protects against adjacent segment disease is also currently unknown. In dogs, it has been reported that a disc prosthesis has been well tolerated with few complications and good functional outcome in a limited case series [90] (Chapter 40). In the longer term, however, the same concerns remain that pseudoankylosis might ensue which might have important clinical consequences.

Further work is warranted to establish if disc disease in DAWS is primary or if it is associated with other osseous anomalies, whether instability truly exists, and if dynamic forces contribute to clinically significant spinal cord and nerve root pathology. Evidence-based surgical treatment algorithms should accompany more refined understanding of the entities treated, for example, with regard to disc replacement versus distraction–stabilization. This is especially true for dogs affected by OAWS where the evolution and effect of osseous compression must be understood in symbiosis with efforts to surgically alleviate resultant clinical symptoms by stabilization or decompressive techniques.

In conclusion, "wobbler" disease is related to disc disease, but the nature and extent of this relationship are complex and incompletely understood at this time. More complete understanding of disease mechanisms should parallel targeted advances in surgical treatments.

References

1. Seim H, III, Withrow S. 1982. Pathophysiology and diagnosis of caudal cervical spondylo-myelopathy with emphasis on the Doberman Pinscher [Dogs]. *J Am Anim Hosp Assoc* 1982;18:241–51.
2. Read R, Robins G, Carlisle CH. 1983. Caudal cervical spondylo-myelopathy (wobbler syndrome) in the dog: a review of thirty cases. *J Small Anim Pract* 24:605–21.
3. Gray M, Kirberger R, Spotswood T. 2003. Cervical spondylomyelopathy (wobbler syndrome) in the Boerboel. *J S Afr Vet Assoc* 74:104–10.
4. da Costa RC. 2010. Cervical spondylomyelopathy (wobbler syndrome) in dogs. *Vet Clin North Am Small Anim Pract* 40:881–913.
5. Jeffery N, McKee W. 2001. Surgery for disc-associated wobbler syndrome in the dog—an examination of the controversy. *J Small Anim Pract* 42:574–81.
6. Adamo PF, Kobayashi H, Markel M, Vanderby R, Jr. 2007. In vitro biomechanical comparison of cervical disk arthroplasty, ventral slot procedure, and smooth pins with polymethylmethacrylate fixation at treated and adjacent canine cervical motion units. *Vet Surg* 36:729–41.
7. Bergknut N, Egenvall A, Hagman R, Gustas P, Hazewinkel HA, *et al.* 2012. Incidence of intervertebral disk degeneration-related diseases and associated mortality rates in dogs. *J Am Vet Med Assoc* 240:1300–9.
8. Trotter E, DeLahunta A, Geary J, Brasmer T. 1976. Caudal cervical vertebral malformation-malarticulation in Great Danes and Doberman Pinschers. *J Am Vet Med Assoc* 168:917.
9. Jaggy A, Gaillard C, Lang J, Vandevelde M. 1988. Hereditary cervical spondylopathy (wobbler syndrome) in the Borzoi dog. *J Am Anim Hosp Assoc* 4:453–60.
10. Lewis D, Hosgood G. 1992. Complications associated with the use of iohexol for myelography of the cervical vertebral column in dogs: 66 cases (1988–1990). *J Am Vet Med Assoc* 200:1381.

11. Trotter EJ. 2009. Cervical spine locking plate fixation for treatment of cervical spondylotic myelopathy in large breed dogs. *Vet Surg* 38:705–18.

12. da Costa RC, Parent JM, Holmberg DL, Sinclair D, Monteith G. 2008. Outcome of medical and surgical treatment in dogs with cervical spondylomyelopathy: 104 cases (1988–2004). *J Am Vet Med Assoc* 233:1284–90.

13. VanGundy T. 1989. Canine wobbler syndrome. 1. Patho-physiology and diagnosis. *Compend Contin Educ Pract Vet* 11:144–57.

14. da Costa RC, Parent JM. 2007. One-year clinical and magnetic resonance imaging follow-up of Doberman Pinschers with cervical spondylomyelopathy treated medically or surgically. *J Am Vet Med Assoc* 231:243–50.

15. Swinkels RA, Oostendorp RA. 1996. Upper cervical instability: fact or fiction? *J Manipulative Physiol Ther* 19:185–94.

16. Parke WW. 1988. Correlative anatomy of cervical spondylotic myelopathy. *Spine (Phila Pa 1976)* 13:831–7.

17. Palmer AC, Wallace ME. 1967. Deformation of cervical vertebrae in Basset hounds. *Vet Rec* 80:430–3.

18. Mason TA. 1979. Cervical vertebral instability (wobbler syndrome) in the dog. *Vet Rec* 104:142–5.

19. Lewis D. 1989. Cervical spondylomyelopathy ('wobbler' syndrome) in the dog: a study based on 224 cases. *J Small Anim Pract* 30:657–65.

20. Lewis D. 1991. Radiological assessment of the cervical spine of the dobermann with reference to cervical spondylo-myelopathy. *J Small Anim Pract* 32:75–82.

21. Burbidge HM. 1999. *Caudal cervical vertebral malformation in the Dobermann pinscher* (Doctor of Philosophy). Massey University, New Zealand.

22. Wright F, Rest JR, Palmer AC. 1973. Ataxia of the Great Dane caused by stenosis of the cervical vertebral canal: comparison with similar conditions in the Basset Hound, Doberman Pinscher, Ridgeback and the Thoroughbred horse. *Vet Rec* 92:1–6.

23. Hedhammar A, deLahunta A, Whalen JP, Kallfelz KA, Nunez EA, *et al.* 1974. Overnutrition and skeletal disease. An experimental study in growing Great Dane dogs. *Cornell Vet* 64:1–160.

24. Hazewinkel HAW. 1985. *Influences of different calcium intakes on calcium metabolism and skeletal development in young Great Danes (PhD Dissertation)*. Rijksuniversiteit te Utrecht, Utrecht, the Netherlands..

25. Seim H. 2002. Wobbler syndrome. In Small animal surgery, ed. T Fossum. St. Louis: Mosby. Number of 1237–49 pp.

26. Rusbridge C, Wheeler SJ, Torrington AM, Pead MJ, Carmichael S. 1998. Comparison of two surgical techniques for the management of cervical spondylomyelopathy in dobermanns. *J Small Anim Pract* 39:425–31.

27. McKee WM, Butterworth SJ, Scott HW. 1999. Management of cervical spondylopathy-associated intervertebral, disc protrusions using metal washers in 78 dogs. *J Small Anim Pract* 40:465–72.

28. da Costa RC, Echandi RL, Beauchamp D. 2012. Computed tomography myelographic findings in dogs with cervical spondylomyelopathy. *Vet Radiol Ultrasound* 53:64–70.

29. Lipsitz D, Levitski RE, Chauvet AE, Berry WL. 2001. Magnetic resonance imaging features of cervical stenotic myelopathy in 21 dogs. *Vet Radiol Ultrasound* 42:20–7.

30. Levitski RE, Chauvet AE, Lipsitz D. 1999. Cervical myelopathy associated with extradural synovial cysts in 4 dogs. *J Vet Intern Med* 13:181–6.

31. Gray MJ, Kirberger RM, Spotswood TC. 2003. Cervical spondylomyelopathy (wobbler syndrome) in the Boerboel. *J S Afr Vet Assoc* 74:104–10.

32. da Costa RC, Johnson J, Parent J. 2010. Are cervical vertebral ratios useful in the diagnosis of cervical spondylomyelopathy in Dobermans? *Proc. ACVIM Forum Proceedings*, Anaheim, CA, 332.

33. da Costa RC, Parent J, Dobson H, Holmberg D, Partlow G. 2006. Comparison of magnetic resonance imaging and myelography in 18 Doberman pinscher dogs with cervical spondylomyelopathy. *Vet Radiol Ultrasound* 47:523–31.

34. Bernhardt M, Hynes RA, Blume HW, White AA, 3rd. 1993. Cervical spondylotic myelopathy. *J Bone Joint Surg Am* 75:119–28.

35. Yu YL, du Boulay GH, Stevens JM, Kendall BE. 1986. Computed tomography in cervical spondylotic myelopathy and radiculopathy: visualisation of structures, myelographic comparison, cord measurements and clinical utility. *Neuroradiology* 28:221–36.

36. White AA, 3rd, Panjabi MM. 1988. Biomechanical considerations in the surgical management of cervical spondylotic myelopathy. *Spine (Phila Pa 1976)* 13:856–60.

37. Okada Y, Ikata T, Katoh S, Yamada H. 1994. Morphologic analysis of the cervical spinal cord, dural tube, and spinal canal by magnetic resonance imaging in normal adults and patients with cervical spondylotic myelopathy. *Spine (Phila Pa 1976)* 19:2331–5.

38. Hamburger C, Buttner A, Uhl E. 1997. The cross-sectional area of the cervical spinal canal in patients with cervical spondylotic myelopathy. Correlation of preoperative and postoperative area with clinical symptoms. *Spine (Phila Pa 1976)* 22:1990–4; discussion 5.

39. Yue WM, Tan SB, Tan MH, Koh DC, Tan CT. 2001. The Torg—Pavlov ratio in cervical spondylotic myelopathy: a comparative study between patients with cervical spondylotic myelopathy and a non-spondylotic, nonmyelopathic population. *Spine (Phila Pa 1976)* 26:1760–4.

40. Tsurumi T, Goto N, Shibata M, Goto J, Kamiyama A. 2005. A morphological comparison of cervical spondylotic myelopathy: MRI and dissection findings. *Okajimas Folia Anat Jpn* 81:119–22.

41. De Decker S, Gielen IMVL, Duchateau L, Polis I, Van Bree HJJ, Van Ham LML. 2010. Agreement and repeatability of linear vertebral body and canal measurements using computed tomography (CT) and low field magnetic resonance imaging (MRI). *Vet Surg* 39:28–34.

42. Mandigers PJ, Senders T, Rothuizen J. 2006. Morbidity and mortality in 928 Dobermanns born in the Netherlands between 1993 and 1999. *Vet Rec* 158:226–9.

43. Boden SD, McCowin PR, Davis DO, Dina TS, Mark AS, Wiesel S. 1990. Abnormal magnetic-resonance scans of the cervical spine in asymptomatic subjects. A prospective investigation. *J Bone Joint Surg Am* 72:1178–84.

44. Watkins R, Williams L, Watkins R. 2005. Cervical spine injuries in athletes. In *The Cervical spine*, ed. CR Clark. Philadelphia: Lippincott Williams & Watkins. Number of 576–86 pp.

45. Fehlings MG, Skaf G. 1998. A review of the pathophysiology of cervical spondylotic myelopathy with insights for potential novel mechanisms drawn from traumatic spinal cord injury. *Spine (Phila Pa 1976)* 23:2730–7.

46. Lu J, Ebraheim NA, Huntoon M, Haman SP. 2000. Cervical intervertebral disc space narrowing and size of intervertebral foramina. *Clinical Orthop Relat Res* 370:259–64.

47. Breit S, Kunzel W. 2004. A morphometric investigation on breed-specific features affecting sagittal rotational and lateral bending mobility in the canine cervical spine (c3-c7). *Anat Histol Embryol* 33:244–50.

48. Rao R. 2003. Neck pain, cervical radiculopathy, and cervical myelopathy: pathophysiology, natural history, and clinical evaluation. *Instr Course Lect* 52:479–88.

49. Panjabi M, Yue J, Dvorak J. 2005. Cervical spine kinematics and clinical instability. In *The cervical spine*, ed. CR Clark. Philadelphia: Lippincott Williams & Wilkins. Number of 55–78 pp.

50. Waltz TA. 1967. Physical factors in the production of the myelopathy of cervical spondylosis. *Brain* 90:395–404.

51. Morgan JP, Miyabayashi T, Choy S. 1986. Cervical spine motion: radiographic study. *Am J Vet Res* 47:2165–9.

52. Penning L, Badoux DM. 1987. Radiological study of the movements of the cervical spine in the dog compared with those in man. *Anat Histol Embryol* 16:1–20.

53. Kumaresan S, Yoganandan N, Pintar FA, Maiman DJ, Goel VK. 2001. Contribution of disc degeneration to osteophyte formation in the cervical spine: a biomechanical investigation. *J Orthop Res* 19: 977–84.

54. Levine DN. 1997. Pathogenesis of cervical spondylotic myelopathy. *J Neurol Neurosurg Psychiatry* 62:334–40.

55. Ichihara K, Taguchi T, Sakuramoto I, Kawano S, Kawai S. 2003. Mechanism of the spinal cord injury and the cervical spondylotic myelopathy: new approach based on the mechanical features of the spinal cord white and gray matter. *J Neurosurg* 99:278–85.

56. Henderson FC, Geddes JF, Vaccaro AR, Woodard E, Berry KJ, Benzel EC. 2005. Stretch-associated injury in cervical spondylotic myelopathy: new concept and review. *Neurosurgery* 56:1101–13; discussion 1101–13.

57. Zhao F, Pollintine P, Hole BD, Dolan P, Adams MA. 2005. Discogenic origins of spinal instability. *Spine (Phila Pa 1976)* 30:2621–30.

58. Parker AJ, Park RD, Cusick PK, Small E, Jeffers CB. 1973. Cervical vertebral instability in the dog. *J Am Vet Med Assoc* 163:71–4.

59. Read RA, Robins GM, Carlize CH. 1983. Caudal cervical spondylo-myelopathy (wobbler syndrome) in the dog: a review of thirty cases. *J Small Anim Pract* 24:605–21.

60. Van Mameren H. 1988. *Motion patterns in the cervical spine* (PhD Thesis). University of Limburg, Maastricht, The Netherlands.

61. Roozmon P, Gracovetsky SA, Gouw GJ, Newman N. 1993. Examining motion in the cervical spine. II: Characterization of coupled joint motion using an opto-electronic device to track skin markers. *J Biomed Eng* 15:13–22.

62. Antonaci F, Ghirmai S, Bono G, Nappi G. 2000. Current methods for cervical spine movement evaluation: a review. *Clin Exp Rheumatol* 18:S45–52.

63. Amevo B, Worth D, Bogduk N. 1991. Instantaneous axes of rotation of the typical cervical motion segments: a study in normal volunteers. *Clinical Biomech* 6:111–7.

64. Lang B. 1972. Die bewegungsmoeglichkeiten der wilbelsaeule von hund und katze. *Kleintierpraxis* 17:217–44.

65. Johnson JA, da Costa RC, Bhattacharya S, Goel V, Allen MJ. 2011. Kinematic motion patterns of the cranial and caudal canine cervical spine. *Vet Surg* 40:720–7.

66. Farfan HF, Cossette JW, Robertson GH, Wells RV, Kraus H. 1970. The effects of torsion on the lumbar intervertebral joints: the role of torsion in the production of disc degeneration. *J Bone Joint Surg Am* 52:468–97.

67. Cheng CH, Chen PJ, Kuo YW, Wang JL. 2011. The effects of disc degeneration and muscle dysfunction on cervical spine stability from a biomechanical study. *Proc Inst Mech Eng H* 225:149–57.

68. Kirkaldy-Willis WH, Farfan HF. 1982. Instability of the lumbar spine. *Clin Orthop Relat Res* 165:110–23.

69. Dai L. 1998. Disc degeneration and cervical instability. Correlation of magnetic resonance imaging with radiography. *Spine (Phila Pa 1976)* 23:1734–8.

70. Kuwazawa Y, Bashir W, Pope MH, Takahashi K, Smith FW. 2006. Biomechanical aspects of the cervical cord: effects of postural changes in healthy volunteers using positional magnetic resonance imaging. *J Spinal Disord Tech* 19:348–52.

71. Hirasawa Y, Bashir WA, Smith FW, Magnusson ML, Pope MH, Takahashi K. 2007. Postural changes of the dural sac in the lumbar spines of asymptomatic individuals using positional stand-up magnetic resonance imaging. *Spine (Phila Pa 1976)* 32:E136–40.

72. Miyazaki M, Hong SW, Yoon SH, Zou J, Tow B, et al. 2008. Kinematic analysis of the relationship between the grade of disc degeneration and motion unit of the cervical spine. *Spine (Phila Pa 1976)* 33:187–93.

73. Axelsson P, Karlsson BS. 2004. Intervertebral mobility in the progressive degenerative process. A radiostereometric analysis. *Eur Spine J* 13:567–72.

74. Sharp NJH, Wheeler SJ, Cofone M. 1992. Radiological evaluation of 'wobbler' syndrome-caudal cervical spondylomyelopathy. *J Small Anim Pract* 33:491–9.

75. Newcomb B, Arble J, Rochat M, Pechman R, Payton M. 2012. Comparison of computed tomography and myelography to a reference standard of computed tomographic myelography for evaluation of dogs with intervertebral disc disease. *Vet Surg* 41:207–14.

76. Penderis J, Dennis R. 2004. Use of traction during magnetic resonance imaging of caudal cervical spondylomyelopathy ("wobbler syndrome") in the dog. *Vet Radiol Ultrasound* 45:216–9.

77. Guillem Gallach R, Suran J, Caceres AV, Reetz JA, Brown DC, Mai W. 2011. Reliability of T2-weighted sagittal magnetic resonance images for determining the location of compressive disk herniation in dogs. *Vet Radiol Ultrasound* 52:479–86.

78. Budzik JF, Balbi V, Le Thuc V, Duhamel A, Assaker R, Cotten A. 2011. Diffusion tensor imaging and fibre tracking in cervical spondylotic myelopathy. *Eur Radiol* 21:426–33.

79. Neuhold A, Stiskal M, Platzer C, Pernecky G, Brainin M. 1991. Combined use of spin-echo and gradient-echo MR-imaging in cervical disk disease. Comparison with myelography and intraoperative findings. *Neuroradiology* 33:422–6.

80. Perneczky G, Bock FW, Neuhold A, Stiskal M. 1992. Diagnosis of cervical disc disease. MRI versus cervical myelography. *Acta Neurochir (Wien)* 116:44–8.

81. De Decker S, Van Soens I, Duchateau L, Gielen IM, van Bree HJ, et al. 2011. Transcranial magnetic stimulation in Doberman Pinschers with clinically relevant and clinically irrelevant spinal cord compression on magnetic resonance imaging. *J Am Vet Med Assoc* 238:81–8.

82. Buchli R. 1975. Successful acupuncture treatment of a cervical disc syndrome in a dog. *Vet Med Small Anim Clin* 70:1302.

83. Janssens LA. 1992. Acupuncture for the treatment of thoracolumbar and cervical disc disease in the dog. *Probl Vet Med* 4:107–16.

84. Levine JM, Levine GJ, Johnson SI, Kerwin SC, Hettlich BF, Fosgate GT. 2007. Evaluation of the success of medical management for presumptive cervical intervertebral disk herniation in dogs. *Vet Surg* 36:492–9.

85. Liang ZH, Di Z, Jiang S, Xu SJ, Zhu XP, et al. 2012. The optimized acupuncture treatment for neck pain caused by cervical spondylosis: a study protocol of a multicentre randomized controlled trial. *Trials* 13:107.

86. Speciale J, Fingeroth JM. 2000. Use of physiatry as the sole treatment for three paretic or paralyzed dogs with chronic compressive conditions of the caudal portion of the cervical spinal cord. *J Am Vet Med Assoc* 217:43–7, 29.

87. Janssens L. 1985. The treatment of canine cervical disc disease by acupuncture: a review of thirty-two cases. *J Small Anim Pract* 26:203–12.

88. Laim A, Jaggy A, Forterre F, Doherr MG, Aeschbacher G, Glardon O. 2009. Effects of adjunct electroacupuncture on severity of postoperative pain in dogs undergoing hemilaminectomy because of acute thoracolumbar intervertebral disk disease. *J Am Vet Med Assoc* 234:1141–6.

89. Sharp NJH, Wheeler SJ. 2005. Cervical spondylomyelopathy. In Small animal spinal disorders diagnosis and surgery, ed. NJH Sharp, SJ Wheeler. Philadelphia: Elsevier Mosby. Number of 211–46 pp.

90. Adamo PF. 2011. Cervical arthroplasty in two dogs with disk-associated cervical spondylomyelopathy. *J Am Vet Med Assoc* 239:808–17.

91. Goring RL, Beale BS, Faulkner RF. 1991. The inverted cone decompression technique: a surgical treatment for cervical vertebral instability "wobbler syndrome" in Doberman Pinschers. *J Am Anim Hosp Assoc* 27:403–9.

92. McCartney W. 2007. Comparison of recovery times and complication rates between a modified slanted slot and the standard ventral slot for the treatment of cervical disc disease in 20 dogs. *J Small Anim Pract* 48:498–501.

93. Smith BA, Hosgood G, Kerwin SC. 1997. Ventral slot decompression for cervical intervertebral disc disease in 112 dogs. *Aust Vet Pract* 27:58–64.

94. Bergman RL, Levine JM, Coates JR, Bahr A, Hettlich BF, Kerwin SC. 2008. Cervical spinal locking plate in combination with cortical ring allograft for a one level fusion in dogs with cervical spondylotic myelopathy. *Vet Surg* 37:530–6.

95. Koehler CL, Stover SM, LeCouteur RA, Schulz KS, Hawkins DA. 2005. Effect of a ventral slot procedure and of smooth or positive-profile threaded pins with polymethylmethacrylate fixation on intervertebral biomechanics at treated and adjacent canine cervical vertebral motion units. *Am J Vet Res* 66:678–87.

96. Schulte K, Clark CR, Goel VK. 1989. Kinematics of the cervical spine following discectomy and stabilization. *Spine (Phila Pa 1976)* 14:1116–21.

97. Macy NB, Les CM, Stover SM, Kass PH. 1999. Effect of disk fenestration on sagittal kinematics of the canine C5–C6 intervertebral space. *Vet Surg* 28:171–9.

98. De Risio L, Munana K, Murray M, Olby N, Sharp NJ, Cuddon P. 2002. Dorsal laminectomy for caudal cervical spondylomyelopathy: postoperative recovery and long-term follow-up in 20 dogs. *Vet Surg* 31:418–27.

99. Rossmeisl JH, Jr., Lanz OI, Inzana KD, Bergman RL. 2005. A modified lateral approach to the canine cervical spine: procedural description and clinical application in 16 dogs with lateralized compressive myelopathy or radiculopathy. *Vet Surg* 34:436–44.

100. Downes CJ, Gemmill TJ, Gibbons SE, McKee WM. 2009. Hemilaminectomy and vertebral stabilisation for the treatment of thoracolumbar disc protrusion in 28 dogs. *J Small Anim Pract* 50:525–35.

101. Bruecker KA, Seim HB, 3rd, Withrow SJ. 1989. Clinical evaluation of three surgical methods for treatment of caudal cervical spondylomyelopathy of dogs. *Vet Surg* 18:197–203.

102. Fransson BA, Zhu Q, Bagley RS, Tucker R, Oxland TR. 2007. Biomechanical evaluation of cervical intervertebral plug stabilization in an ovine model. *Vet Surg* 36:449–57.

103. Adrega da Silva C, Bernard F, Bardet JF. 2010. Caudal cervical arthrodesis using a distractable fusion cage in a dog. *Vet Comp Orthop Traumatol* 23:209–13.

104. De Decker S, Caemaert J, Tshamala MC, Gielen IM, Van Bree HJ, et al. 2011. Surgical treatment of disk-associated wobbler syndrome by a distractable vertebral titanium cage in seven dogs. *Vet Surg* 40:544–54.

105. Steffen F, Voss K, Morgan JP. 2011. Distraction-fusion for caudal cervical spondylomyelopathy using an intervertebral cage and locking plates in 14 dogs. *Vet Surg* 40:743–52.

106. Voss K, Steffen F, Montavon PM. 2006. Use of the ComPact UniLock System for ventral stabilization procedures of the cervical spine: a retrospective study. *Vet Comp Orthop Traumatol* 19:21–8.

107. Jeffery ND, McKee WM. 2001. Surgery for disc-associated wobbler syndrome in the dog—an examination of the controversy. *J Small Anim Pract* 42:574–81.

108. Shamir MH, Chai O, Loeb E. 2008. A method for intervertebral space distraction before stabilization combined with complete ventral slot for treatment of disc-associated wobbler syndrome in dogs. *Vet Surg* 37:186–92.

109. Pfeil T. 2012. Treatment of 65 dogs with wobbler syndrome by distraction and fusion with TTA cages. *Proceedings 16th ESVOT congress*, Bologna, Italy.

110. Fitzpatrick N, Solano M. 2012. Cervical distraction and stabilization using a novel intervertebral spacer and 3.5 mm string-of-pearl (SOP™) plates in 16 dogs affected by disc associated wobbler syndrome (DAWS). *Proceedings WSAVA-BSAVA congress*, Birmingham, UK.

111. Matsunaga S, Kabayama S, Yamamoto T, Yone K, Sakou T, Nakanishi K. 1999. Strain on intervertebral discs after anterior cervical decompression and fusion. *Spine (Phila Pa 1976)* 24:670–5.

112. Hilibrand AS, Robbins M. 2004. Adjacent segment degeneration and adjacent segment disease: the consequences of spinal fusion? *Spine J* 4:190S–4S.

113. Eck JC, Humphreys SC, Lim TH, Jeong ST, Kim JG, et al. 2002. Biomechanical study on the effect of cervical spine fusion on adjacent-level intradiscal pressure and segmental motion. *Spine (Phila Pa 1976)* 27:2431–4.

114. Lund T, Oxland TR. 2011. Adjacent level disk disease—is it really a fusion disease? *Orthop Clin N Am* 42:529–41, viii.

115. Faizan A, Goel VK, Biyani A, Garfin SR, Bono CM. 2012. Adjacent level effects of bi level disc replacement, bi level fusion and disc replacement plus fusion in cervical spine—a finite element based study. *Clin Biomech* 27:226–33.

116. Yue JJ, Bertagnoli R, McAfee PC, An HS. 2008. *Motion preservation surgery of the spine: advanced techniques and controversies.* Elsevier Health Sciences, Philadelphia, PA.

117. Ramadan A, Mitulescu A, Champain S. 2008. Cervical arthroplasty with Discocerv™ "Cervidisc Evolution" surgical procedure and clinical experience 9 years after the first implantation of the first generation. *Interact Surg* 3:187–200.

8

Spondylosis Deformans

William B. Thomas and James M. Fingeroth

Several disorders are characterized by new bone formation on the spine of people and animals, including spondylosis deformans, diffuse idiopathic skeletal hyperostosis (DISH), and osteoarthritis of the facet joints. The nomenclature of these disorders is confusing for several reasons. The terms used to describe these conditions have often been used indiscriminately rather than adhering to precise diagnostic criteria. For example, in the past, the term spondylosis deformans was sometimes used to also refer to what is more properly called DISH. Another example is that clinicians may interchange the terms "spondylitis," which indicates an inflammatory condition, and "spondylosis," which is not inflammatory. Finally, it is not certain that the canine diseases are always identical to those in human patients.

Another point of confusion relates to the tendency to erroneously attribute a patient's clinical signs to one of these conditions when in fact the patient is suffering from an unrelated spinal lesion. This arises because the new bone formation is often so obvious and sometimes even dramatic on radiographs. On the other hand, more clinically significant lesions such as intervertebral disc herniations result in subtle changes on plain radiographs and may not even be apparent without more advanced imaging techniques such as magnetic resonance imaging (MRI).

Spondylosis deformans

Spondylosis deformans is a noninflammatory condition characterized by the formation of bony projections at the location where the annulus fibrosus is attached to the cortical surface of adjacent vertebral bodies (Sharpey fibers). Although these bony growths are often referred to as osteophytes, true osteophytes occur at the osteochondral junction of synovial joints. The correct term for the bony proliferation in spondylosis deformans is enthesophyte [1]. These enthesophytes are located several millimeters away from the junction between the disc and the vertebra (Figure 8.1). They typically expand ventrally and laterally but not dorsally. Enthesophytes vary from small spurs to bony bridges across the disc space leaving at least part of the ventral surface of the vertebral body unaffected. Spondylosis deformans can be classified as follows (Figure 8.2) [2, 3]:

Advances in Intervertebral Disc Disease in Dogs and Cats, First Edition. Edited by James M. Fingeroth and William B. Thomas.
© 2015 ACVS Foundation. Published 2015 by John Wiley & Sons, Inc.

Grade 0: No enthesophytes.

Grade 1: Small enthesophyte at the edge of the epiphysis that does not extend past the end plate.

Grade 2: Enthesophyte extends beyond the end plate but does not connect to enthesophyte on the adjacent vertebra.

Grade 3: Enthesophytes on adjacent vertebrae connected to each other forming a radiographic bony bridge between the two.

Pathophysiology

While the exact pathogenesis of spondylosis deformans is unclear, changes in the peripheral fibers of the annulus appear to be the most important inciting cause. In most cases, age-related breakdown

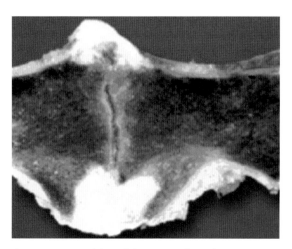

Figure 8.1   Spondylosis deformans. Enthesophytes are located on the ventral aspect of the vertebral body, several millimeters away from the junction between the disc and the vertebra.

of the peripheral annular fibers (Sharpey fibers) lead to discontinuity and weakening of the attachment of the disc to the vertebra. This leads to stress on the ventral longitudinal ligament where it attaches to the vertebral body. Enthesophytes develop at the stressed area and grow by a process of endochondral ossification. Bone growth extends ventrally and then laterally but rarely dorsally, probably because of the differences in the attachments of the ventral and dorsal longitudinal ligaments and the ventral and dorsal attachments of the annulus and vertebral bodies [4]. Spondylosis deformans can also develop subsequent to other causes of disc injury, such as spinal trauma, ventral slot surgery, or discospondylitis. With regard to the latter, this is often a point of confusion for clinicians, with occasional misinterpretation of noninflammatory spondylosis with the inflammatory (usually infectious) lesions in the disc space seen with discospondylitis. This is addressed further in Chapter 20. This confusion is sometimes compounded by the fact as noted previously that discospondylitis, because of its degradative effect on the disc and end plates, usually induces spondylosis (i.e., enthesophytes on the involved adjacent vertebrae). Hence, radiographic interpretation requires the clinician to distinguish between benign spondylosis from that which has resulted from inflammatory destruction of the intervertebral disc.

Clinical features

Spondylosis deformans is common in dogs, with the reported incidence varying depending on the age and breed distribution of the studied population and the method of diagnosis [4]. It is uncommon in

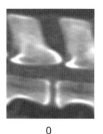
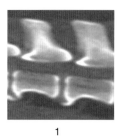
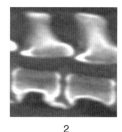
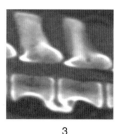

| 0 | 1 | 2 | 3 |

Figure 8.2   Grades of spondylosis deformans. Grade 0: no enthesophytes. Grade 1: small enthesophyte at the edge of the epiphysis that does not extend past the end plate. Grade 2: enthesophyte extends beyond the end plate but does not connect to enthesophyte on the adjacent vertebra. Grade 3: enthesophytes on adjacent vertebrae connected to each other forming radiographic bony bridges between vertebrae.

dogs less than 2 years of age and after that the prevalence and the grade of spondylosis increase with age. By the age of 9 years, approximately 25–70% of dogs are affected [5, 6]. Large-breed dogs are at increased risk but any size dog can be affected [3, 5, 7]. The prevalence of spondylosis deformans is especially high in boxers (approximately 40–85%, depending on age), and a genetic predisposition has been identified in this breed [2, 3, 7]. The L7–S1 disc space is most commonly affected with the thoracolumbar region (T12–L3) being the next most commonly affected level. Affected patients often have multiple sites of involvement [5, 7, 8]. Spondylosis in the cervical region is less common. Spondylosis deformans is also common in cats, and as with dogs, the prevalence increases with age [6, 9].

Spondylosis deformans is usually an incidental finding, and there is no clear correlation between the presence of spondylosis and clinical signs of spinal disease [5, 8]. In two studies, there was no significant difference in pain, lameness, or neurologic deficits in dogs with spondylosis compared to dogs without spondylosis [10, 11]. This is similar to lumbar spondylosis in people, where the frequency of signs or symptoms among individuals with enthesophytes is no greater than among those individuals without enthesophytes [12]. Bony spurs typically do not expand into the vertebral canal and therefore do not compress the spinal cord to cause neurologic deficits (Figure 8.3). Because new bone formation can protrude dorsolaterally, it is possible for the nerve root or spinal nerve to be compressed. However, the resulting compression occurs slowly, and clinical signs associated with spondylosis deformans are difficult to confirm [5, 8, 13]. In a study of cats, spondylosis deformans was found to be related with behavioral changes such as decreased willingness to greet their owners, reluctance to being petted, increased aggressiveness, and a poorer quality of life as perceived by the clients [14]. However, since this study did not include any advanced imaging of the spine, it is unclear whether the clinical differences seen in cats with greater degrees of spondylosis might have been due to concomitant intervertebral disc herniation. Since disc degeneration is associated with both increased prevalence of spondylosis and (for cats and nonchondrodystrophoid dogs) the potential development of disc herniation, it is possible that a population of animals with more dramatic spondylosis may also have a higher rate of disc herniation

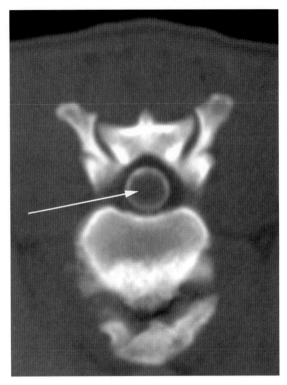

Figure 8.3   CT myelogram of spondylosis deformans. Enthesophytes form ventrally and therefore do not affect the spinal cord (arrow).

and that it is the latter that results in observed clinical signs rather than the spondylosis itself.

Diagnosis

Radiographically, the enthesophytes associated with spondylosis deformans begin as smooth-bordered triangular outgrowths located several millimeters from the edge of the end plate (Figure 8.4). As the condition progresses, the enthesophytes may appear to bridge the intervertebral disc space, although true ankylosis is rare. Spondylosis deformans can also be identified on computed tomography (CT) and MRI (Figure 8.5).

Treatment

In patients with apparent spinal pain and stiffness, a course of conservative therapy is appropriate, consisting of nonsteroidal anti-inflammatory drugs or analgesics and weight loss as needed. In patients

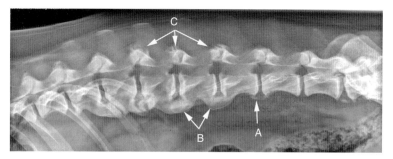

Figure 8.4   Spondylosis deformans, radiograph. Grade 1 spondylosis involves the L4–L5 vertebrae (A), and grade 3 spondylosis (B) is evident at T13–L1 through L3–L4. There is also osteoarthritis of the facet joints (C).

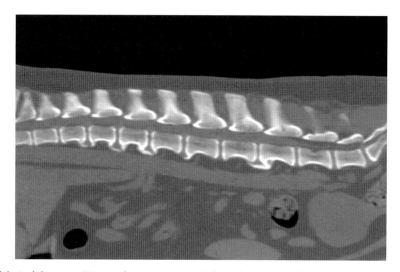

Figure 8.5   Spondylosis deformans, CT sagittal reconstruction. Enthesophytes are evident at multiple sites.

with neurologic deficits or severe or persistent spinal pain, further diagnostic testing such as CT, MRI, and analysis of cerebrospinal fluid is indicated in an attempt to identify the cause of the clinical signs, rather than assuming that the spondylosis seen on radiographs is the culprit.

DISH

DISH, also known as ankylosing hyperostosis or Forestier disease in humans, is characterized by calcification and ossification at entheses, the sites where a ligament, tendon, or joint capsule inserts into bone.

DISH in human patients

DISH is common in older people and is usually asymptomatic although it can be associated with

pain, limited range of spinal motion, and increased susceptibility to spinal fracture after trivial trauma [15]. In human patients, the anterolateral aspect of the thoracic spine is most commonly affected, although the lumbar and cervical regions are also commonly involved. The majority of affected people also have hyperostosis at other locations, including the elbows, wrists, ankles, and shoulders [15]. In human patients, the propensity for new bone formation has a metabolic cause, and DISH is associated with obesity, type 2 diabetes, hyperinsulinemia, and other features of metabolic syndrome [16].

Diagnostic criteria for DISH rely on new bone formation that bridges four contiguous vertebral bodies in the absence of inflammatory sacroiliac or facet joint change. However, clinically DISH often occurs in patients with concurrent age-related disc or facet joint degeneration. The earliest change is ossification at the site of attachment of the dorsal longitudinal ligament in the middle of the vertebral body, well away from the annulus. Later, the ossification bridges the disc space. Eventually, the new bone "flows" from one vertebra to the next. This is most characteristic on the right side of the thoracic vertebrae, possibly because pressure from the aorta limits bone formation on the left side. As the term "diffuse" indicates, new bone formation is not limited to the spine and can affect the hands, feet, knees and elbows.

DISH in dogs

Wright in 1982 was the first to identify a condition similar to human DISH in dogs and to separate this disorder from spondylosis deformans [13, 17]. Since then, there have been several publications describing DISH in dogs [7, 18–21]. Various authors have used different diagnostic criteria. Considering the risk of error inherent in extrapolating clinical features from a human disease to veterinary medicine, it is still unclear as to what are the best diagnostic criteria to use in dogs [22]. Nevertheless, most authors have used the radiographic criteria proposed by Resnick for the diagnosis of DISH in human patients:

1. Presence of flowing calcification and ossification along the ventrolateral aspects of at least four contiguous vertebral bodies with or without associated localized pointed excrescences at the intervening vertebral body–disc junctions
2. Relative preservation of intervertebral disc width in the involved vertebral segments and the absence of extensive radiographic changes of disc disease, including vacuum phenomena and vertebral body marginal sclerosis
3. Absence of facet joint bony ankylosis and sacroiliac joint erosion, sclerosis, or bony fusion [23]

Clinical features

In one radiographic study of dogs older than 1 year, the prevalence of DISH was 3.8% and the prevalence increased with age. As with spondylosis, boxers were at increased risk

with 40% of boxers affected. The thoracic and lumbar vertebrae were most commonly affected [7]. Extraspinal manifestations have not been reported commonly, but periarticular ossifications of appendicular joints and the pelvis have been described [18, 19].

It is unclear how often DISH results in clinical signs and many patients appear to be asymptomatic. However, spinal pain and stiffness have been reported [7]. Human patients are at increased risk of spinal fracture after trivial trauma due to altered biomechanical properties of the spine [24]. Kornmayer *et al.* described a weimaraner with DISH that suffered two separate spinal fractures coincident with minor trauma over a period of 2 years [21]. Altered biomechanics due to fusion of multiple consecutive disc spaces can also increase degeneration of adjacent, unfused disc spaces resulting in intervertebral disc disease at these sites [20].

Diagnosis

The new bone formation in DISH consists of enthesophytes affecting the ventral longitudinal ligament continuing along the entire ventral aspect of at least four contiguous vertebral bodies. This is in contrast to spondylosis deformans in which the bone formation originates from the region adjacent to the ventral end plate and is mostly confined to region of the intervertebral disc (Figure 8.6).

Osteoarthritis of the facet joints

The facet (zygapophyseal) joints are paired, true synovial joints that comprise the dorsolateral articulation between adjacent vertebrae. Facet joints play an important role in stabilizing the spine in flexion and extension, and restricting axial rotation. Osteoarthritis of the facet joints is similar to that of all diarthrodial joints. Cartilage degradation leads to erosions with sclerosis of the subchondral bone. The facet joint capsule is richly innervated with nociceptive fibers and may be a source of a spinal pain. Also, facet hypertrophy, malalignment, and osteophyte formation may narrow the vertebral canal or intervertebral foramen. Although osteoarthritis of the facet joints can occur coincident with

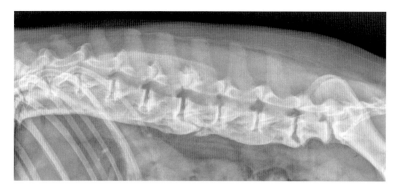

Figure 8.6   Diffuse idiopathic skeletal hyperostosis. This radiograph of a 5-year-old boxer with no clinical signs shows flowing bone formation along the ventral aspect of contiguous thoracic and lumbar vertebrae.

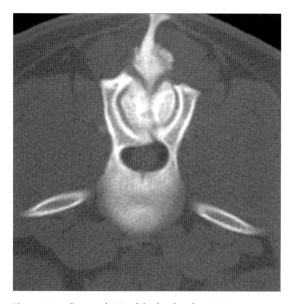

Figure 8.7   Osteoarthritis of the lumbar facet joints. Transverse CT showing enlargement of the facets with osteophyte formation.

spondylosis deformans, they are separate processes [1]. In human patients, osteoarthritis of the facet joints is a potential source of spinal pain although there is a poor correlation between spinal pain and the degree of osteoarthritis seen on imaging [25].

In dogs, facet joint osteoarthritis is often an incidental finding, but spinal pain is possible. Radiographs show enlargement of the facets and osteophytes (Figure 8.4). CT is helpful is characterizing specific changes and identifying any compression of the vertebral canal or intervertebral foramen (Figure 8.7). Treatment consists of anti-inflammatory and analgesic medication and rest for acute cases. Weight loss is helpful for overweight dogs.

Baastrup's sign

Baastrup's sign or kissing spines is characterized by the close approximation of adjacent spinous processes with resultant enlargement, flattening, and sclerosis of the apposing interspinous surfaces [26]. The cause is repetitive strain on the interspinous ligaments that leads to degeneration and collapse of the ligaments, allowing contact between adjacent spinous processes. This abnormal contact between spinous processes can result in neoarthrosis and formation of an adventitious bursa [26]. In the original description in 1933, Baastrup described clinical features in people consisting of lumbar tenderness and pain on extension that was relieved by spinal flexion. Recent studies indicate Baastrup's sign is common in elderly people and is usually concurrent with other degenerative changes such as facet joint osteoarthritis. It is probably part of the expected degenerative changes in the aging spine with questionable clinical significance [26].

While there are no published clinical studies of Baastrup's sign in dogs, similar radiographic changes are occasionally seen in older dogs. Diagnostic criteria on radiographs or CT consist of (i) close approximation and contact between apposing spinous processes and (ii) sclerosis of the cranial and caudal portions of adjacent processes (Figure 8.8). Affected dogs often also have signs of facet joint osteoarthritis.

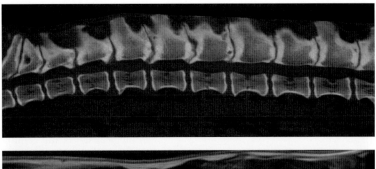

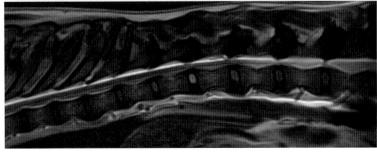

Figure 8.8   Baastrup's sign. CT (top) and MRI (bottom) show close approximation and sclerosis of adjacent spinous processes. There is also facet joint osteoarthritis.

References

1. Widmer WR, Thrall DE. The canine and feline vertebrae. In: Thrall DE, editor. Textbook of Veterinary Diagnostic Radiology. 6th ed. St. Louis: Elsevier; 2013. pp. 186–7.
2. Langeland M, Lingaas F. Spondylosis deformans in the boxer: Estimates of heritability. J Small Anim Pract. 1995;36:166–9.
3. Carnier P, Gallo L, Sturaro E, Piccinini P, Bittante G. Prevalence of spondylosis deformans and estimates of genetic parameters for the degree of osteophytes development in Italian Boxer dogs. J Anim Sci. 2004 Jan;82(1):85–92.
4. Romatowski J. Spondylosis deformans in the dog. Compend Contin Educ Pract Vet. 1986;8:531–4.
5. Morgan JP, Ljunggren G, Read R. Spondylosis deformans (vertebral osteophytosis) in the dog. J Small Anim Pract. 1967;8:57–66.
6. Read RM, Smith RN. A comparison of spondylosis deformans in the English and Swedish cat and in the English dog. J Small Anim Pract. 1968;9:159–66.
7. Kranenburg HC, Voorhout G, Grinwis GC, Hazewinkel HA, Meij BP. Diffuse idiopathic skeletal hyperostosis (DISH) and spondylosis deformans in purebred dogs: a retrospective radiographic study. Vet J. 2011 Nov;190(2):e84–90.
8. Morgan JP, Hansson K, Miyabayashi T. Spondylosis deformans in the female beagle dog: A radiographic study. J Small Anim Pract. 1989;30:457–60.
9. Lascelles BD, Henry JB, 3rd, Brown J, Robertson I, Sumrell AT, Simpson W, et al. Cross-sectional study of the prevalence of radiographic degenerative joint disease in domesticated cats. Vet Surg. 2010 Jul;39(5):535–44.
10. Morgan JP. Spondylosis derformans in the dog. A morphologic study with some clinical and experimental observations. Acta Orthop Scand. 1967;7:7–87.
11. Wright JA. Spondylosis deforms of the lumbo-sacral joint in dogs. J Small Anim Pract. 1980;21:45–58.
12. O'Neill TW, McCloskey EV, Kanis JA, Bhalla AK, Reeve J, Reid DM, et al. The distribution, determinants, and clinical correlates of vertebral osteophytosis: a population based survey. J Rheumatol. 1999 Apr;26(4):842–8.
13. Wright JA. A study of vertebral osteophyte formation in the canine spine. II. Radiographic survey. J Small Anim Pract. 1982;23:747–61.
14. Kranenburg HC, Meij BP, van Hofwegen EM, Voorhout G, Slingerland LI, Picavet P, et al. Prevalence of spondylosis deformans in the feline spine and correlation with owner-perceived behavioural changes. Vet Comp Orthop Traumatol. 2012 May 15;25(3):217–23.
15. Mader R, Sarzi-Puttini P, Atzeni F, Olivieri I, Pappone N, Verlaan JJ, et al. Extraspinal manifestations of diffuse idiopathic skeletal hyperostosis. Rheumatology. 2009 Dec;48(12):1478–81.
16. Littlejohn G. Diffuse idiopathic skeletal hyperostosis. In: Hochberg MC, Silman AJ, Smolen JS,

Weinblatt ME, Weisman MH, editors. Rheumatology. 5th ed. Philadelphia: Mosby Elsevier; 2011. pp. 1801–6.

17. Wright JA. A study of vertebral osteophyte formation in the canine spine. I. Spinal survey. J Small Anim Pract. 1982;23:697–711.

18. Woodard JC, Poulos PW, Parker RB, Jackson RI, Eurell JC. Canine diffuse idiopathic skeletal hyperostosis. Vet Pathol. 1985;22:317–26.

19. Morgan JP, Stavenborn M. Disseminated idiopathic skeletal hyperostosis (DISH) in a dog. Vet Radiol Ultrasound. 1991;32:65–70.

20. Ortega M, Goncalves R, Haley A, Wessmann A, Penderis J. Spondylosis deformans and diffuse idiopathic skeletal hyperostosis (dish) resulting in adjacent segment disease. Vet Radiol Ultrasound. 2012 Mar–Apr;53(2):128–34.

21. Kornmayer M, Burger M, Amort K, Brunnberg L. Spinal fracture in a dog with diffuse idiopathic skeletal hyperostosis. Vet Comp Orthop Traumatol. 2013;26(1):76–81.

22. Greatting HH, Young BD, Pool RR, Levine JM. Diffuse idiopathic skeletal hyperostosis (DISH). Vet Radiol Ultrasound. 2011 Jul–Aug;52(4):472–3.

23. Resnick D, Niwayama G. Radiographic and pathologic features of spinal involvement in diffuse idiopathic skeletal hyperostosis (DISH). Radiology. 1976 Jun;119(3):559–68.

24. Westerveld LA, Verlaan JJ, Oner FC. Spinal fractures in patients with ankylosing spinal disorders: a systematic review of the literature on treatment, neurological status and complications. Eur Spine J. 2009 Feb;18(2):145–56.

25. Kalichman L, Hunter DJ. Lumbar facet joint osteoarthritis: a review. Seminars in arthritis and rheumatism. 2007 Oct;37(2):69–80.

26. Kwong Y, Rao N, Latief K. MDCT findings in Baastrup disease: disease or normal feature of the aging spine? Am J Roentgenol. 2011 May;196(5):1156–9.

9 What is Fibrocartilaginous Embolism and Is It Related to IVDD?

Luisa De Risio

Overview

Embolization of spinal vasculature with fibrocartilaginous material histochemically identical to the nucleus pulposus of the intervertebral disc is the most common cause of ischemic myelopathy in dogs and cats. This condition is called "fibrocartilaginous embolism" (FCE) or "fibrocartilaginous embolic myelopathy" (FCEM). The intraparenchymal (intrinsic) spinal cord arteries are functional end arteries and their occlusion results in ischemic necrosis of the territory supplied. This typically results in peracute (<6h) onset of neurological signs, with distribution and severity referable to the site and extent of the infarction. Neurologic deficits typically do not progress beyond the first 24 h.

Pathophysiology

The source of the fibrocartilaginous material is assumed to be the nucleus pulposus that is undergoing degeneration in adult animals. This hypothesis is supported by the observation that FCE occurs primarily in the spinal cord and the lesion commonly extends over a few spinal cord segments, suggesting that the emboli arise from one degenerated intervertebral disc. The intervertebral disc is normally avascular in adults. Exactly how the fibrocartilaginous material gains access to the spinal cord vasculature is not known, but several theories have been proposed [1, 2]. These include:

- Direct penetration of nucleus pulposus fragments into the spinal vasculature. Injection of nucleus through the arterial wall is unlikely due to the relatively thick arterial muscular wall and direct penetration into the venous system is more likely. Extruded disc material has been identified in the ventral internal vertebral venous plexus adjacent to the affected spinal cord segment in dogs with histologically confirmed FCEM [3–5]. Arteriovenous anastomoses have been shown in the epidural and periradicular space in dogs and humans and could explain the presence of emboli on either

Advances in Intervertebral Disc Disease in Dogs and Cats, First Edition. Edited by James M. Fingeroth and William B. Thomas.

side of the circulation, regardless of whether the entry point is arterial or venous. Reverse venous blood flow associated with the Valsalva maneuver (such as during straining or exercise) may have a role in the distribution of the fibrocartilaginous emboli into the spinal cord arteries and veins.

- Protrusion of nucleus pulposus material into sinusoidal venous channels within the adjacent vertebral bone marrow, with subsequent retrograde entrance into the basivertebral vein and into the ventral internal vertebral venous plexus. As in the previous hypothesis, retrograde venous flow associated with the Valsalva maneuver may have a role in the distribution of the fibrocartilaginous emboli into the spinal cord vasculature. Protrusion of degenerated disc material into the adjacent vertebral bone marrow is referred to as Schmorl's nodes in humans. In dogs, this type of intravertebral disc herniation appears rare, possibly because of dogs' quadrupedal posture and

the thickness of the cortical bone adjacent to the intervertebral disc.

- Penetration of nucleus pulposus material into newly formed inflammatory blood vessels within a degenerated intervertebral disc. Following chronic inflammation, ingrowth of blood vessels within the degenerated annulus fibrosus has been documented in nonchondrodystrophoid dogs and in humans. A sudden rise in intervertebral disc internal pressure exceeding arterial blood pressure may result in penetration of nucleus pulposus fibrocartilage into the degenerated annulus and into the newly formed intervertebral disc vessels with progression into the intrinsic spinal cord vasculature. Fibrocartilage has been identified within newly formed blood vessels in the degenerated intervertebral disc in two dogs with histologically confirmed FCEM [3, 4].
- Penetration of nucleus pulposus fibrocartilage into embryonic remnant vessels within the

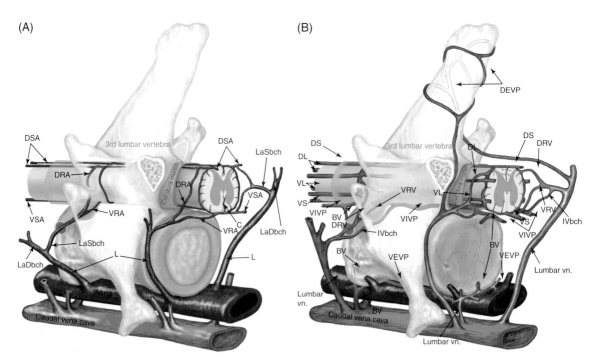

Figure 9.1 (A) Arterial supply to the lumbar spinal cord. C, central artery; DRA, dorsal radicular artery; DSA, dorsal spinal artery (paired); L, lumbar artery; LaDbch, lumbar artery dorsal branch; LaSbch, lumbar artery spinal branch; VSA, ventral spinal artery; VR, ventral radicular artery. (B) Venous drainage of the lumbar spinal cord. BV, basivertebral vein; DEVP, dorsal external vertebral venous plexus; DL, dorsolateral vein (paired); DRV, dorsal radicular vein; DS, dorsal spinal vein; IVbch, intervertebral vein branch; VEVP, ventral external vertebral venous plexus; VIVP, ventral internal vertebral venous plexus; VL, ventrolateral vein (paired); VRV, ventral radicular vein; VS, ventral spinal vein. *Source:* With permission from De Risio L, Platt SR. 2010. Fibrocartilaginous embolic myelopathy in small animals. *Vet Clin North Am Small Anim Pract.* 40(5):859–69. © Elsevier.

nucleus pulposus. As in the previous hypothesis, a sudden rise in intradiscal pressure exceeding arterial blood pressure may result in penetration of nucleus pulposus fibrocartilage into the embryonic remnant intervertebral disc vessels and progression into the intrinsic spinal cord vasculature.

In immature animals, the annulus fibrosus is vascularized, and the semiliquid nucleus pulposus could be injected in the annulus fibrosus blood vessels when the intradiscal pressure suddenly increases during exercise or minor trauma [6]. The vertebral growth-plate cartilage (which is vascularized) could also be the source of the fibrocartilaginous material in immature dogs [7]. Another hypothesis on the source of the fibrocartilaginous material suggests that it may arise from metaplasia of the vascular endothelium, which later ruptures into the lumen and embolizes within the intrinsic spinal cord vasculature [1]. The vascular anatomy of the spinal cord is illustrated in Figure 9.1.

The ischemic injury caused by the arterial obstruction initiates a series of biochemical and metabolic events (similar to the secondary injury phenomenon described in Chapters 15 and 25), which result in neuronal and glial cell death. The gray matter, due to its greater metabolic demand, is generally affected more severely than the white matter.

Clinical presentation

FCEM has been reported in dogs more commonly than in cats. At the time of writing, there are several studies including 24 or more dogs with FCEM (Table 9.1). The literature on feline FCEM is limited to case reports, and three case series for a total of 38 cats are reported in the literature (Table 9.2).

FCEM has been reported in large and giant breed dogs more commonly than in small- to medium-sized dogs [5, 8–13], and it is most common in nonchondrodystrophoid canine breeds. The reported male to female ratio in dogs ranges from 1:1 [8] to approximately 2.5:1 [9, 12]. The age at diagnosis in dogs ranges from 2 months [6] to 13 years and 5 months [13], with a median of 4–6 years in most studies [5, 8, 10, 12, 13].

Combining the data available on all the cats reported with FCEM in the literature, the domestic short hair is the most represented breed, the male to female ratio is 1.3:1, and the age at diagnosis ranges from 2 to 16 years (median, 10 years) [3, 14–22].

The typical clinical presentation is characterized by peracute (<6h) onset of nonprogressive and nonpainful (after the first 24h) and often lateralized neurological deficits consistent with the location, extent, and severity of the spinal cord infarction [12]. Rarely, neurologic dysfunction can progress for longer than 24h, possibly as a result of additional embolizations or secondary spinal cord injury. In up to 80% of dogs diagnosed with FCEM, the dog was performing some type of physical activity, such as running, jumping, or playing, at onset of neurologic signs [8]. Signs of sudden and transient hyperalgesia (e.g., yelping as in pain) are observed by the owners at the onset of neurologic signs in up to 61.5% of affected dogs [8]. This transient hyperalgesia may be the result of stimulation of nociceptors in the endothelium of embolized spinal blood vessels [23]. This focal spinal hyperalgesia generally resolves in a few minutes to hours. Lateralization of neurologic signs has been reported in 52.8–86.5% of dogs with FCEM [5, 8, 10, 12, 13]. The asymmetry of signs can be very marked and often result in severely paretic or plegic limb/s on one side, while the contralateral limb/s has/have minimal deficits. This marked lateralization of signs is uncommon with other myelopathies and results from asymmetric branching of the intrinsic spinal cord vasculature, particularly the central branches of the ventral spinal artery, which have an asymmetric distribution in several spinal cord segments (Figure 9.1). The central arteries supply most of the gray matter and part of the lateral and ventral white matter of the spinal cord, sending branches to each side, or alternatively and irregularly to the left or right side of the spinal cord. The mean percentage of central arteries that send branches unilaterally is 79% in the cervical region, 58% in the thoracic region, and 37% in the lumbar region [24]. FCEM can also result in bilateral and symmetrical neurologic deficits. FCEM most commonly affects the L4–S3 and C6–T2 spinal cord segments in dogs with a histologic diagnosis [8, 10] and L4–S3 and T3–L3 in dogs with an antemortem diagnosis (Table 9.1) [5, 8, 10, 12, 13]. Neurologic deficits

Table 9.1 Summary of studies including ≥24 dogs of different breeds with a diagnosis of FCEM

Reference	Total Number of Dogs	Number of Dogs with AD and HD	Percentage of Large or Giant Breed Dogs	Age (Years, Median, and Range)	Male to Female Ratio	Percentage of Dogs with each Neuroanatomic Localization and/or Site of the Lesion based on Histology or MRI				Percentage of Dogs with Lateralization of Neurologic Signs	Percentage of Dogs with Nociception	Percentage of Dogs with Partial or Complete Recovery
						C1–C5	C6–T2	T3–L3	L4–S3			
[5]	24	AD[a] 19 HD 5	79	5 (0.5–10)	1.2:1	16.7	20.8	33.3	29.2	70.8	NR	58.3
[8]	72	AD[a] 26 HD 36	54 75	5 (1–10) 4 (0.3–7)	1:1 1.3:1	3.8 2.8	3.8 30.6	42.3 19.4	50.0 47.2	80.8 52.8	88.0 50.0	73.9
[10]	75	AD[a] 54 HD 21	74 81	6 (1–11) 5 (5–9)	1.7:1 1.6:1	5.6 9.5	11.1 33.4	37.0 14.3	43.3 42.8	64.8 55.0	90.7 33.3	65.3
[23]	26	AD[b] 26	54	4 (0.5–10)	1.4:1	15.4	19.2	34.6	30.8	73.1	96.2	66.7
[12]	52	AD[c] 50 HD 2	81	6 (0.4–11.9)	2.5:1	0.0	28.9	26.9	44.2	86.5	94.2	84.0
[13]	26	AD[c] 26	16	5.6 (0.4–13.4)	1.3:1	19.2	23.0	50.0	7.8	61.5	92.3	80.8

AD, antemortem diagnosis only; HD, histological diagnosis; NR, not reported.

[a]Antemortem diagnosis of FCEM based on clinical presentation, myelography, ± CSF analysis.

[b]Antemortem diagnosis of FCEM based on clinical presentation, ± myelography, ± CSF analysis (myelography was performed in 14 dogs, Dunie-Meringot 2007).

[c]Antemortem diagnosis of FCEM based on clinical presentation, MRI, ± CSF analysis (1.5 tesla MRI [12]; 0.3 tesla MRI [13]).

Table 9.2 Summary of case reports of cats diagnosed with FCEM

Case Report/ Series	Number of Cats	Breed	Sex	Age (Years)	Duration of Progression of Clinical Signs	Neuroanatomic Localization	Neurological Dysfunction	Diagnostic Imaging	Follow-up	Histologic Diagnosis	Site of the Lesion based on Histology or MRI
[22]	1	DSH	FS	10	<24 h	L4–S3 right sided	Paraparesis, urinary, and fecal incontinence	Survey radiographs	Euthanized 6 days after presentation due to lack of improvement	Yes	L6–S3
[14]	1	NR	NR	12	NR	L4–S3	Paraplegia	NR	Euthanized	Yes	Lumbar intumescence
[15]	1	DSH	ME	12	48 h	C6–T2 left sided	Tetraparesis	Survey radiographs	Euthanized 2 days after presentation due to lack of improvement	Yes	Cervical intumescence
[16]	1	DSH	MN	12	<24 h	C6–T2 left sided	Hemiparesis	Myelography	Nearly complete recovery 7 weeks after diagnosis	No	Caudal cervical spinal cord
[17]	1	DSH	FS	9	<24 hours	L4–S3 left sided	Paraplegia, urinary incontinence, loss of nociception in the left pelvic limb	Myelography	Euthanized 12 days after diagnosis due to incomplete improvement	Yes	L4–S3
[18]	1	DSH	MN	8	5 days	C6–T2 left sided	Nonambulatory tetraparesis	Survey radiographs	Euthanized 7 days after presentation due to lack of improvement	Yes	C6–C7

(Continued)

Table 9.2 (Cont'd)

Case Report/ Series	Number of Cats	Breed	Sex	Age (Years)	Duration of Progression of Clinical Signs	Neuroanatomic Localization	Neurological Dysfunction	Diagnostic Imaging	Follow-up	Histologic Diagnosis	Site of the Lesion based on Histology or MRI
[19]	2	Persian	MN	10	<24h	C1–C5 left sided	Plegia of the left thoracic and both pelvic limbs, paresis of the right thoracic limb	MRI	Significant improvement 6 weeks after presentation. No recurrence in 4 years of follow-up available	No	C1–C3 left sided
		DSH	FS	4	A few hours	C6–T2 left sided	Left-sided hemiplegia, mild right-sided hemiparesis	MRI	Full neurological recovery 2 weeks after presentation	No	C7 left sided
[20]	5	DSH	FS	10	24h	T3–L3 left sided	Nonambulatory paraparesis	Myelography	Euthanized 1 day after diagnosis	Yes	L1
		DSH	FS	11	36h	C1–C5 left sided	Nonambulatory tetraparesis	None	Euthanized 3 days after diagnosis	Yes	C4
		Maine coon	MN	7	<5h	C6–T2 left sided	Tetraparesis	MRI	Euthanized 7 days after diagnosis due to lack of improvement	Yes	C6–C7
		DSH	MN	10	2h	C6–T2 right sided	Nonambulatory tetraparesis	MRI	Ambulatory 14 days after diagnosis	No	C5–C6
		DSH	MN	7	<5h	T3–L3	Paraplegia	MRI	Ambulatory 2 days after diagnosis	No	L2–L3–L4

Reference	n	Breed	Sex	Age	Duration	Neurolocalization	Neurologic signs	Imaging	Outcome	Recurrence	MRI lesion location
[21]	6	Persian	FS	16	NR	C1–C5	Tetraparesis	MRI	Ambulatory 10 days after diagnosis	No	C2–C3
		DSH	FS	13	NR	C6–T2 left sided	Paraparesis	MRI	Ambulatory 13 days after diagnosis	No	C7–T1 left sided
		DSH	FS	8	NR	L4–S1 left sided	Paraparesis	MRI	Ambulatory 27 days after diagnosis	No	L5–L6 left sided
		DSH	MN	13	NR	C1–C5	Tetraparesis	MRI	Ambulatory 7 days after diagnosis	No	C3–C4
		DSH	MN	12	NR	C6–T2 left sided	Tetraparesis	MRI	Ambulatory 21 days after diagnosis	No	C7–T1 left sided
		DSH	ME	2	NR	C1–C5 right sided	Tetraparesis	MRI	Ambulatory 10 days after diagnosis	No	C1–C2 right sided
[33]	19	14 DSH, 2 DLH, 2 Persian, 1 British SH	11 MN, 7 FS, 1F	Median 10	Median <24h	In all but 1 cat with 2 lesions on MRI, clinical and MRI neurolocalizations corresponded	Median and mean neurologic score of 3 (nonambulatory paresis)	MRI	Median time to recovery of ambulation was 3.5 days (3–19 days) 15/19 (79%) cats had a favorable outcome with a medial follow-up of 3 years and 1 month	Yes (1 cat)	C1–C5 (6 cats), C6–T2 (6 cats), T3–L3 (5 cats), L4–S1 (3 cats) with 1 cat affected by 2 separate lesions

NR, not reported.

usually refer to the affected spinal cord segment (C1–C5, C6–T2, T3–L3, or L4–S3). However, in the acute stage of the disease, a decreased withdrawal reflex has been reported in severely paraparetic and paraplegic dogs with magnetic resonance imaging (MRI) changes consistent with FCEM within the T3–L3 spinal cord segment [12]. The majority of these dogs had an interruption of the cutaneous trunci reflex consistent with the site of FCEM on MRI [12]. It has been suggested that the transient decrease of the pelvic limb withdrawal reflex in dogs with acute thoracolumbar spinal cord injury is due to sudden interruption of descending supraspinal input on motor neurons and interneurons, fusimotor depression, and increased segmental inhibition [25]. This phenomenon is clinically relevant, as it may lead to an incorrect neuroanatomic localization, site of diagnostic investigation, and prognosis.

FCEM most commonly affects the cervical spinal cord in cats. Lesion distribution in the 38 cats reported in the literature is C1–C5 in 11 cats, C6–T2 in 14 cats, T3–L3 in 7 cats, and L4–S3 in 7 cats. Lateralization of neurologic signs has been reported in 26 of 38 (68%) cats in which this information is available (Table 9.2).

Differential diagnoses

The main differential diagnoses for peracute, non-progressive, lateralized myelopathy include ischemic myelopathy due to obstruction of the intrinsic spinal vasculature by material other than fibrocartilage, such as thrombi, or bacterial, parasitic, neoplastic, or fat emboli and acute noncompressive nucleus pulposus extrusion (ANNPE) (see Chapter 13). Underlying medical conditions that may predispose to embolization or thrombosis, including cardiomyopathy, endocarditis, hypothyroidism, hyperthyroidism, hyperadrenocorticism, chronic renal failure, and hypertension, should be considered and investigated, particularly in cats with peracute onset nonpainful and nonprogressive myelopathy. ANNPE occurs when nondegenerated nucleus pulposus extrudes during strenuous exercise or trauma, contuses the spinal cord, and dissipates within the epidural space, causing minimal to no spinal cord compression. The clinical presentation of dogs with ANNPE is often very similar to one of dogs with

FCEM. Lateralization of neurological deficits has been reported in 62% of dogs with ANNPE [26]. The main clinical difference between ANNPE and FCEM is discomfort or hyperesthesia during palpation of the affected spinal segments, which has been reported in 57% of dogs with ANNPE, while it is uncommon in dogs with FCEM [12, 26]. High-field MRI and experience in neuroimaging also may help differentiate these two diseases [2, 12, 26].

Other differential diagnoses include compressive intervertebral disc extrusion, infectious and noninfectious meningomyelitis, neoplasia, hemorrhage (e.g., secondary to coagulopathy), and vertebral fracture, subluxation, or luxation. The history, onset, and progression of signs and the presence/absence of spinal hyperesthesia on clinical examination help to expand or narrow the list of differential diagnoses. Animals with FCEM may show discomfort on palpation of the affected spinal segment when examined within a few hours of onset of neurological dysfunction or anytime after onset of signs in case of concurrent spinal pathology such as spondylosis deformans. Alternatively, animals with spinal disorders commonly associated with some degree of spinal hyperesthesia (such as intervertebral disc extrusion) may show no obvious signs of hyperesthesia on palpation of the affected spinal segment because they are very stoic or due to recent administration of anti-inflammatory and/or analgesic medications. Pharmacological treatment may also interfere with progression of signs resulting in clinical stabilization or improvement of animals with disorders that would be progressive if untreated. Therefore, diagnostic investigations are needed to support the clinical suspicion of FCEM.

Diagnosis

The antemortem diagnosis of FCEM is based on history, clinical findings, exclusion of other etiologies of myelopathy (through diagnostic imaging and cerebrospinal fluid (CSF) analysis), and visualization of a lesion compatible with spinal cord ischemia on MRI. The definitive diagnosis of FCEM can only be reached through histological examination of the affected spinal cord segments.

Diagnostic investigations

Plain radiographs

Plain radiographs of the spine help to exclude vertebral fracture, subluxation/luxation, neoplasia, and osteomyelitis/discospondylitis.

Myelography

Myelography helps exclude causes of myelopathy resulting in spinal cord compression, such as intervertebral disc extrusion. In dogs and cats with FCEM, myelography can be normal or may show an intramedullary pattern consistent with focal spinal cord swelling in the acute stage of the disease. An intramedullary myelographic pattern has been reported in 39–47% of dogs with histologically confirmed FCEM [8, 10]; however, this pattern can occur also with other myelopathies, including focal myelitis, intramedullary neoplasia, intraparenchymal hemorrhage, and ANNPE. A narrowed intervertebral disc space (on good-quality radiographs with optimal patient positioning) underlying the area of intramedullary myelographic pattern should prompt the suspicion of ANNPE.

Computed tomography and CT myelography

As with myelography, computed tomography (CT) and particularly CT myelography help rule out other causes of myelopathy, particularly those resulting in spinal cord compression. An intramedullary pattern of spinal cord swelling may be detected in the acute stage of FCEM; however, this pattern can occur also with other types of myelopathies.

MRI

MRI of the affected spinal segments is the diagnostic imaging modality of choice to achieve an antemortem diagnosis of FCEM. In addition to excluding other causes of myelopathy, it allows visualization of signal intensity changes suggestive of spinal cord infarction. The MRI features suggestive of FCEM include a focal, relatively sharply demarcated intramedullary and often lateralized lesion (edematous infarcted tissue), predominantly involving the gray matter that is hyperintense to normal gray matter on T2-weighted fast spin echo (FSE) and FLAIR images and iso- or hypointense to normal gray matter on T1-weighted FSE images (Figure 9.2). Postcontrast T1-weighted FSE images may show mild and heterogeneous enhancement of the affected area, generally on the fifth to seventh day of disease [2, 12, 19, 27]. The lesion is often present in spinal cord segments near an intervertebral disc in which the nucleus pulposus has undergone degenerative changes resulting in a loss of signal intensity on T2W images.

MRI performed 24–72 h after onset of neurologic signs may reveal no intraparenchymal signal intensity changes in dogs with FCEM [12]. Dogs that are ambulatory in the acute stage of the disease are more likely to have a normal MRI than nonambulatory dogs [12]. The extent of the lesion on both sagittal and transverse T2-weighted MR images has been reported to be associated with the severity of clinical signs on presentation and with outcome [12, 28]. The degree and extent of the ischemic injury and the availability of high contrast resolution MRI influence the ability to detect signal intensity changes in the early stage of FCEM [12, 29].

Diffusion-weighted imaging can reveal abnormalities within a few hours of spinal cord ischemia, before the appearance of T2-weighted signal changes, and can help differentiating cytotoxic ischemic edema from the vasogenic edema associated with inflammatory lesions [30].

MRI can help to differentiate between FCEM and ANNPE. The MRI findings suggestive of ANNPE include a focal intramedullary hyperintensity overlying an intervertebral disc, with reduced volume and signal intensity of the nucleus pulposus on T2-weighted FSE images; narrowed intervertebral disc space; and presence of extraneous material or signal change within the epidural space dorsal to the affected disc, with absent or minimal spinal cord compression (Figure 9.3) [26, 31].

CSF analysis

CSF analysis may be normal or may reveal nonspecific abnormalities including xanthochromia, elevated protein concentration, and mild to

(A)   (B)

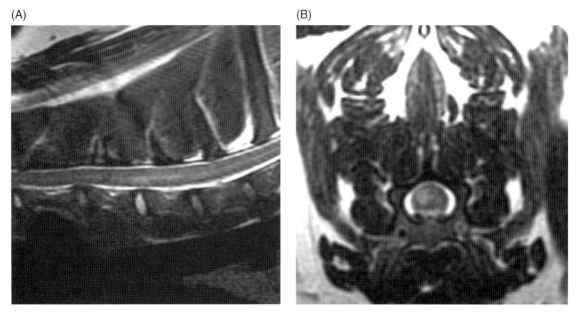

Figure 9.2   Sagittal (A) and transverse (B) T2-weighted FSE MRI of a 5-year-old border collie cross with peracute onset right-sided hemiparesis. Note the intramedullary hyperintensity dorsal to the C6 vertebral body (A) and (B) and C5–C6 intervertebral disc (A), affecting mainly the gray matter on the right side (B). There are no abnormalities within the epidural space (B). The intervertebral discs C4–C4, C6–C7, and C7–T1 show degenerative changes.

(A)   (B)

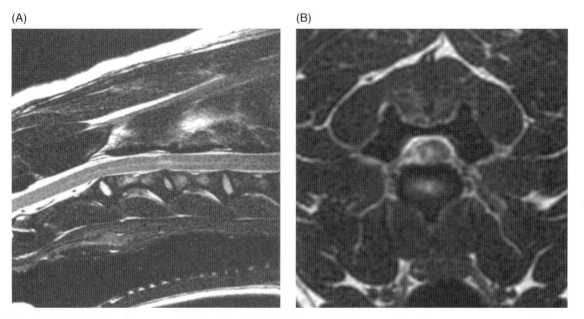

Figure 9.3   Sagittal (A) and transverse (B) T2-weighted MRI of a 9-year-old Wheaten terrier with peracute onset nonambulatory tetraparesis. Note the intramedullary hyperintensity above the C3–C4 intervertebral disc (A) and (B), the reduction in volume and signal intensity of the C3–C4 intervertebral disc nucleus pulposus (A), the narrowed C3–C4 intervertebral disc space (A), and the presence of extraneous material within the epidural space (mainly on the right side) dorsal to the affected disc (B). This MRI appearance is more consistent with ANNPE than FCEM.

(A)

(B)

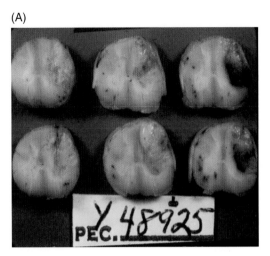 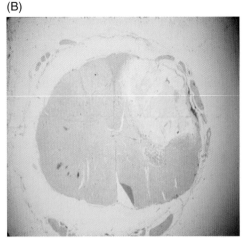

Figure 9.4   Gross (A) and histologic (B) sections of a spinal cord depicting the typical changes seen after fibrocartilagenous embolization and infarction. (Courtesy of Dr. Alexander de Lahunta.)

moderate neutrophilic or mixed pleocytosis. Polymerase chain reaction for different infectious agents on CSF may help to rule out specific causes of meningomyelitis.

Histological examination

The definitive diagnosis of FCEM can be reached only by histological examination of the affected spinal cord segments. This reveals fibrocartilaginous material in spinal arteries or veins within or near an area of focal myelomalacia (Figure 9.4). The margins of the lesion tend to be well delineated from normal tissue. The lesion distribution reflects the territory of the embolized vessels and is therefore often asymmetric. The gray matter is generally more severely affected than the white matter. The lesion is initially ischemic but sometimes may become hemorrhagic.

Treatment

To date, there is no evidence of any beneficial medical treatment for FCEM including methylprednisolone sodium succinate (in dogs and in people), and other types of glucocorticoids or NSAIDs (in dogs) [13, 28, 32]. However, no prospective randomized controlled clinical trial has been performed to investigate the value of these or other types of medical treatment in patients with FCEM.

Nursing care and physiotherapy play an important role in the management of dogs and cats with FCEM, particularly of those that are recumbent, by promoting recovery and help preventing complications. Nursing care and physiotherapy are described in detail in Chapters 27 and 38.

Recently, percutaneous transplantation of human umbilical cord-derived mesenchymal stem cells has been reported in a dog with loss of nociception due to suspected fibrocartilaginous embolic myelopathy [34]. Nociception did not recover at 1 year post mesenchymal stem cell transplantation; however, pelvic limb motor function and voluntary urination were observed since 4 weeks post transplantation [34].

Prognosis

The prognosis of FCEM depends on the severity and the extent of the ischemic injury. These can be estimated clinically based on the distribution and severity of neurological dysfunction and with MRI that shows the longitudinal and transverse extent of the lesion.

Negative clinical prognostic factors include loss of nociception [5, 8, 10], lower motor neuron signs [5, 8], and symmetrical neurological deficits [8, 10]. The severity of neurological signs at the time of initial examination has been reported to be significantly associated with the extent of the intramedullary lesion on MRI and with outcome [28]. The longitudinal extent of the lesion on MRI was defined as the ratio between the length of the intramedullary hyperintensity on midsagittal T2-weighted images and the length of the vertebral body (referred to as lesion length–vertebral length ratio) of C6 (in dogs with cervical lesions) or L2 (in dogs with thoracolumbar lesions). The transverse extent of the lesion was defined as the cross-sectional area of the largest intramedullary hyperintensity on transverse T2-weighted images expressed as a percentage of the cross-sectional area of the spinal cord at the same level (referred to as percent cross-sectional area of the lesion). The lesion length–vertebral length ratio and the percent cross-sectional area of the lesion were both significantly associated with outcome. Dogs with a lesion length–vertebral length ratio greater than 2.0 or a percent cross-sectional area of 67% or greater were significantly more likely to have an unsuccessful outcome than those with lower values [28].

Two studies have suggested that the presence of CSF abnormalities (increased protein concentration ± pleocytosis) may be associated with a poorer outcome in dogs with FCEM [8, 10]. However, another study identified no association between the presence of CSF abnormalities and outcome [28]. Another factor reported to influence prognosis in dogs (particularly large or giant breed dogs) is the owner's commitment to pursue nursing care and physiotherapy [8].

Time intervals between onset of neurological signs and recovery of voluntary motor activity, unassisted ambulation, and maximal recovery have been reported as 6 days (range, 2.5–15 days), 11 days (range, 4–136 days), and 3.75 months (range, 1–12 months), respectively [28]. No statistically significant association has been identified between recovery times and neuroanatomical localization, severity of motor dysfunction, involvement of an intumescence and site or extent of the lesion on MRI.

Recovery rates vary among studies (Table 9.1), ranging from 58.3% to 84% in dogs with FCEM. This variability is most likely due to differences in inclusion criteria, severity and distribution of ischemic lesions, definition of outcome, and owner's commitment.

There is limited information on recovery rate and prognosis in cats with FCEM (Table 9.2). Of the 38 cats reported with FCEM in the literature, 26 had a favorable outcome. The majority of cats with unfavorable outcomes were euthanized within a week after onset of neurologic signs. Time to ambulation for nonambulatory cats has been reported to range from 2 to 27 days after diagnosis [20, 21, 33].

References

1. Cauzinille L. Fibrocartilaginous embolism in dogs. *Vet Clin North Am Small Anim Pract*. 2000 Jan;30(1): 155–67.
2. De Risio L, Platt SR. Fibrocartilaginous embolic myelopathy in small animals. *Vet Clin North Am Small Anim Pract*. 2010 Sep;40(5):859–69.
3. Zaki FA, Prata RG. Necrotizing myelopathy secondary to embolization of herniated intervertebral disk material in the dog. *J Am Vet Med Assoc*. 1976 Jul 15;169(2):222–8.
4. Hayes MA, Creighton SR, Boysen BG, Holfeld N. Acute necrotizing myelopathy from nucleus pulposus embolism in dogs with intervertebral disk degeneration. *J Am Vet Med Assoc*. 1978 Aug 1;173 (3):289–5.
5. Gilmore DR, de Lahunta A. Necrotizing myelopathy secondary to presumed or confirmed fibrocartilaginous embolism in 24 dogs. *J Am Anim Hosp Assoc*. 1986;23:373–6.
6. Junker K, van den Ingh TS, Bossard MM, van Nes JJ. Fibrocartilaginous embolism of the spinal cord (FCE) in juvenile Irish Wolfhounds. *The Veterinary Quarterly*. 2000 Jul;22(3):154–6.
7. de Lahunta A, Glass E. *Veterinary Neuroanatomy and Clinical Neurology*. 3rd ed. St.Louis: Saunders Elsevier; 2009.
8. Cauzinille L, Kornegay JN. Fibrocartilaginous embolism in dogs: review of 36 histologically confirmed cases and retrospective study of 26 suspected cases. *J Vet Intern Med*. 1996 Jul–Aug;10(4):241–5.
9. Hawthorne JC, Wallace LJ, Fenner WR, Waters DJ. Fibrocartilaginous embolic myelopathy in miniature schnauzers. *J Am Anim Hosp Assoc*. 2001 Jul–Aug; 37(4):374–83.
10. Gandini G, Cizinauskas S, Lang J, Fatzer R, Jaggy A. Fibrocartilaginous embolism in 75 dogs: clinical findings and factors influencing the recovery rate. *J Small Anim Pract*. 2003 Feb;44(2):76–80.
11. Grunenfelder FI, Weishaupt D, Green R, Steffen F. Magnetic resonance imaging findings in spinal cord infarction in three small breed dogs. *Vet Radiol Ultrasound*. 2005 Mar–Apr;46(2):91–6.
12. De Risio L, Adams V, Dennis R, McConnell F, Platt S. Magnetic resonance imaging findings and clinical associations in 52 dogs with suspected ischemic myelopathy. *J Vet Intern Med*. 2007 Nov–Dec;21(6): 1290–8.

13. Nakamoto Y, Ozawa T, Katakabe K, Nishiya K, Yasuda N, Mashita T, et al. Fibrocartilaginous embolism of the spinal cord diagnosed by characteristic clinical findings and magnetic resonance imaging in 26 dogs. *J Vet Med Sci.* 2009 Feb;71(2):171–6.

14. Bischel P, Vandevelde M, Lang J. L'infarctus de la moelle epiniere a la suite d'embolies fibrocartilagineuses chez le chien et la chat. *Schweiz Arc Tierheilkd.* 1984;126:387–97.

15. Turner PV, Percy DH, Allyson K. Fibrocartilaginous embolic myelopathy in a cat. *Can Vet J.* 1995 Nov; 36(11):712–3.

16. Coradini M, Johnstone I, Filippich LJ, Armit S. Suspected fibrocartilaginous embolism in a cat. *Aust Vet J.* 2005 Sep;83(9):550–1.

17. Scott HW, O'Leary MT. Fibrocartilaginous embolism in a cat. *J Small Anim Pract.* 1996;37:228–31.

18. Abramson CJ, Platt SR, Stedman NL. Tetraparesis in a cat with fibrocartilaginous emboli. *J Am Anim Hosp Assoc.* 2002 Mar–Apr;38(2):153–6.

19. MacKay AD, Rusbridge C, Sparkes AH, Platt SR. MRI characteristics of suspected acute spinal cord infarction in two cats, and a review of the literature. *J Feline Med Surg.* 2005 Apr;7(2):101–7.

20. Mikszewski JS, Van Winkle TJ, Troxel MT. Fibrocartilaginous embolic myelopathy in five cats. *J Am Anim Hosp Assoc.* 2006 May–Jun;42(3):226–33.

21. Nakamoto Y, Ozawa T, Mashita T, Mitsuda M, Katakabe K, Nakaichi M. Clinical outcomes of suspected ischemic myelopathy in cats. *J Vet Med Sci.* 2010 Dec;72(12):1657–60.

22. Zaki FA, Prata RG, Werner LL. Necrotizing myelopathy in a cat. *J Am Vet Med Assoc.* 1976 Jul 15;169(2): 228–9.

23. Dunié-Mérigot A, Huneault L, Parent J. L'embolie fibrocartilagineuse chez le chien: une étude retrospective. *Can Vet J.* 2007;48:63–8.

24. Caulkins SE, Purinton PT, Oliver JE, Jr. Arterial supply to the spinal cord of dogs and cats. *Am J Vet Res.* 1989 Mar;50(3):425–30.

25. Smith PM, Jeffery ND. Spinal shock—comparative aspects and clinical relevance. *J Vet Intern Med.* 2005; 19:788–93.

26. De Risio L, Adams V, Dennis R, McConnell FJ. Association of clinical and magnetic resonance imaging findings with outcome in dogs with presumptive acute noncompressive nucleus pulposus extrusion: 42 cases (2000-2007). *J Am Vet Med Assoc.* 2009 Feb 15;234(4):495–504.

27. Abramson CJ, Garosi L, Platt SR, Dennis R, McConnell JF. Magnetic resonance imaging appearance of suspected ischemic myelopathy in dogs. *Vet Radiol Ultrasound.* 2005 May–Jun;46(3):225–9.

28. De Risio L, Adams V, Dennis R, McConnell F, Platt SR. Association of clinical and magnetic resonance imaging findings with outcome in dogs suspected to have ischemic myelopathy: 50 cases (2000–2006). *J Am Vet Med Assoc.* 2008;233:129–35.

29. Luo CB, Chang FC, Teng MN, Chen SS, Lirng JF, Chang CY. Magnetic resonance imaging as a guide in the diagnosis and follow-up of spinal cord infarction. *J Chin Med Assoc.* 2003;66:89–95.

30. Manara R, Calderone M, Severino MS, Citton V, Toldo I, Laverda AM, et al. Spinal cord infarction due to fibrocartilaginous embolization: the role of diffusion weighted imaging and short-tau inversion recovery sequences. *J Child Neurol.* 2010; 25:1024–8.

31. Chang Y, Dennis R, Platt S, Penderis J. Magnetic resonance imaging features of traumatic intervertebral disc extrusion in dogs. *Vet Rec.* 2007;160:795–9.

32. Mateen FJ, Monrad PA, Hunderfund AN, Robertson CE, Sorenson EJ. Clinically suspected fibrocartilaginous embolism: clinical characteristics, treatments, and outcomes. *Eur J Neurol.* 2011 Feb;18(2):218–25.

33. Theobald A, Volk HA, Dennis R, De Risio L. Clinical outcome in 19 cats with clinical and magnetic resonance imaging diagnosis of ischaemic myelopathy (2000-2011). *J Feline Med Surg.* 2013 Feb;15(2):132–41.

34. Chung WH, Park SA, Lee JH, Chung DJ, Choi CB, Kim DH, Han H, Kim HY. Percutaneous transplantation of human umbilical cord-derived mesenchymal stem cells in a dog with suspected fibrocartilaginous embolic myelopathy. *J Vet Sci.* 2013;14(4):495–7.

Section III

Clinical Features of Intervertebral Disc Disease and Important Differentials

Veterinarians confronted with patients exhibiting a range of clinical signs must sort through a variety of issues, ranging from differential diagnosis, selection of diagnostic procedures, determining which patients might best be treated via surgery, the urgency of any therapeutic interventions, prognosis, and potential complications or consequences of IVDD. In this section, we address some of the key concepts that can assist veterinarians with their understanding of the pathological events in affected patients, help guide decision making, and improve communications with clients. We also seek to address and possibly dispel some of the mistaken ideas that have long swirled around IVDD, and remind ourselves that not all clinical disc *disease* is necessarily related to disc *herniation*.

10 History, Neurologic Examination, and Neuroanatomic Localization for Spinal Cord and Nerve Root Disease

William B. Thomas and Luisa De Risio

The importance of the history and examination in patients with spinal pain or neurologic deficits cannot be overemphasized. At times, the diagnosis may seem straightforward, for example, when a middle-aged dachshund presents with back pain and paraparesis. But focusing prematurely on a particular diagnosis to the exclusion of other possibilities is the single most common cause of diagnostic error [1]. After all, dachshunds can suffer other causes of spinal pain or neurologic deficits.

With the increasing availability of sophisticated diagnostic techniques such as magnetic resonance imaging (MRI), clinicians may wonder if the neurologic examination has become obsolete [2]. However, recommendations regarding diagnostic tests should be based on the results of the history and examination. Not every dachshund with back pain needs diagnostic imaging. Also, it is important to focus diagnostic testing on the appropriate region as determined by the neurologic examination. Imaging the thoracolumbar region in a patient with a cervical lesion would result in a missed diagnosis. Though uncommon and typically very brief in domestic animals compared to human patients, the occurrence of spinal shock could

mislead the localization if not recognized. Finally, modern imaging techniques have become so sensitive that they often show incidental lesions that are not relevant to the patient's current condition. So, accurate interpretation of diagnostic tests always requires correlation with the history and examination.

Clinicians who do not specialize in neurology are often intimidated by the neurologic examination and may feel all patients with neurologic disease belong to the realm of the specialist. But most practitioners can manage many patients with spinal disease and they should know how to examine the nervous system and interpret the results. The aim of this chapter is to present a practical guide that can be applied to any patient presenting with possible spinal cord disease. This is based on an orderly process of clinical reasoning. First, determine the patient's clinical signs by obtaining a history and performing an examination. Then interpret these signs in the context of anatomy and physiology to localize the disease to a particular region of the nervous system, the neuroanatomic localization. Next, formulate a list of possible etiologic diagnoses considering the

Advances in Intervertebral Disc Disease in Dogs and Cats, First Edition. Edited by James M. Fingeroth and William B. Thomas.
© 2015 ACVS Foundation. Published 2015 by John Wiley & Sons, Inc.

signalment, history, and examination. Based on this list of differential diagnoses, the clinician recommends appropriate laboratory and imaging studies to confirm or exclude the diagnostic possibilities and allow appropriate treatment.

History

The history is the most essential part of the evaluation. An accurate history allows the clinician to formulate an appropriate differential list, if not the actual diagnosis. The history also allows the veterinarian to develop empathy for the client and patient and encourages the client to develop confidence in the veterinarian. Patience, kindness, and a manner that conveys interest and compassion facilitate this process [3].

Signalment

The signalment, including the patient's age, breed, and sex, may provide clues to the diagnosis. For example, chondrodystrophic breeds are at increased risk of intervertebral disc extrusions compared to other breeds, although any breed dog and cat can suffer disc disease [4–6]. Disc herniation is uncommon in patients less than 1 year of age, and the incidence increases with age to a peak of 4–6 years for chondrodystrophic breeds and 6–8 years for other breeds of dog [4–6].

Presenting concern

The presenting concern, also called the chief complaint, is the starting point of the diagnostic process because it allows the clinician to focus the questioning. Ask the client to describe the signs they observed that brought them to the hospital. Open-ended questions are best, such as "What seems to be the problem with Gretchen today?" You should not interrupt. Later, the clinician can augment the client's account with specific questions.

It is important to understand the difference between observations and conclusions. Consider the client's statement, "My dog is in pain." Pain is a purely subjective phenomenon and cannot be directly observed. Rather the client has arrived at this conclusion based on certain observations. So

ask about the specific things the client has noticed that led him or her to conclude that their pet is in pain. Examples might include, "She cries when I pick her up" and "She no longer jumps on the bed." Be aware that clients may not use words in a medically specific manner. For example, a client may say "lameness" when they are really observing paresis. Such ambiguity must be clarified early to avoid wasting time exploring an unlikely diagnosis.

Once the presenting concern is clarified, explore the details. Ask when the problem started and what has changed since the onset. Anything that may have precipitated the signs such as trauma is noted. Realize that clients are prone to assume that some recent event is the cause for the pet's current problem. Avoid the error of concluding that temporal relationships always imply a cause-and-effect relationship. Fairly trivial trauma may be coincidental or even a result of spinal cord disease rather than the cause. For example, the patient fell off the bed because of impending ataxia or paresis, and not "the patient became weak after falling off the bed," as the client might report.

In patients with substantial paraparesis or paraplegia, it is important to ask about voluntary urination. The most reliable historical evidence that the patient is able to urinate voluntarily is the observation that the pet postures and urinates when taken outside. The client may mistake finding urine in bedding or other places as evidence of voluntary urination when this is actually involuntary leakage of urine due to an overly full bladder.

Review any available records from other veterinarians including results of examinations and laboratory studies. If imaging studies have been performed previously, try to obtain copies to evaluate rather than rely on written reports.

After the presenting concern is characterized fully, it helps to summarize this for the client. This reassures the client that the veterinarian has heard and understood their concerns and allows the clinician to determine if there are other concerns that were not mentioned.

Past medical history

Ask if the pet has suffered previous bouts of spinal disease, such as neck pain, back pain, or weakness. If so, find out whether the patient recovered completely so as not to confuse residual deficits with those caused by the current condition. It is important to know about any concurrent or past systemic disease. For example, a history of carcinoma suggests metastatic disease as the cause of any neurologic signs. Considering the zoonotic potential of rabies, always determine the vaccination status before handling any dog or cat with acute neurologic disease. Vaccinations against canine distemper and feline leukemia also influence the likelihood of certain neurologic diseases. Even if other medical issues are not directly related to the current problem, they might affect long-term prognosis or alter the risk of general anesthesia required for imaging studies or surgery.

Review any previous or current treatments. Having the client bring in all medication bottles is helpful as they may not accurately recall drug names or dosages. Always ask specifically about over-the-counter drugs such as aspirin, acetaminophen, or ibuprofen because many clients do not consider these as "medication."

Other body systems are reviewed to identify any other abnormalities. Gastrointestinal signs are of particular importance, so ask if the client has noticed decreased appetite, vomiting, diarrhea, or blood in the feces. Patients with spinal cord disease are at increased risk of these signs due to altered autonomic function affecting the gastrointestinal tract. Additionally, these patients may have been treated with corticosteroids and nonsteroidal anti-inflammatory drugs that have gastrointestinal side effects [7–9].

Physical examination

The physical examination may identify a systemic disease affecting the nervous system. An example would be fever associated with meningitis or discospondylitis. An efficient approach is to incorporate the physical examination with the neurologic examination. For example, examination of the head, eyes, ears, and mouth can be performed while testing cranial nerves. Lymph nodes can be palpated at the same time the head, spine, and limbs are palpated. The skin is examined to identify any dermatitis affecting potential surgery sites when the neck and back are assessed. At the end of a thorough neurologic examination, one has to only auscult the chest, palpate the abdomen, and record temperature, pulse, and respiration to have performed a suitable physical examination.

Neurologic examination

The general components of the neurologic examination are listed in Table 10.1. Every conceivable test is not necessary in every patient. Rather, the history allows the clinician to focus on the examination. A patient with spinal disease does not need an intricate evaluation of cranial nerves and mapping of sensation throughout all dermatomes. Ambulatory animals do not need to be subjected to assessment of deep pain perception. Take care when manipulating patients with potential spinal instability. For example, withhold postural reaction testing in a nonambulatory patient with recent trauma until an unstable spinal fracture or luxation has been ruled out by imaging. Flexing the neck in toy breed dogs that may have atlantoaxial instability can be disastrous. A neurologic examination form is helpful in recording the results and prompting the clinician to not miss key components. An example is provided in Figure 10.1.

More than any other type of examination, the neurologic examination requires patient cooperation. Sedating an unmanageable patient is a good approach for procedures such as joint palpation or chest auscultation. But sedatives and tranquilizers alter the results of much of the neurologic examination. So anything the clinician can do to foster cooperation of the patient is time well spent. Start by observing the patient while obtaining the history. Ambulatory patients are allowed to move freely about the examination room. This allows a chance to assess mental status, behavior, posture, and gait. Also many patients are calmer after they have investigated their surroundings. When it is time for the hands-on portion of the examination, gentle petting is useful and helps establish a pleasant

Table 10.1 Major components of the neurologic examination

Mental status and behavior
Posture
Gait
Postural reactions
Spinal reflexes and muscle tone
Cranial nerves
Palpation
Sensory testing

Observations (Circle all that apply)	
Mental status	Normal Delirious Lethargic Stupor Coma
Behavior	Normal Aggressive Excited Anxious Apathetic
Posture	Normal Head tilt L R Schiff-Sherrington Decerebrate Decerebellate Torticollis Kyphosis Wide-based
Gait	Normal Circling L R Lameness Ataxia: General proprioceptive, Vestibular, Cerebellar Monoparesis Paraparesis Baraplegia Tetraparesis Tetraplegia Hemiharesis L R

Cranial nerves	Left	Right
I. Olfactory		
II, VII. Menace		
II,III, Pupillary light reflexes		
II. Cotton-ball tracking		
III, IV, VI,VIII. Vestibulo-ocular		
III, IV, VI. Strabismus		
V. Facial sensation		
V. Jaw movement		
V, VI. Corneal reflex		
V, VII. Palpebral reflex		
VII. Facial muscles		
VIII. Head tilt		
VIII. Hearing		
VIII. Abnormal nystagmus Fast phase L R Horizontal Vertical Rotary		
IX, X. Swallowing, Gag		
XII. Neck musculature		
XII. Tongue		

Postural reactions		Left	Right
Proprioceptive positioning			
	Thoracic		
	Pelvic		
Hopping			
	Thoracic		
	Pelvic		
Placing			
	Thoracic		
	Pelvic		
Hemiwalking			
	Thoracic		
	Pelvic		

Spinal reflexes		Left	Right
Patellar			
Withdrawal	Thoracic		
	Pelvic		
Crossed extensor	Thoracic		
	Pelvic		
Cutaneous trunci	Normal		
	cut-off		
Perineal			

Palpation
Hyperesthesia:

Sensation		Left	Right
Superficial pain			
	Tail		
	Pelvic limb		
	Thoracic limb		
Deep pain			
	Tail		
	Pelvic limb		
	Thoracic limb		

Neuroanatomic localization	
Brain	Forebrain
	Cerebellum
	Brainstem
Spinal cord	C1-5
	C6-T2
	T3-L3
	L4-S3
Neuromuscular	Nerve
	Neuromuscular junction
	Muscle

Figure 10.1   Neurologic examination form.

tone. Start with procedures least likely to upset the patient and delay disagreeable tests until the end of the examination. Many patients do not like being held down for reflex testing and obviously eliciting spinal pain and testing for pain perception are uncomfortable, so save these for last.

Mental status and behavior

Normal consciousness implies wakefulness and awareness and is assessed by observing for response to the environment. Lethargy is characterized by inattention and decreased spontaneous activity. It can be caused by systemic illness or brain disease. With delirium, the patient is alert but overactive and responds inappropriately. A patient in a stupor is unconscious but can be aroused with stimuli, such as sound or pain. With coma, the patient is unconscious and cannot be aroused even with painful stimuli. Stupor and coma are commonly caused by a brain stem lesion or severe, diffuse disease of the forebrain.

Abnormal behavior is identified by comparing the patient's behavior to expected behavior for animals of a similar breed and age. The client is often able to bring subtle changes in behavior to the veterinarian's attention. Behavioral abnormalities suggest a forebrain lesion.

Posture

The posture should be upright with the head held straight. Animals with neck pain often carry the head lower than normal. In some cases, the thoracolumbar region is arched (kyphosis), mimicking the posture seen with back pain. Patients with thoracolumbar pain often exhibit thoracolumbar kyphosis and rigidity. With caudal lumbar or lumbosacral pain, the patient may stand with the lumbosacral region flexed and the thoracic limbs placed caudally, shifting weight cranially. A wide-based stance is common in patients with ataxia.

Head tilt, where one ear is held lower than the other, usually indicates vestibular dysfunction. Head tilt must be differentiated from head turn or torticollis. A head turn is when the head is held level (one ear is not lower than the other) but the nose is turned right or left. An animal with forebrain lesions may tend to turn the head and circle in one direction. Torticollis is an abnormal curving or twisting of the neck and can occur with developmental vertebral

abnormalities or spinal cord lesions that affect the gray matter or the vestibulospinal tract in the white matter [10].

Animals with severe paresis or paralysis can exhibit several different postures. Patients with mid- to caudal lumbar lesions often sit upright with their pelvic limbs extended cranially, bearing weight on their ischium. With lesions near the thoracolumbar junction, the patient sits up with the pelvic limbs placed caudally. With cranial thoracic lesions, the patient may not be able to sit upright because of paresis of the paraspinal muscles in the thoracic and lumbar region. With tetraparesis caused by a cervical lesion, the patient may be recumbent, on their side, and unable to sit up, and with severe tetraplegia there may be respiratory compromise.

Acute lesions of the thoracic or lumbar segments can result in Schiff–Sherrington posture, characterized by extension of the thoracic limbs and paralysis of the pelvic limbs. There may also be extension of the head and neck (opisthotonus). Despite the increased extensor tone, the thoracic limbs are not paralyzed and exhibit normal voluntary movement. Schiff–Sherrington posture should not be confused with two other causes of increased extensor tone. Decerebrate rigidity produces extension and paresis of all limbs and opisthotonus. This posture is caused by a brain stem lesion and affected patients typically have decreased consciousness. Decerebellate rigidity occurs with acute cerebellar lesions and is characterized by opisthotonus, thoracic limb extension, and flexion or extension of the hips without paresis. In addition, animals with back pain and fear/stress associated with coming to the hospital may exhibit what appears to be extensor rigidity in the thoracic limbs, and this is often over-interpreted as Schiff–Sherrington posture.

Gait

A nonslick surface, such as carpet, grass, or pavement, is used to assess gait. Observe the gait from the side, front, and rear. The patient, if able, should be walked, trotted, turned in circles, and walked up and down a short flight of stairs. Cats may be motivated to move by employing toys they can follow/chase, or by moving their carrier to different locations because cats will often want to hide back inside the carrier. Videotaping the patient and reviewing the tape in slow motion is helpful in characterizing subtle abnormalities.

Each foot should come off the ground crisply with no scraping or dragging, clear the ground evenly, and land smoothly without slapping the ground. Each stride should cover approximately the same distance. Mild abnormalities are often most evident when the patient is turning. Subtle neurologic deficits are often more evident at the walk, while orthopedic disease is usually more apparent when the patient is trotting.

Limb pain can cause a limp when the patient tries to bear weight briefly and gingerly on a painful limb and then quickly and forcefully plants the contralateral limb to relieve the pain. As a result, the stride of the painful limb has a shortened weight-bearing phase. When a single limb is severely painful, it is often carried. This is in contrast to a paretic limb, which dragged. Patients with bilateral limb pain, such as from hip disease or ruptured cruciate ligaments may not walk at all or have short-strided, stilted gaits, which might be confused with neurologic disease. Supporting the patient and evaluating proprioceptive positioning will often resolve this confusion. Likewise, some neurologic disorders cause lameness suggestive of orthopedic disease. For example, attenuation of a nerve root or spinal nerve by intervertebral disc extrusion often results in lameness of the limb innervated by the damaged nerve, called nerve root signature.

The ability to stand and move requires intact motor and proprioceptive systems. Proprioception detects the position or movement of body parts. Receptors sensitive to movement and stretch are located in muscles, tendons, and joints. This information is conveyed by peripheral nerves to the spinal cord, which integrates local reflexes involved in posture and movement. Proprioceptive information also travels through ascending spinal tracts to the brain stem, cerebellum, and forebrain, which integrate coordinated movement. A lesion affecting the proprioceptive pathways causes ataxia.

Ataxia is an inability to perform normal, coordinated motor activity that is not caused by weakness, musculoskeletal abnormality, or abnormal movements, such as tremor. The three types of ataxia are general proprioceptive, cerebellar, and vestibular. Spinal cord lesions cause general proprioceptive ataxia, characterized by a swaying, staggering gait. There is a delay in the onset of the swing phase of gait (protraction). The limb may adduct or abduct during protraction and there may be scuffing or dragging of the foot.

Cerebellar ataxia is caused by cerebellar disease and is characterized by errors in the rate and range of movement, especially hypermetria. Limb movements are abrupt in onset with overflexion of the limbs on protraction. The limbs are placed inappropriately and there is swaying of the trunk and head. Vestibular ataxia is caused by a lesion in the inner ear or brain stem/cerebellum. It is characterized by leaning, falling, or rolling to one side. Other signs of vestibular disease, such as head tilt and abnormal nystagmus, may be evident. With bilateral vestibular dysfunction, the patient maintains a crouched position, is reluctant to move, and exhibits side-to-side head movements.

Normal function of the motor system requires a complex interplay between the brain, descending motor tracts in the brain stem and spinal cord, motor neurons, peripheral nerves, neuromuscular junctions, and muscles. Any lesion in this system can cause paresis, a deficiency in the generation of gait or ability to support weight. Paresis is evident as a decreased rate or range of motion, increased fatigability, or inability to perform certain motor acts. Paralysis is a complete loss of voluntary motor function, while paresis indicates a partial loss of voluntary motor function.

Lesions compromising the motor system affect either the upper motor neuron (UMN) or the lower motor neuron (LMN). This scheme is a physiologic one, not an anatomic one, particularly in the case of the UMN, which is functionally composed of a series of neurons extending from their origin in different regions of the brain to their termination on the LMN in the spinal cord. Disruption of the UMN pathway causes paresis or paralysis, normal or exaggerated spinal cord reflexes, and normal or increased muscle tone (spasticity). With spinal cord disease, UMN paresis is compounded by ataxia. When walking, the combination of a delay in the onset of protraction, overextension of the limb in protraction and spasticity result in an increased stride length and a "floating" gait. This is distinct from the overflexion of the limb seen with cerebellar lesions.

The LMN is the final common pathway to the effector muscle. The LMN consists of the cell body in the ventral gray matter of the spinal cord, the ventral nerve root, and peripheral nerve up to and including the neuromuscular junction. Damage to the LMN anywhere along this pathway causes paresis or paralysis, decreased or absent spinal cord reflexes, decreased muscle tone (hypotonia), and early and severe muscle atrophy (denervation atrophy). With LMN paresis, the decreased ability to support weight causes a shortened stride that can be confused with lameness. The patient may tend to collapse after a few steps, move the pelvic limbs together (bunny hop), and exhibit muscle tremor.

The differentiation between a UMN lesion and an LMN lesion cannot be based on the severity of the weakness alone. The degree of weakness can be as severe with a UMN lesion as with an LMN lesion. Assessment of muscle tone and spinal cord reflexes allows discrimination between the two types of lesion.

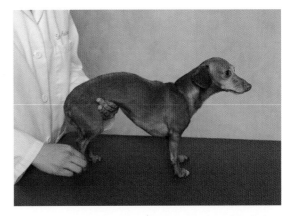

Figure 10.2   Proprioceptive positioning in the pelvic limb.

Postural reactions

Postural reactions assess the same neurologic pathways involved in gait, namely the proprioceptive and motor systems. Their main value is detecting subtle deficits or inconspicuous asymmetry that may not be obvious during the observation of gait. Postural reactions are also useful in discriminating between orthopedic and neurological disorders. Bear in mind that some dogs and cats are not always best evaluated by doing these tests using an examination table, and more accurate assessments may be achieved by doing them on the floor.

Proprioceptive positioning

Proprioceptive positioning is often referred to as conscious proprioception (CP). This is somewhat of a misnomer for two reasons. In animals, it is impossible to know how much of the response is truly conscious. And in addition to proprioception, some degree of motor function is necessary for a normal response. To test proprioceptive positioning, the patient stands on a nonslippery surface. Support the animal to avoid body tilt, which would stimulate a vestibular mediated response. Supporting most of the patient's weight is also helpful in those animals reluctant to bear weight because of a painful limb. The paw is turned over so that the dorsal surface is in contact with the ground (Figures 10.2 and 10.3). The patient should immediately return the paw to a normal position. This maneuver is a sensitive test of general proprioception in the distal limb in animals that still have some motor function. Another test of proprioceptive positioning is to

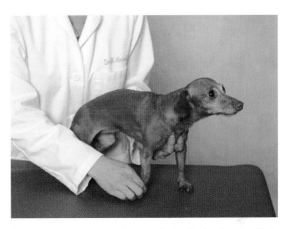

Figure 10.3   Proprioceptive positioning in the thoracic limb.

place a towel or piece of paper under the weight-bearing limb and slowly pull the towel or paper laterally. Healthy animals will return the limb to a normal position. This evaluates proprioception in the proximal region of the limb. When properly supported, most patients with orthopedic disease will have normal proprioceptive positioning.

Hopping

To test hopping in the thoracic limbs, stand over the patient and with one hand under the pelvis and lift the pelvic limbs off the ground. With the other hand, hold up one thoracic limb such that most the patient's weight is supported by the other thoracic limb. Move the animal laterally (Figure 10.4). Normal animals will hop on the limb while keeping the paw under their body for support. To test pelvic

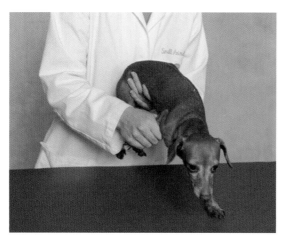

Figure 10.4   Hopping in the thoracic limb.

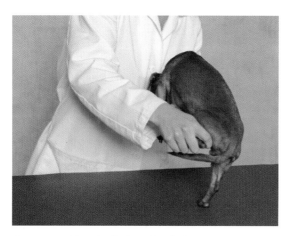

Figure 10.5   Hopping in the pelvic limb.

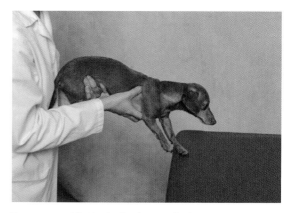

Figure 10.6   Placing in the thoracic limbs.

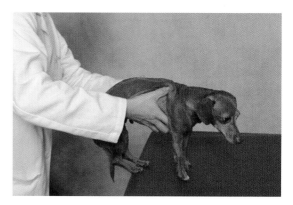

Figure 10.7   Placing in the pelvic limbs.

limbs, place one hand under the sternum, and with the other hand, pick up on pelvic limb and move the patient laterally (Figure 10.5). Each limb is tested individually and responses on the left and right are compared. This is a sensitive test for subtle weakness or asymmetry. Hypermetria is often evident as an exaggerated limb movement. Many normal animals cannot hop when moved medially so only try to hop the patient laterally.

Placing response

This test is most practical for smaller animals that can be held. Pick the animal up and move it toward the edge of a table (Figure 10.6). The normal response is to place the paws of the thoracic limbs on the surface as the table is approached. Continue moving

the patient forward to assess placing of the pelvic limbs (Figure 10.7). The left and right sides are compared to detect any unilateral or asymmetric deficits. Some smaller pets accustomed to being held may not respond normally. This can usually be overcome by holding the animal away from the examiner's body. The resulting insecurity will often convince the animal to make an effort to stand on the table. The placing response can be checked both with visual cues and also with just tactile cues (the latter done by covering the animal's eyes while the limbs are brought into contact with the table edge). Checking tactile placing is helpful in distinguishing neurologic and orthopedic causes for limb dysfunction.

Hemiwalking and wheelbarrowing

These tests are performed if other postural reactions are equivocal or in large dogs when eliciting the hopping response is physically difficult for the examiner. For hemiwalking, the clinician holds up the limbs on one side of the body and moves the patient laterally. The normal reaction is as described for the hopping response. Wheelbarrowing in the thoracic limbs is done by supporting the patient under the abdomen so that the pelvic limbs do not touch the ground and moving the patient forward. Normal animals will walk with symmetrical, alternate movements of the thoracic limbs. The pelvic limbs can be tested similarly by supporting the patient under the thorax.

Muscle tone

Muscle tone is the velocity-dependent resistance of muscle to passive stretch and is maintained by intrinsic muscle stiffness and the muscle stretch reflex mediated by the LMN. LMN lesions cause loss of normal muscle tone resulting in decreased resistance to passive movement called hypotonia.

Descending UMN pathways normally attenuate the muscle stretch reflex. Lesions of the UMN pathway cause changes in the excitability of motor neurons, interneuronal connections, and local reflex pathways that over time lead to hyperexcitable muscle stretch reflexes and increased muscle tone, called spasticity. The interval between injury and the appearance of spasticity varies from days to months. Once spasticity develops, the chronic shortening of muscle results in enhancement of the intrinsic muscle stiffness and changes in collagen tissue and tendons that lead to subclinical contractures and exacerbation of spasticity. Increased muscle tone predominates in the antigravity (extensor) muscles and results in a spastic gait characterized by decreased limb flexion. At rest, there is increased resistance to passive flexion of the limb.

Muscle tone is assessed with the patient in lateral recumbency. The limb muscles are flexed and extended throughout the normal range of motion, feeling for resistance to flexion and extension.

Spinal cord reflexes

Spinal cord reflexes assess the integrity of the sensory and motor components of the reflex arc and the influence of descending UMN pathways.

Muscle stretch reflexes

Muscle stretch reflexes, also called myotatic or deep tendon reflexes, are best elicited by using a rubber-tipped reflex hammer with a weighted head so that a brisk, accurately placed stimulus is applied. Use of other instruments, such as scissors, is not recommended because these do not provide a consistent stimulus and appear less professional to the client. A relaxed patient is important. This can be difficult when patients are fearful or in pain. Having an assistant distract the patient by gentle petting and soothing talk is often helpful. Assessing muscle tone first, by passively moving the limb, also helps relax the patient. Also, by first checking muscle tone and joint mobility, one can determine if there are musculoskeletal alterations that might influence the excursion seen when reflexes are subsequently tested. For an optimal response, the muscle must be passively maintained in a state of appropriate tension with plenty of room for contraction. A position midway between flexion and extension is best.

The most reliable muscle stretch reflex is the patellar reflex. With the patient in lateral recumbency place one hand under the thigh to support the limb with the stifle in a partially flexed position. With the other hand, briskly strike the patellar tendon with a reflex hammer (Figure 10.8). The normal response is a single, quick extension of the stifle. Results can be graded as 0 for absent, 1 for present but reduced, 2 for normal, 3 for exaggerated, and 4 for exaggerated with clonus. Clonus is repetitive flexion and extension of the joint in response to a single stimulus.

A weak or absent patellar reflex indicates a lesion of the femoral nerve or the L4–L6 spinal

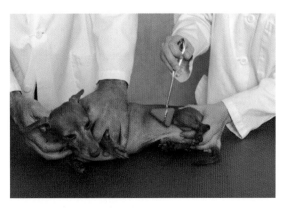

Figure 10.8   Patellar reflex.

segments. A lesion in the UMN system cranial to L4 will result in a normal or exaggerated reflex. Exaggerated reflexes are more common with chronic than with acute UMN lesions. It is important to realize that any UMN lesion severe enough to cause an exaggerated reflex will almost always cause some degree of weakness. An exaggerated reflex in the face of normal gait and postural reactions is usually due to examiner error or a tense, excited patient.

There are several other potential causes of abnormal patellar reflexes. Severe rigidity or muscle contraction that limits joint movement, such as fibrosis of a joint or muscle can physically limit the response. Structural abnormalities of the joint, such as cranial cruciate rupture, can also cause a diminished response. In these patients, other signs of LMN weakness are absent. In dogs 10 years of age or older, one or both patellar reflexes may be absent with no other signs of neurologic disease [11].

Normal animals that are anxious or unable to relax may have increased or decreased patellar reflexes. In some cases, the down limb is more relaxed and testing that limb is more reliable. Another technique for anxious patients that are small enough is for the examiner to sit down and hold the patient in dorsal recumbency between the examiner's thighs to test the reflex. Never diagnose a UMN or an LMN lesion based on reflexes alone when the gait and postural reactions are normal.

A state of "spinal shock" can occur immediately after severe spinal cord injury. This is characterized by paralysis, areflexia, hypotonia, and loss of sensation caudal to the level of injury. In dogs and cats, reflexes usually return within a few hours. But the hypotonia can persist for a few weeks, eventually giving way to normal tone and then increased tone.

A lesion of the L6–S1 spinal segments or sciatic nerve can cause an exaggerated patellar reflex. This is due to decreased tone in the muscles that flex the stifle and normally dampen stifle extension when the patellar reflex is elicited. Such lesions also cause other abnormalities, such as a decreased withdrawal reflex.

Other muscle stretch reflexes have been described and include the gastrocnemius, cranial tibial, extensor carpi, biceps brachii, and triceps reflexes. In our experience, these reflexes are unreliable in many dogs and cats and serve little useful purpose.

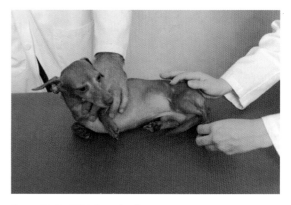

Figure 10.9   Withdrawal reflex.

Withdrawal (flexor) reflex

To test the withdrawal reflex in the pelvic limb, the patient is maintained in lateral recumbency with the uppermost pelvic limb extended. Gently pinch a toe with the fingers. The normal response is flexion of the hip, stifle, and hock (Figure 10.9). When motor function is not completely lost, the response is often attenuated by voluntary movement such that withdrawal of the limb is a combination of spinal mediated reflex and voluntary movement. Similarly, patients may voluntarily inhibit withdrawal of their limb making it necessary to use a strong stimulus to elicit flexion. Therefore, the withdrawal reflex should always be interpreted in the context of other neurologic findings [10]. As with the patellar reflex, the presence of confounding musculoskeletal lesions that limit joint movement should be assessed prior to reflex testing.

Medial and lateral digits should be tested. When testing the third through fifth digit, a weak or absent reflex suggests an LMN lesion involving the sciatic nerve or L7–S1 spinal segments. With mild lesions, there is often weak flexion of the hock with preservation of stifle and hip flexion, so flexion of all three joints should be noticed. Sensation from the medial aspect of the foot, including the second digit, is conveyed by the medial saphenous nerve, a branch of the femoral nerve originating in the L4–L6 spinal segments.

When testing the withdrawal reflex, the contralateral limb is observed for extension. Extension of the opposite limb, called a crossed extensor reflex, is abnormal and indicates a UMN lesion cranial to L4. With severe UMN lesions, after the initial state of injury, a mass reflex may develop. In these patients, pinching a toe or the tail may elicit alternating flexion and extension of the pelvic limbs similar to running movements, wagging of the tail, urination, and defecation.

The withdrawal reflex in the thoracic limb is tested in a similar manner. A weak or absent reflex suggests a lesion of the C6–T1 spinal segments or related nerves (axillary, musculocutaneous, median, and ulnar nerves). However, a dog with a focal C1– C5 lesion will often have a weak withdrawal reflex in the thoracic limb, so this finding alone is not accurate enough to allow precise neuroanatomic localization [12].

Because the withdrawal reflex is mediated at the level of the spinal cord, a positive withdrawal reflex does not establish that the patient is aware of the stimulus. It is critical for the veterinarian to understand the difference between reflex flexion of the limb and conscious perception of the stimulus. The conscious perception of pain is also evaluated at the same time as the withdrawal reflex; this is discussed in the section on sensory testing.

Perineal reflex

The perineal reflex is elicited by lightly touching or stroking the perineum with the end of a closed hemostat. The left and right sides are tested. Normal response is contraction of the anal sphincter and flexion of the tail. A weak or absent reflex indicates a lesion affecting the S1–S3 spinal segments, nerve roots, spinal nerves, or pudendal nerve.

Cutaneous trunci reflex

This reflex is commonly and erroneously referred to as the panniculus reflex, but the term panniculus refers to a subcutaneous layer of fat, which is not involved in this reflex. To elicit the cutaneous trunci reflex, use a hemostat to gently squeeze the skin 1–2cm lateral to the spine (Figure 10.10). The opposite side is tested similarly. Start over the lumbosacral region and proceed cranially, one vertebral level at a time. The normal response is a bilateral contraction of the cutaneous trunci muscle, resulting in a twitch of the skin over the thorax and abdomen. This reflex is present in the thoracic and lumbar region caudally to the level of L5 or L6 in most dogs [13]. The LMN for this reflex is via the lateral thoracic nerve, originating in the C8–T2 segments and

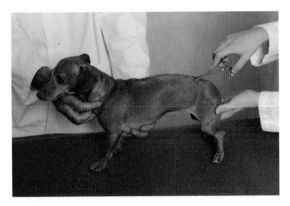

Figure 10.10 Cutaneous trunci reflex.

coursing through the brachial plexus. A lesion affecting the thoracolumbar region of the spinal cord may cause a loss of this reflex when the skin caudal to the level of the lesion is stimulated; pinching the skin cranial to the lesion results in a normal response. Loss of the reflex correlates with the severity of the lesion and usually occurs before ambulation is lost. When there is a clear cutoff of the reflex, the spinal cord lesion is usually 2–3 vertebra cranial to the cutoff. Asymmetric lesions can result in an ipsilateral loss of the reflex caudal to the lesion [14].

A lesion affecting the brachial plexus may cause a loss of the ipsilateral cutaneous trunci reflex with a normal response on the other side, regardless of the level at which the skin is stimulated.

Cranial nerve examination

The cranial nerves are evaluated as described in Table 10.2. Spinal cord lesions will not affect cranial nerves, so deficits in cranial nerve function indicate a multifocal lesion or a separate process. However, severe lesions of the cervical or T1–T3 spinal segments can interfere with sympathetic innervation to the face, which is technically not a cranial nerve. This is seen as a Horner's syndrome, characterized by ipsilateral drooping of the upper eyelid (ptosis), sunken globe (enophthalmos), small pupil (miosis), and elevation of the third eyelid.

Palpation

Light palpation helps detect swelling, atrophy, or changes in surface temperature. Atrophy is

Table 10.2 Important cranial nerve tests

Test	Elicited by	Response	Afferent (sensory) nerve	Efferent (motor) nerve
Menace	Menacing gesture	Blink	II (optic)	VII (facial)
Pupillary light	Shining light in eye	Pupillary constriction	II (optic)	III (oculomotor)
Vestibulo-ocular	Moving head	Physiologic nystagmus	VIII (vestibular branch)	III, IV, VI (oculomotor, trochlear, abducens)
Palpebral	Touching medial canthus	Blink	V (trigeminal)	VII (facial)
Hearing	Unexpected noise	Head and ears orient toward sound	VIII (cochlear branch)	NA
Gag	Touch pharynx	Contraction of pharynx	IX, X (glossopharyngeal, vagus)	IX, X (glossopharyngeal, vagus)

characterized by loss of muscle bulk, most apparent when the muscle is compared to its contralateral counterpart. Deep palpation and manipulation detect painful regions. If crying, whimpering, or muscle tensing occur on palpation, more vigorous maneuvers, such as manipulation, are unnecessary and may be dangerous in patients with unstable fractures or luxations. Also, palpation is usually more specific, because manipulation of one region often produces movement in other areas.

Palpate the spine to detect any curvature, displacement, masses, swelling, paraspinal muscle atrophy, or pain. In patients with a presenting concern suggesting a thoracolumbar lesion, start with palpating the neck and save palpating a potentially painful region until last. In patients with cervical lesions, start caudally. The tail is palpated, extended, and flexed. Downward pressure on the sacrum often elicits pain in animals with lumbosacral lesions. When palpating the thoracolumbar spine, lightly place one hand on the abdomen to detect tensing of the abdominal muscles as the affected area is palpated. The spinous processes, articular processes, and transverse processes or ribs are palpated separately (Figure 10.11). If palpation is not painful, the spine can be gently manipulated by applying ventral and lateral pressure to extend and flex the spine, respectively. To extend the lumbosacral joint, place one hand under the pelvis while the animal is standing. Raise the pelvis and press downward on the seventh lumbar vertebra with the other hand.

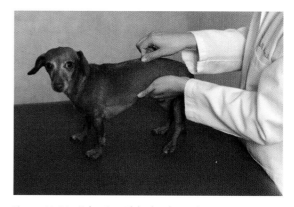

Figure 10.11 Palpation of the lumbar spine.

Cervical pain is often manifested by tensing of the cervical muscles and twitching of the ears during palpation or manipulation (Figure 10.12). If palpation does not induce pain, gently extend and flex the head with one hand while placing the other hand on the cervical muscles to detect muscle tensing. Caudal neck pain can often be detected by gently rocking the large transverse processes of the sixth cervical vertebra.

Focal spinal pain is localizing, and in many patients with disc herniation and spinal pain, it may be the only abnormality on examination. The presence or absence of spinal pain is also helpful in determining etiology. Neck or back pain results from bone, disc, spinal nerve/root, vertebral diarthrodial joint, or meningeal involvement and possibly from muscle pain/spasm. On the other

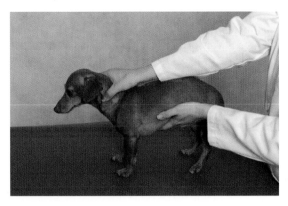

Figure 10.12   Palpation of the cervical spine.

hand, lesions affecting only the spinal cord parenchyma are usually not painful. Examples of the latter include fibrocartilaginous embolism and degenerative myelopathy.

Limbs

Limbs are initially palpated with the patient standing, if possible. Contralateral limbs are compared for symmetry. The limbs are more closely examined with the animal in lateral recumbency, when the spinal reflexes are tested. A thorough orthopedic examination is important in patients presenting for gait abnormalities, and where the neurologic examination does not disclose deficits that can be ascribed to central nervous system or peripheral nerve disease. The most common example is acute bilateral cranial cruciate ligament rupture, which can be mistaken for spinal cord disease because the patient is often unwilling to use the pelvic limbs, or has difficulty maintaining the knees in extension.

Sensory evaluation

Cutaneous sensation includes touch, pain, heat, cold, and vibratory senses. Of these, only pain is routinely tested in animals. Pain is defined as an unpleasant sensory and emotional experience associated with actual or potential tissue damage. It is a conscious experience that involves the sensory, emotional, and cognitive functions of the brain. Since pain is subjective and only appreciated by the patient, what we test in animals may be more accurately referred to as nociception.

This is the process by which information about a noxious stimulus is conveyed to the brain [15].

Superficial pain originates in receptors in the skin and travels to the brain primarily by the ipsilateral spinocervicothalamic tract in the spinal cord. Deep pain originates in receptors in deeper structures, such as bone. Deep pain is conveyed primarily by the spinoreticular pathway. The axons transmitting deep pain sensation are small, unmyelinated fibers located diffusely in the lateral and ventral funiculi of the spinal cord with frequent decussations. This pathway is the least susceptible to damage from compression, which explains the clinical observation that deep pain perception is the last function to be lost in spinal cord injury (see Chapter 11) [16].

The purpose of testing pain perception is to detect and map out any areas of sensory loss. This aids anatomic localization and determination of prognosis. Altered states of consciousness and certain drugs, such as analgesics and sedatives, may alter results and have to be considered when testing sensation.

Superficial pain

Specific cutaneous areas are chosen for testing based on anatomy of the cutaneous nerves (Table 10.3). A two-step pinch technique is used for stimulation [17]. With a hemostat, lift and grasp a small fold of skin at the test site. When the patient is quiet, lightly and briefly pinch the skin until a response is elicited. This two-step technique avoids stimulation of adjacent areas and ensures that only the skin at the test site is stimulated. Two types of response may be seen: (i) a reflex flexion of the limb or skin twitch indicating the sensory neurons and spinal segments are intact and (ii) a behavioral response, such as crying or biting, which indicates that the ascending pain pathways in the spinal cord and brain stem to the forebrain are intact.

Deep pain sensation

Testing deep pain perception is necessary only if superficial pain is absent. When there is no response to pinching with the fingers, use a hemostat to compress the digits or tail. The degree of compression is gradually increased until a response is elicited. Withdrawal of the limb indicates only an intact

Table 10.3 Cutaneous test sites for nerves of the thoracic and pelvic limbs [17]

Nerve	Site
Axillary	Lateral surface of the brachium, slightly caudal to the shoulder joint
Radial	Dorsal surface of third or fourth digit
Musculocutaneous	Medial surface of the antebrachium, slightly distal to the medial condyle of the humerus
Ulnar, dorsal branch	Lateral surface of the fifth digit
Saphenous (branch of femoral)	Medial surface of the pelvic limb, 4 cm distal to the medial epicondyle of the femur
Peroneal	Dorsal surface of the third digit
Tibial	Ventral surface of foot, at the proximal border of the metatarsal pad
Perineal	Males: lateral surface of the scrotum Females: slightly cranial to the vulva and lateral to ventral midline

reflex arc. A behavioral response such as turning the head or vocalization indicates conscious perception. In patients with severe spinal cord injuries, the presence or absence of deep pain perception is important in assessing prognosis for recovery, so it is critical not to confuse reflex withdrawal with conscious perception (see Chapters 11 and 19).

Neuroanatomic localization

Based on the history and examination, the veterinarian decides if the patient suffers from a neurologic disease and, if so, localizes the lesion within the nervous system. This can rarely be done on the basis of a single finding. Rather, accurate anatomic diagnosis requires consideration of all findings, including normal as well as abnormal results. Neurologic deficits depend primarily on the location of the lesion rather than the cause of the lesion.

Regardless of the specific disease affecting the spinal cord, loss of neurologic function occurs in a predictable sequence. Ataxia is the first to appear, because the general proprioceptive fibers are the most sensitive to compression due to their large diameter and heavy reliance on myelin for saltatory conduction. As the disease progresses, motor fibers (smaller diameter and less myelinated) are affected, causing paresis then paralysis. Superficial pain perception is lost next and finally deep pain perception. Certain combinations of neurological deficits are recognized as characteristic of lesions in certain locations, and knowledge of these combinations aids in proper localization.

C1–C5

Dogs with cervical disc herniation often present with signs of cervical pain without neurologic deficits. This is typically manifested as a low head carriage, neck rigidity and spasms of the cervical muscles. When looking up, they move their eyes only, not their head. Signs of neck pain from cervical disc herniation can wax and wane to a remarkable degree. The patient may behave normally throughout most of the day only to suffer bouts of screaming and muscle spasms that at times can be misinterpreted as seizures.

Unilateral or bilateral lameness caused by nerve root attenuation (nerve root signature) has been reported in 15–50% of cases of intervertebral disc herniation. This is more common with caudal cervical lesions but may on occasion be observed with disc extrusion at C4–C5 or C5–C6, since nerve roots from these levels contribute to nerves of the brachial plexus.

Neurologic deficits due to lesions of the C1–C5 spinal segments can range from mild ataxia to paresis or even paralysis of all limbs. Ambulatory patients have swaying and scuffing of all limbs with a normal to increased stride length. In some cases the pelvic limb deficits are more obvious than those in the thoracic limbs. Much less common is weakness of the thoracic limbs with relatively normal pelvic limbs, referred to as a central cord syndrome. This occurs with selective damage to the more medial pathways in the spinal cord that are involved with thoracic limb function. Asymmetric lesions can result in ipsilateral hemiparesis or hemiplegia. Mentation and cranial nerves are normal, although an ipsilateral Horner's syndrome is possible. Spinal reflexes are normal or exaggerated in all limbs, although weak withdrawal reflexes in the pelvic limbs are occasionally observed. Severe lesions can cause respiratory paresis, manifested as abdominal breathing with weak to absent intercostal movement and preserved diaphragm function. In some cases this results in paradoxical chest movement where the chest wall moves inward on inspiration, instead of outward. Compromise of breathing muscles may be subtle, and might be discerned via a history from the client of dysphonia (voice change and weak bark). More severe injury can cause paralysis of the diaphragm as well, resulting in fatal apnea.

C6–T2

Lesions affecting the C6–T2 spinal segments can cause neck pain similar to more cranial cervical lesions. Lesions affecting a nerve root or spinal nerve often cause thoracic limb lameness (nerve root signature). Neurologic deficits include ataxia, tetraparesis, tetraplegia, and ipsilateral hemiparesis/hemiplegia. Ambulatory patients often have a characteristic gait, with short strides in the thoracic limb (LMN paresis) and normal or increased strides in the pelvic limbs (UMN paresis). This has been described elsewhere as a "two-engine gait" [18]. Mental status and cranial nerves are normal, although ipsilateral or bilateral Horner's syndrome is possible in severe cases. Spinal reflexes are normal to exaggerated in the pelvic limbs. Thoracic limbs reflexes may be weak to absent with hypotonia and rapid muscle atrophy. However, the withdrawal reflex is not reliable in differentiating between a C1–C5 and a C6–T2 lesion, and the myotatic reflexes in the thoracic limbs are more generally unreliable as noted previously.

T3–L3

Lesions compromising the T3–L3 spinal segments may cause focal spinal pain and varying degrees of weakness in the pelvic limbs with normal thoracic limbs. Reflexes in the pelvic limbs are normal or exaggerated. Voluntary urination and defecation are usually lost around the time the patient becomes nonambulatory. Acute, severe lesions affecting this region may cause Schiff–Sherrington posture or spinal shock as described earlier. The cutaneous trunci reflex may be absent caudal to the lesion and in severe cases, conscious perception of deep pain is absent caudal to the lesion.

L4–S3

Lesions affecting the L4–S3 spinal segments cause LMN weakness in the pelvic limbs. The patellar, withdrawal, and perineal reflexes may be weak or absent with hypotonia. With lesions of one or more week's duration, there may be atrophy of the muscles of the pelvic limbs. If the lesion is caudal enough to affect the sacral segments but spare the L4–L6 spinal segments, patients may develop LMN urinary and fecal incontinence when they are still ambulatory. Severe lesions will cause a loss of deep pain perception in the pelvic limbs and tail.

Brain

The presence of abnormal behavior, altered mental status, seizures, or cranial nerve deficits indicates a brain lesion. Such lesions can also cause gait deficits ranging from mild ataxia to tetraplegia, so it is important to recognize deficits that indicate brain involvement instead of or in addition to a spinal lesion.

Peripheral nerve

Most peripheral nerve lesions cause motor and sensory deficits. There is weakness with decreased postural reactions, decreased muscle tone, and weak or absent spinal reflexes. Cranial nerves may be affected as well as spinal nerves. Superficial and deep pain sensation may be absent. Polyneuropathies usually cause deficits in all limbs, although the pelvic limbs may be affected first. With mononeuropathies, deficits are restricted to regions innervated by the affected nerve.

Neuromuscular junction

Lesions of the neuromuscular junction cause weakness without ataxia or loss of proprioception. Most junctionopathies, such as tick paralysis, cause persistent weakness in all limbs with weak to absent spinal reflexes and hypotonia. Myasthenia gravis is often characterized by exercise-induced weakness that improves or resolves with rest. However, the weakness can affect only the pelvic limbs and does not always worsen with exercise, features that can be confused with spinal cord disease [19].

Muscle

Muscle disorders are often characterized by weakness, fatigability, and stiff, stilted gait. A postural tremor is possible. Palpation may reveal muscle atrophy or pain. A few myopathies cause enlargement of affected muscles due to hypertrophy, swelling, or infiltration with fat or other tissue. Proprioception and other sensations are preserved. Spinal reflexes are usually normal but may be weak.

Conclusions

If one adheres to the clinical process outlined here, it is usually possible to define the location of a neurologic lesion. Based on this anatomic diagnosis in conjunction with careful consideration of the history the veterinarian should be able to identify several potential causes of the illness and recommend appropriate diagnostic tests. An accurate diagnosis enables the veterinarian to recommend the proper treatment and is helpful in predicting prognosis. Most important, and as stressed elsewhere throughout this text, it is inappropriate to assume that signs of spinal cord disease are in fact always due to spinal cord disease (hence the caveats in this chapter and the need for a detailed history and examination before jumping to conclusions) and, where spinal cord disease has been established, to simply lump all patients with these signs as "IVDD," without due consideration of other potential etiologies or without regard to distinguishing IVDD from actual herniation (see Chapters 4, 20, 21, and 22).

References

1. Graber ML, Franklin N, Gordon R. Diagnostic error in internal medicine. *Arch Intern Med* 2005;165:1493–1499.
2. Ziegler DK. Is the neurologic examination becoming obsolete? *Neurology* 1985;35:559.
3. Campbell WW. The neurologic history. In: *DeJong's The Neurologic Examination*. 6th ed. Philadelphia: Lippincott Williams and Wilkins, 2005;19–31.
4. Goggin JE, Li AS, Franti CE. Canine intervertebral disk disease: characterization by age, sex, breed, and anatomic site of involvement. *Am J Vet Res* 1970;31: 1687–1692.
5. Priester WA. Canine intervertebral disk disease—occurrence by age, breed, and sex among 8,117 cases. *Theriogenology* 1976;6:293–303.
6. Bergknut N, Egenvall A, Hagman R, *et al*. Incidence of intervertebral disk degeneration-related diseases and associated mortality rates in dogs. *J Am Vet Med Assoc* 2012;240:1300–1309.
7. Levine JM, Levine GJ, Boozer L, *et al*. Adverse effects and outcome associated with dexamethasone administration in dogs with acute thoracolumbar intervertebral disk herniation: 161 cases (2000-2006). *J Am Vet Med Assoc* 2008;232:411–417.
8. Toombs JP, Caywood DD, Lipowitz AJ, *et al*. Colonic perforation following neurosurgical procedures and corticosteroid therapy in four dogs. *J Am Vet Med Assoc* 1980;177:68–72.
9. KuKanich B, Bidgood T, Knesl O. Clinical pharmacology of nonsteroidal anti-inflammatory drugs in dogs. *Vet Anaesth Analg* 2012;39:69–90.
10. Parent J. Clinical approach and lesion localization in patients with spinal diseases. *Vet Clin North Am Small Anim Pract* 2010;40:733–753.
11. Levine JM, Hillman RB, Erb HN, *et al*. The influence of age on patellar reflex response in the dog. *J Vet Intern Med* 2002;16:244–246.
12. Forterre F, Konar M, Tomek A, *et al*. Accuracy of the withdrawal reflex for localization of the site of cervical disk herniation in dogs: 35 cases (2004–2007). *J Am Vet Med Assoc* 2008;232:559–563.
13. Muguet-Chanoit AC, Olby NJ, Babb KM, *et al*. The sensory field and repeatability of the cutaneous trunci muscle reflex of the dog. *Vet Surg* 2011;40: 781–785.
14. Gutierrez-Quintana R, Edgar J, Wessmann A, Cherubini GB, Penderis J. The cutaneous trunci reflex for localising and grading thoracolumbar spinal cord injuries in dogs. *J Small Anim Pract* 2012;53:470–475.
15. Lamont LA, Tranquilli WJ, Grimm KA. Physiology of pain. *Vet Clin North Am Small Anim Pract* 2000;30: 703–728, v.
16. Hellyer PW, Robertson SA, Fails AD. Pain and its management. In: Tranquilli WJ, Thurman JC, Grimm KA, eds. *Lumb & Jones' Veterinary Anesthesia and Analgesia*. 4th ed. Ames, IA: Blackwell, 2007; 31–57.
17. Bailey CS, Kitchell RL. Cutaneous sensory testing in the dog. *J Vet Intern Med* 1987;1:128–135.
18. de Lahunta A, Glass E. *Veterinary Neuroanatomy and Clinical Neurology*. 3rd ed. St. Louis, MO: Saunders Elsevier, 2009.
19. Dewey CW, Bailey CS, Shelton GD, *et al*. Clinical forms of acquired myasthenia gravis in dogs: 25 cases (1988–1995). *J Vet Intern Med* 1997;11: 50–57.

11 Deep Pain: How Should We Test and Interpret Nociception?

James M. Fingeroth, William B. Thomas, and Luisa De Risio

One of the goals when examining patients with clinical signs due to intervertebral disc herniation (IVDH) is to suggest a prognosis to the client and also to determine the acuteness of any emergency situation. Unfortunately, in the absence of an imaging study that irrefutably demonstrates a nonreversible transverse myelopathy, we base such prognostic and treatment determinations mostly on the neurologic examination and history. As discussed elsewhere in this text, there are some imaging findings and cerebrospinal fluid markers that can be helpful in suggesting the prognosis, but these are usually unavailable to primary care clinicians. Moreover, as shown by Olby *et al.*, functional recovery is yet possible in some patients despite loss of up to 90% of ascending and descending axons in the affected spinal cord segment [1].

As discussed elsewhere in this text, spinal cord contusion and compression have their earliest and most deleterious effects on the myelin sheathing that surrounds neurons subserving ascending proprioceptive and descending motor pathways (see Chapter 15). Compromise of proprioception and/or voluntary motor function can therefore occur even though the axons themselves remain intact. Assessing these functions alone cannot determine the degree or reversibility of any underlying spinal cord injury, since we cannot easily distinguish between loss of saltatory conduction (myelin loss) and actual axonal transection. In contrast, those axons that subserve the conduction of deep pain are typically small diameter with minimal to no myelin sheathing. Consequently, the absence of deep pain caudal to the level of the spinal cord lesion suggests a more severe spinal cord injury, and possibly one that is irreversible.

In dogs with thoracolumbar disc extrusions, deep pain perception is the most important prognostic factor for neurologic recovery. For example, in one study, 92% of patients with intact deep pain perception regained the ability to walk after surgery, whereas only 69% of patients with absent or questionable deep pain perception became ambulatory postoperatively [2]. This study demonstrated a 1.7 times better chance for return to ambulation in dogs with preserved deep pain perception than in those dogs without deep pain perception. Therefore the accurate testing of deep pain perception is critical. However, the assessment of deep pain perception is subjective

Advances in Intervertebral Disc Disease in Dogs and Cats, First Edition. Edited by James M. Fingeroth and William B. Thomas.

and requires the clinician understand the functional neuroanatomy and clinical techniques involved. Determining deep pain status is generally only germane to dogs with thoracic, thoracolumbar, or lumbar spinal cord lesions. Dogs with cervical spinal cord lesions and loss of nociception will usually suffer respiratory paralysis, and therefore die unless intubated and mechanically ventilated. The respiratory paralysis will provide much better prognostic information than determining if the animal retains sensation caudal to the lesion.

Pain versus nociception

The International Association for the Study of Pain (IASP) defines pain as an unpleasant sensory and emotional experience that is associated with actual or potential tissue damage or described in such terms [3]. Because sensory experiences and emotions are always subjective, pain can never be measured directly, even in human patients. Instead, the person's communication of his or her own pain is used as a proxy measure. Therefore, assessing pain in veterinary patients that cannot express their subjective experiences is especially challenging [4].

The IASP defines nociception as the neural process of encoding noxious stimuli [3]. The term nociception was introduced over 100 years ago by Sherrington to distinguish between detection of a noxious stimulus and the psychological and emotional response to it. This was based on studies of laboratory cats in which the cerebral hemispheres and portions of the thalamus were ablated. In these decerebrate animals, pinching a foot elicited responses including turning the head toward the stimulus, dilation of the pupils, and crying or snarling [5]. De Lahunta reports similar findings in a newborn calf with congenital aplasia of the cerebrum and thalamus. Noxious stimuli applied to the hoof elicited signs of discomfort including turning the head toward the stimulus [6]. Certain regions of the forebrain are thought to be responsible for the conscious perception of pain, including the location of the stimulus, as well as the unpleasant, emotional aspects associated with pain. Because behavioral responses such as vocalization and turning the head toward the noxious stimulus may occur in animals without

a functional forebrain, these responses may not indicate conscious pain. Accordingly, some authors suggest that it is most accurate to describe what we assess as "pain" in veterinary patients as nociception [3, 7, 8].

On the other hand, although a nonhuman animal cannot express in words the psychological and emotional consequences of a noxious stimulus, it is imperative to acknowledge that unless it is established to the contrary, we should assume that those procedures that produce pain in us might also produce pain in animals [7]. And veterinary patients with IVDH typically do not have a diffuse, severe forebrain lesion; they are not decerebrate. Therefore, one can argue that using the term "pain" in this circumstance is appropriate. In recognizing both sides of this semantic debate, the authors have made the editorial decision to use the phrase "deep pain" in this chapter when referring to the clinical assessment of veterinary patients because that is the phrase used in most veterinary literature concerning intervertebral disc disease. The term "nociception" is used in accordance with the IASP definition to refer to the unconscious neural process of encoding noxious stimuli. From a clinical perspective, the two terms can be used somewhat interchangeably and synonymously however.

Neuroanatomy

The first step in nociception is activation of receptors that respond to stimuli that are actually or potentially damaging to body tissue. Activation of nociceptors associated with fast-conducting nerve fibers (A-δ fibers) is associated with sharp, pricking pain. Nociceptors associated with slow-conducting fibers (C fibers) are associated with a slower, burning type of pain. Both types of receptors innervate the skin (superficial pain) and deep somatic or visceral structures (deep pain). The distinction between superficial and deep pain is not just based on location. Each is associated with an anatomically and functionally segregated pathway, varies in the susceptibility to damage, and is tested separately in the neurologic examination [9].

Superficial pain is transmitted primarily by the spinothalamic pathway. Axons ascend in the ipsilateral lateral funiculus of the spinal cord to the contralateral thalamus and somatosensory cortex. This pathway is discriminative in that the precise location of the stimulus is perceived [7].

Deep pain is conveyed primarily by the spino-reticular pathway. The primary sensory axons enter the spinal cord and immediately diverge to send collaterals across several spinal cord segments. The ascending pathway is located diffusely in the lateral and ventral funiculi on both sides of the spinal cord. This pathway projects to the cerebral cortex through diffuse projections from the reticular formation in the brain stem and thalamus. Activation of this pathway increases arousal and activates the limbic system, which is involved in the emotional component of pain. Due to the diffuse nature of this pathway, the perception of deep pain is poorly localized [7]. Because this pathway is so diffuse and involves small, unmyelinated fibers which are the least susceptible to damage by compression, deep pain perception is the last function to be lost in spinal cord injury caused by IVDH.

Testing pain perception

Because of the predictable pattern of functional loss associated with spinal cord compression, and the correlation of this pattern with degree of neuronal myelination, it is generally safe to conclude that a patient that retains some voluntary motor function must *ipso facto* retain nociception. It is therefore unnecessary to test sensation in such a patient, and one should expect preservation of both superficial and deep pain perception.

The superficial pain pathway is tested by lightly and briefly pinching the skin to preferentially activate the superficial pain pathway. Perception of the stimulus is assesses by observing for a response such as turning the head toward the stimulus. If there is no behavioral response to pinching the toes or the tail, start caudally and pinch the skin just lateral to each vertebra to determine if there is a level at which pain is perceived. This may allow more precise localization of the lesion.

Testing for deep pain perception is only necessary in nonambulatory patients exhibiting no voluntary motor function that also have no response to superficial pain testing. A hemostat is applied across the base of a toenail, the toe, or vertebra of the tail. Gradually increase the pressure to stimulate nociceptors in the periosteum. Observe for a behavioral response such as turning the head toward the stimulus, crying, or licking or a physiological response such as increased heart rate, increased respiratory rate, or pupil dilation [10]. Because deep pain is poorly localized, sometimes the only indication of perception is the patient becoming anxious or agitated. Any of these responses is considered evidence of intact deep pain perception. However, some ambulatory dogs appear not to respond appropriately to noxious stimulation. This is apparent when we sometimes stimulate a digit on a thoracic limb or skin cranial to the lesion in a patient with disc herniation affecting the thoracolumbar spinal cord segments, wherein there should be no compromise whatsoever of the nociceptive pathways cranial to the lesion, and yet the dog does not respond. There are several possible explanations for this phenomenon, such as insufficient stimulation by the examiner, altered perception by the patient, or the examiner's failure to recognize the patient's conscious reaction. Most importantly, we must always remember when testing nociception in veterinary medicine that it is a subjective test and, with an animal's inability to verbally communicate subjective emotions, we are at a disadvantage when effectively asking the question (with our fingers, hemostat, pin, or other noxious instrument), "Can you feel this?" In humans, sensory testing can be far more layered, as human patients can verbally report different types of sensation such as hot/cold, sharp/dull, vibration, as well as actual discomfort.

The implications of the subjectivity during nociceptive assessment of animals, and the finding on occasion of apparent diminished or absent response to stimulation of anatomic areas well cranial to any spinal cord lesion, are that it is quite possible that there are instances when we test body areas caudal to the spinal cord lesion and do not observe a response that we falsely conclude that there has been "loss of deep pain."

Pain is both a sensory and an emotional experience. Therefore an animal's emotional state can affect results when performing nociceptive testing. It is not uncommon for a dog, on initial assessment in the exam room, to be judged as having no deep pain, yet on subsequent examination (in an altered environment, after having some initial therapy, or by a different examiner) to now exhibit a conscious reaction to noxious stimulation caudal to the spinal cord lesion. The explanation for this is speculative, but it seems plausible that an animal, flooded with anxiety and discomfort, might literally "tune out" new stimuli even though we would expect to be able to override any stoicism by squeezing or pinching hard enough.

Based on this, there are several recommendations when trying to assess deep pain:

1. If there is voluntary motor function and/or superficial pain sensation present, it is unnecessary to induce more discomfort by producing a deep pain reaction.
2. When presented with a paralyzed dog, it may be beneficial to check pain sensation as the very first thing, before doing any other examinations or manipulations. While this does not preclude the possibility of a false-negative finding, it may lessen the odds for such when compared to the patient that is rendered more anxious after being handled and prodded by a stranger.
3. When an examination indicates a loss of deep pain, retest the dog subsequently to determine if there has been any change in status once the dog is calmer and has possibly been given sedating or anxiolytic medication.
4. For hospitalized patients (those having non-surgical management or those recovering from spinal surgery), try to assess pain perception before getting the animal out of its cage or run and doing any other manipulations. If the patient is sleeping, try to sneak into its cage or run and observe whether noxious stimulation causes arousal. Similarly, if the patient is eating, one can observe whether it stops in response to noxious stimulation.
5. Always remember that in addition to false negatives, we can have false positives when testing nociception. A true false positive would occur when the animal appears to react to noxious stimulation despite not truly feeling discomfort. This could occur because the animal moves or vocalizes coincidental to our stimulation. For example, patients with severe back pain may exhibit a painful response when a withdrawal reflex is elicited if flexion of the limb also moves the lumbar spine, even if pain perception is absent in the limb. It should

be quickly apparent by repeat testing with the limb still flexed whether there is a reliable correlation between any patient movement or other reaction and the application of the noxious stimulus. Another "false positive" is in reality the misinterpretation by the examiner of limb movement as an indication of conscious perception by the patient. Veterinarians must be cognizant of the withdrawal reflex when digits are stimulated and that they themselves consciously ignore such limb movement when assessing nociception (see Chapter 10). The focus should always be on the animal's eyes and head, looking for pupillary dilation or active turning of the head toward the noxious stimulation, or other clear signs of conscious recognition of the stimulus. Mistaking an intact withdrawal reflex for intact pain perception is a cardinal error and might result in an inappropriate delay in treatment that, in turn, could determine whether the patient recovers or is rendered permanently paraplegic.

Reliability of clinical testing of pain perception

Although testing of pain perception is subjective, Levine *et al.* studied the interrater variability of several components of the neurologic examination, including pain perception, in 49 dogs with spinal cord injury [10]. Each patient was examined by two different veterinarians who made blinded independent assessments. The veterinarians included interns, surgery residents, a board-certified neurologist, and board-certified surgeons. Dogs were scored as having normal superficial and deep pain perception, no superficial pain perception but intact deep pain perception, or neither superficial nor deep pain perception. Interrater agreement ranged from 94 to 100% with a weighted kappa value of 0.89–1.0, respectively. A kappa value of 0.8–1.0 is considered as almost perfect agreement beyond chance [10]. Based on these results, assessment of superficial and deep pain perception in dogs with IVDH can be a reliable clinical assessment when performed and interpreted properly.

Electrophysiologic testing

Given the subjectivity of both the patient's response to noxious stimulation and our ability to apply and interpret nociceptive testing, one might wonder whether there could be more objective methods for determining the integrity of the spinal cord. In theory, the use of somatosensory evoked potentials (SSEP) might be one method. SSEP are electrical events elicited from neurons, synapses, or axons in response to stimulation of peripheral nerves. They can be recorded from electrodes on the scalp or near the spine. The recordings are time locked to the stimulus, and several recordings are averaged to exclude nonspecific electrical activity such as that arising from muscle and cerebral cortex. The most commonly used stimulus is electrical stimulation through a needle electrode placed in the skin of the distal portion of the pelvic limb. Recordings from electrodes placed cranial to the lumbar intumescence and caudal to the first cervical vertebra reveal ascending evoked potentials transmitted in spinal cord sensory pathways [11]. The SSEP recorded from the scalp are fragments of electroencephalographic activity time locked to the somatosensory stimulus. This primarily reflects conduction of A-δ fibers involved in nociception [12].

Shores recorded SSEP at the T10–11 space in response to tibial nerve stimulation in 30 dogs with acute disc extrusions affecting the T11–L7 vertebral levels. In all six dogs with paraplegia and loss of pain perception caudal to the lesion, there was no electrophysiologic evidence of transmission through the site of injury [13]. Poncelet *et al.* recorded SSEP from the scalp and at various levels along the spine in response to tibial nerve stimulation in 20 dogs with disc extrusions caudal to T9. SSEP could not be recorded cranial to the lesion in all six dogs with paraplegia and loss of pain perception and in three of seven dogs with paraplegia and intact pain sensation [14]. Holliday also reports the inability to demonstrate SSEP cranial to the lesion in patients with unequivocal loss of deep pain perception [11]. Based on these results, SSEP do not provide additional prognostic information in patients with clear loss of pain perception. However, finding SSEP cranial to a lesion in a patient with equivocal pain perception or in a patient that cannot be examined adequately provides objective evidence of some degree of spinal cord integrity [11].

What are the implications of "loss of deep pain"?

Because there is a rough, albeit very imprecise correlation between loss of nociception and severity/ irreversibility of spinal cord injury, the prognosis is always more guarded when an animal is diagnosed as deep pain negative. There are conflicting data in the literature however regarding both how poor the prognosis is, as well as the role that time (between loss of deep pain occurs and permanent paralysis is a certainty) plays in the outcome.

Complete transverse disruption of the spinal cord (whether surgically cut or as a result of focal malacia wherein there fewer than 10% of neurons survive) is unquestionably associated with permanent paralysis caudal to the lesion at our current state-of-the-art in spinal cord injury treatment. Because we cannot objectively determine this from our physical examination other than those rare cases of ascending/descending myelomalacia (see Chapter 12), there will always be some degree of uncertainty in prognosis when animals have loss of deep pain. This uncertainty extends as well to the operating room with respect to utilizing durotomy as a means of assessing spinal cord integrity and odds for functional recovery [15] (see Chapter 33).

There have been several published studies addressing the issue of time delay between onset of nociceptive loss and definitive treatment (usually surgical decompression of the spinal cord) and subsequent rates of functional recovery [16–27]. There are several inherent problems within each of these studies, and in trying to compare one study to another. First, as noted earlier, the determination of the presence or absence of deep pain is subjective and prone to some examiner error. Hence, some animals reported to be without deep pain perception may in reality have had both intact (although reduced) sensation or at least less than a complete, transecting spinal cord injury. We should not be surprised therefore, that some of these patients might recover irrespective of the time delay between *apparent* loss of deep pain and definitive treatment. This might explain the favorable results in one study that concluded that surgery done even 96h after loss of deep pain could lead to functional recovery in a significant number of patients [17]. There are also reported differences in outcome between chondrodystrophoid dogs with loss of deep pain versus large-breed, nonchondrodystrophoid dogs with absent deep pain, wherein up to 76% of the former recovered but only 25% of the latter did [23]. And as also noted earlier, loss of deep pain, even when real, is only a suggestion that the spinal cord might have been irreparably injured. We simply do not know whether prolonged delay in effecting spinal cord decompression in such patients would always be associated with further progression of the spinal cord injury (i.e., progression to functional transection with greater than 90% axonal disruption) or whether some dogs so affected might yet recover with or without surgical intervention. We do know from the studies on acute noncompressive nucleus pulposus extrusions (see Chapters 9 and 13) that some of these dogs, though judged to be deep pain negative initially, do recover ambulation (but not necessarily continence) despite the absence of any surgical intervention.

Another problem with many of these studies is that they involve small numbers of patients, and most have been retrospective in nature. These are inherent problems in much of the veterinary literature, but it underscores the weakness of using such studies as validated predictors of future behavior in subsequent patients.

Finally, one major problem with these various studies and in our clinical practice is that, for the vast majority of patients presented with paralysis and apparent loss of deep pain, *we have no way to accurately determine how long the patient has had loss of deep pain perception.* For example, the client who last observed their pet either normal or at least still with voluntary motor function many hours before discovering the pet paralyzed leaves us unable to know whether the loss of deep pain occurred many hours or only minutes before arriving at our veterinary facility. Similarly in the referral setting, a surgeon or neurologist may receive a pet from another hospital where the animal was misjudged to still have sensation (on the improper premise that limb withdrawal was observed when noxious stimulation was applied), or where loss of

nociception was noted, but again with uncertainty as to when this developed. Only in instances where pets are hospitalized and undergo accurate serial examinations around the clock can we precisely demonstrate a change from positive to negative deep pain perception.

Given all these uncertainties, it is challenging to determine a single conclusion as to the prognostic significance of deep pain absence, or to provide a quantitative prognosis for recovery based either on the absence of deep pain itself, or some number of hours since the (presumed) onset of the condition. Clearly, there are some patients in whom the loss of deep pain reflects acute spinal cord transection and for whom no treatment will restore function even if performed within minutes of the spinal cord injury. Conversely, there are likely to be patients with protracted courses of deep pain absence for whom recovery is yet possible, with or without surgical intervention. However, and despite these uncertainties, we can fairly conclude that the absence of deep pain based on a series of reliable examinations warrants a more guarded prognosis than patients who retain deep pain.

It is also logical and supported by at least some studies that the earlier the compressed spinal cord is treated with disc removal the better the odds are for recovery. Numbers frequently quoted for functional recovery suggest an 80–90% rate in paraplegic dogs with intact deep pain and decompressive surgery and approximately 50% (0–72%) recovery rate in dogs without deep pain [2, 16, 26]. Some would quote lower odds for deep pain-negative dogs or suggest a descending scale of odds based on the number of hours since deep pain was lost [27]. These numbers have some general merit in trying to convey a prognosis to clients or in suggesting the urgency of imaging and decompressive surgery, but with the absence of much larger studies done in a prospective manner, they remain educated guesses and approximations. The key element in discussing prognosis with either referring veterinarians or with clients is to indicate that most dogs will recover if they have surgically managed compressive lesions and intact deep pain sensation, with less regard to any time delay between onset of paraparesis or paraplegia and decompression, whereas dogs with loss of deep pain have a lesser chance of recovery, and that the longer decompressive treatment is delayed the odds for recovery may lessen still.

It is also important to consider how much time is allowed to transpire after surgery before a dog is judged to be permanently paraplegic. Some recoveries can be very prolonged (weeks to months in some cases), suggesting that with sufficient time and supportive care, return to ambulation is possible despite initial pessimism. On the other hand, it has been demonstrated in one study that failure to recover deep pain within 2–4 weeks after surgery was an indication of a poor prognosis for functional recovery [2].

References

1. Olby N, Levine J, Harris T, Munana K, Skeen T, Sharp N. Long-term functional outcome of dogs with severe injuries of the thoracolumbar spinal cord: 87 cases (1996-2001). J Am Vet Med Assoc. 2003 Mar 15;222(6):762–9.

2. Ruddle TL, Allen DA, Schertel ER, Barnhart MD, Wilson ER, Lineberger JA, et al. Outcome and prognostic factors in non-ambulatory Hansen Type I intervertebral disc extrusions: 308 cases. Vet Comp Orthop Traumatol. 2006;19(1):29–34.

3. Loeser JD, Treede R-D. The Kyoto protocol of IASP Basic Pain Terminology. Pain. 2008;137:437–77.

4. Committee on Recognition and Alleviation of Pain in Laboratory Animals NRC. Recognition and Alleviation of Pain in Laboratory Animals. Washington, DC: The National Academies Press; 2009.

5. Sherrington CS. Reflexes as adapted reactions. In: The Integrative Action of the Nervous System. New Haven, CT: Yale University Press; 1920. pp. 235–68.

6. De Lahunta A, Glass E. Veterinary Neuroanatomy and Clinical Neurology. 3rd ed. St. Louis, MO: Saunders Elsevier; 2009.

7. Gebhart GF. Scientific issues of pain and distress. In: Committee on Regulatory Issues in Animal Care and Use IfLAR, National Research Council, editor. Definition of Pain and Distress and Reporting Requirements for Laboratory Animals: Proceedings of the Workshop Held June 22, 2000. Washington, DC: The National Academies Press; 2000. pp. 22–31.

8. Simpson S. Watchwords of the neurologic examination. Prog Vet Neurol. 1990;1(1):18–27.

9. Lamont LA, Tranquilli WJ, Grimm KA. Physiology of pain. Vet Clin North Am Small Anim Pract. [Review]. 2000 Jul;30(4):703–28, v.

10. Levine GJ, Levine JM, Budke CM, Budke CM, Kerwin SC, Au J, et al. Description and repeatability of a newly developed spinal cord injury scale for dogs. Prev Vet Med. 2009;89:121–7.

11. Holliday TA. Electrodiagnostic examination. Somatosensory evoked potentials and electromyography. Vet Clin North Am Small Anim Pract. 1992 Jul;22(4):833–57.

12. van Oostrom H, Stienen PJ, Doornenbal A, Hellebrekers LJ. Nociception-related somatosensory evoked potentials in awake dogs recorded after intra epidermal electrical stimulation. Eur J Pain. 2009 Feb;13(2):154–60.

13. Shores A, Redding RW, Knecht CD. Spinal-evoked potentials in dogs with acute compressive thoracolumbar spinal cord disease. Am J Vet Res. 1987 Oct;48(10):1525–30.

14. Poncelet L, Michaux C, Balligand M. Somatosensory potentials in dogs with naturally acquired thoracolumbar spinal cord disease. Am J Vet Res. 1993 Nov;54(11):1935–41.

15. Loughin CA, Dewey CW, Ringwood PB, Pettigrew RW, Kent M, Budsberg SC. Effect of durotomy on functional outcome of dogs with type I thoracolumbar disc extrusion and absent deep pain perception. Vet Comp Orthop Traumatol. 2005;18(3):141–6.

16. Amsellum PM, Toombs JP, Laverty PH, Breur GJ. Loss of deep pain sensation following thoracolumbar intervertebral disk herniation in dogs: treatment and prognosis. Compend Contin Educ Pract Vet. 2003;24:266–74.

17. Anderson SM, Lippincott CL, Gill PJ. Hemilaminectomy in dogs without deep pain. Calif Vet. 1991;45:24–8.

18. Scott HW. Hemilaminectomy for the treatment of thoracolumbar disc disease in the dog: a follow-up study of 40 cases. J Small Anim Pract. 1997 Nov;38(11): 488–94.

19. Scott HW, McKee WM. Laminectomy for 34 dogs with thoracolumbar intervertebral disc disease and loss of deep pain perception. J Small Anim Pract. 1999 Sep;40(9):417–22.

20. Laitinen OM, Puerto DA. Surgical decompression in dogs with thoracolumbar intervertebral disc disease and loss of deep pain perception: a retrospective study of 46 cases. Acta Vet Scand. 2005;46(1–2):79–85.

21. Olby NJ, De Risio L, Munana KR, Wosar MA, Skeen TM, Sharp NJ, et al. Development of a functional scoring system in dogs with acute spinal cord injuries. Am J Vet Res. 2001 Oct;62(10):1624–8.

22. Gambardelli PC. Dorsal decompressive laminectomy for treatment of thoracolumbar disc disease in dogs: a retrospective study of 98 cases. Vet Surg. 1980;9:24–26.

23. Cudia SP, Duval JM. Thoracolumbar intervertebral disk disease in large, nonchondrodystrophic dogs: a retrospective study. J Am Anim Hosp Assoc. 1997 Sep–Oct;33(5):456–60.

24. Duval J, Dewey C, Roberts R, Aron D. Spinal cord swelling as a myelographic indicator of prognosis: a

retrospective study in dogs with intervertebral disc disease and loss of deep pain perception. Vet Surg. 1996 Jan–Feb;25(1):6–12.

25. Kornegay JN. Intervertebral disk disease: treatment guidelines. In: Kirk RW, Bonagura JD, editors. Kirk's Current Veterinary Therapy XI: Small Animal Practice. Philadelphia, PA: WB Saunders; 1992. pp. 1013–8.

26. Ferreira AJ, Correia JH, Jaggy A. Thoracolumbar disc disease in 71 paraplegic dogs: influence of rate of onset and duration of clinical signs on treatment results. J Small Anim Pract. 2002 Apr;43(4):158–63.

27. Toombs JP. Intervertebral disc disease. In: Slatter DH, editor. Textbook of Small Animal Surgery. 3rd ed. Philadelphia, PA: WB Saunders; 2002. pp. 1202–3.

12 Ascending/Descending Myelomalacia Secondary to Intervertebral Disc Herniation

James M. Fingeroth and Alexander de Lahunta

Thoracolumbar intervertebral disc herniation (IVDH) can result in permanent paraplegia due to irreversible spinal cord injury (SCI). The most common cause for this poor outcome is the result of actual or functional transection of the spinal cord due to the energetic injury to neural parenchyma and microvasculature from the initial contact by the herniated disc and the resultant cascade of *focal* effects elucidated in Chapters 15 and 25. The net effects of such severe SCI may be a focal zone of myelomalacia. Literally meaning "spinal cord softening," myelomalacia is the standard neuropathological term for the gross appearance of focal spinal cord necrosis. However, with the proper combination of client, patient, and nursing care, some animals so affected may continue to enjoy acceptable qualities of life and be managed indefinitely as paraplegics. Functional recovery may yet be possible for some pets with survival of as few as 10% of axons in the malacic zone [1].

In a small subset of dogs afflicted with thoracolumbar IVDH, there may not only be a *focal* myelomalacia but a progressive lesion that results in spreading of myelomalacia cranial and/or caudal from the initial site of IVDH. This phenomenon is defined as *ascending/descending myelomalacia (ADM)*. Other terms used in the literature to describe this phenomenon have included diffuse or progressive hemorrhagic myelomalacia, the ascending syndrome, hematomyelia, and progressive hemorrhagic necrosis of the spinal cord.

Focal myelomalacia is usually confined to an area of four or fewer spinal cord segments [2, 3], whereas ADM may involve larger portions, including the entire spinal cord. Unlike patients suffering from focal myelomalacia, patients with ADM have no chance for survival or return to a humane quality of life. It is therefore important for clinicians to understand this phenomenon and to be able to recognize it, so that they may intervene quickly on their patient's and client's behalf by avoiding unnecessary diagnostic procedures and by recommending humane euthanasia.

Advances in Intervertebral Disc Disease in Dogs and Cats, First Edition. Edited by James M. Fingeroth and William B. Thomas.
© 2015 ACVS Foundation. Published 2015 by John Wiley & Sons, Inc.

Clinical features of ascending/descending myelomalacia

The hallmark of ADM is the progression of an initially focal SCI to one that can no longer be localized to a specific segmental area. The neurological examination and process of neurolocalization (Chapter 10) help first define an anatomic zone where a focal lesion exists, based on evaluation of the gait if present, muscle tone, segmental reflexes, and nociception. These zones include C1–C5, C6–T2 (the cervical intumescence), T3–L3, L4–L5, L6–S1, and S2–caudal (coccygeal) segments. Further refinement of localization is possible in some patients by identifying a deficit in the cutaneous trunci (nee "panniculus") reflex and/or determination of a line of analgesia or sensory level where there is hypoalgesia or analgesia caudal to this line and normal nociception cranial to it. ADM can be recognized when the history or initial neurological examination clearly demonstrated localization to one of these zones (almost always T3–L3), but a subsequent examination discloses deficits that cannot be explained by this localization. ADM can progress bidirectionally, or may only progress cranially (ascend) or only caudally (descend).

Patients with focal T3–L3 IVDH and neurologic deficits will have general proprioceptive ataxia and upper motor neuron paresis in the pelvic limbs or paraplegia. The paresis is usually associated with hyperreflexia and hypertonia in the pelvic limbs. Their breathing and thoracic limb functions will be normal. They may have loss of the cutaneous trunci reflex caudal to the lesion, and in severe cases may have loss of nociception caudal to a line of analgesia or sensory level that corresponds to a level just caudal to the spinal cord lesion. With descending myelomalacia that destroys the lower motor neuron gray matter throughout the lumbar, sacral, and caudal segments, subsequent examination of this patient would reveal loss of tone/flaccidity in the abdominal muscles, pelvic limbs, tail, anus, and bladder. These same areas would be analgesic from the loss of the general somatic afferent pathways. With ascending myelomalacia, the line of analgesia will migrate cranially from the initial localization, intercostal paralysis will be noted, and eventually there may be lower motor neuron paresis or paralysis of the thoracic limbs. A Horner's syndrome may become apparent due to the involvement of the intermediate gray matter in the cranial thoracic spinal cord segments. With further ascension there may be complete respiratory paralysis and death as more of the cervical spinal cord is affected.

Dogs with ADM are typically reported to exhibit signs of excruciating discomfort, and in some cases fever. This is believed to be due to meningeal and subarachnoid hemorrhage at the cranial aspect of the ascending lesion. It has been reported that dogs with ADM have an "anxious" expression or "looking like they know they're going to die." Dogs with ADM have also been described as appearing depressed and may rarely assume an opisthotonic posture [4–6].

The progression of signs usually occurs over a period of hours or up to several days. Most cases of ADM are recognized within 24–72 h after an initial acute onset of SCI, although there have been sporadic reports of occurrence beyond 72 h of initial paralytic signs [6]. The occurrence of ADM appears to be unaffected by any medical and/or surgical intervention that was employed for the paralyzed patient prior to its onset. Hence, it is quite possible to see ADM in a dog that has already undergone decompressive spinal cord surgery or has been treated with pharmaceuticals [7].

Myelography of ADM typically will reveal more than 4 segments where there is disruption of typical subarachnoid columns, and often, there will be contrast seen in the central part of the vertebral canal where the spinal cord should be outlined if it were intact. Magnetic resonance imaging will disclose parenchymal hyperintensity on T2-weighted images and diffuse hypointensity on gradient echo images cranial and caudal to the focal area of extradural mass representing the inciting disc herniation [8, 9].

There is no known effective treatment for ADM. The ascending form is usually fatal, and even the descending-only form would result in diffuse lower motor neuron deficits in the pelvic limbs, bladder, and bowel such that euthanasia is usually the appropriate intervention.

Epidemiology

The true incidence of ADM is not known. Published reports indicate that it may occur in 3–9% of dogs with acute thoracolumbar SCI

[5, 6, 10–18]. Personal experience of the authors and communication with other neurologists and neurosurgeons would suggest a possibly lower incidence, perhaps on the order of 1%. A review of myelograms at one institution identified only five dogs with lesions consistent with ADM (lesions greater than four segments) over a 7-year span, which represented fewer than 1% of all the dogs that underwent myelography there [19]. A retrospective study of 46 dogs with surgical decompression of focal IVDH in the thoracolumbar area identified 1 dog with ADM [20]. Perhaps the fairest statement to make is that ADM is (fortunately) an uncommon sequel to disc herniation but occurs enough and is of such devastating clinical significance that clinicians need to be familiar with the syndrome and recognize it when present. If the characteristic clinical signs are recognized on the initial examination of the patient there is no need for any imaging studies.

There are no data to suggest any gender predilection. Most reported cases have been associated with IVDH, but there are a few instances where other forms of spinal cord trauma have been the initial insult [14]. There have been rare cases of ADM reported with no known inciting cause of SCI, no prior history of surgery or other iatrogenic cause, and no vertebral canal lesions [16, 21]. The majority of reported patients have been dachshunds, but it is unclear if this is a true breed predilection or simply a reflection of the disproportionate number of dachshunds seen in the population of dogs affected with IVDH.

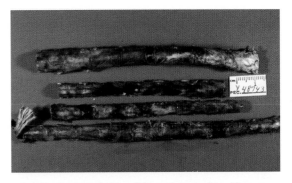

Figure 12.1   Dorsal view of the entire spinal cord from a 4-year-old dachshund with diffuse myelomalacia associated with diffuse meningeal hemorrhage. The cranial ends of each portion face right.

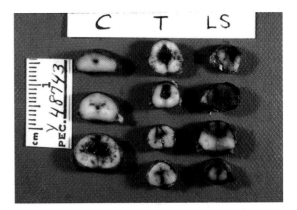

Figure 12.2   Transverse sections from the spinal cord shown in Figure 12.1 demonstrating the extensive hemorrhagic necrosis of the spinal cord parenchyma. Note the tendency of the hemorrhage to localize in the central canal and dorsal funiculus.

Neuropathology

When undergoing necropsy, dogs with ADM will exhibit a variable degree of subarachnoid hemorrhage visible through the dura mater. On removal from the vertebral canal the extensively affected portion of the spinal cord will feel soft (myelomalacia) and this softness will persist even after preservation in formalin.

Usually, it is not possible to open the dura and reflect it from the spinal cord due to adhesions that occurred as a result of the subarachnoid hemorrhage (Figure 12.1). On transecting the affected spinal cord it is very difficult to maintain the integrity of the transverse section due to softening from the spinal cord necrosis. Hemorrhages will appear

as black splotches scattered through the transverse section and will vary considerably from one segment to another. The remaining parenchyma is usually a dull brown color and has the consistency of toothpaste. Typically, at the cranial end of the lesion, there will be a core of softening with or without hemorrhage located in the central canal and the ventral aspect of the dorsal funiculi. In the caudal to midcervical segments, this may be the only lesion that is present (Figure 12.2).

On microscopic examination where the necrosis is the most severe and acute, there is no recognizable parenchyma, just a field of necrotic debris. Where hemorrhage occurs, that will be evident. Occasionally there are a few foci of neutrophils that were able to respond to the inciting acute

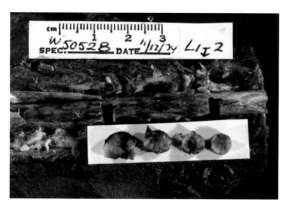

Figure 12.3   Dorsal view and transverse sections of the spinal cord of a 5-year-old dachshund with clinical signs of diffuse myelomalacia. It is difficult to make these transverse sections due to the softening of the spinal cord (malacia) that results from the necrosis. These transverse sections show the discoloration of the necrosis resulting from ischemia more than they show hemorrhage.

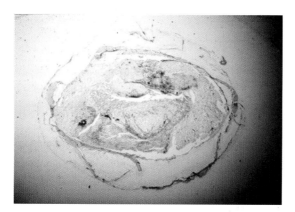

Figure 12.4   Low-power photomicrograph of one of the transverse sections in Figure 12.3. The entire parenchyma exhibits necrosis with a few scattered small hemorrhages.

necrosis, and there may also be small foci of lipid-filled macrophages present. There are no lesions in the spinal nerve roots except for Wallerian degeneration in the ventral roots if a number of days have transpired between the development of myelomalacia and death.

These parenchymal lesions represent a combination of ischemic and hemorrhagic infarction from the extensive vascular compromise that occurs. It should be noted that the term hematomyelia, which has been used as one of the synonyms for this disorder, is a misnomer, since that term defines bleeding that has occurred within the spinal cord, but not the extensive infarction seen with ADM [6] (Figures 12.3 and 12.4).

Another interesting and possibly confusing phenomenon is the finding in some cases of this seemingly centripetal progression to apparently skip some segments, and leave those skipped segments histologically unscathed. This is unlikely to be recognized in the clinical setting, especially since these segments are usually in the thoracic spinal cord.

Pathogenesis

The cascade of events that occurs with acute concussive injury to the spinal cord from a herniated disc and the effects of compression versus concussive SCI are addressed in Chapters 15 and 25 as well as in the literature [3, 11–13, 22–33]. The vascular effects of acute SCI include not only any initial hemorrhage but a progressive course of ischemia and infarction that seems to be unrelated to direct vessel rupture or ongoing compression. This process can even be initiated by kinetic energy that passes near the spinal cord without actually causing any direct mechanical impact or compression. This posttraumatic ischemia/infarction process has been dubbed the "secondary injury" phenomenon and reflects biochemical and pathologic alterations in autoregulation of local spinal cord blood flow. The autodestructive, secondary injury process that produces some degree of focal myelomalacia bears an uncanny similarity to the process we recognize as ADM. However, while a focal injury, even a severe one, may allow this process to extend over a few segments in the typical case, it is usually self-limiting.

Although the exact pathogenic mechanism of the secondary injury phenomenon is not fully elucidated, at its core there seems to be little doubt that it represents a vascular compromise. Since it produces a focal ischemia and infarction identical to that seen in spinal cords with ADM, it is plausible to conjecture that ADM also represents a vascular compromise "writ large," which escapes the local, usually limited zone of myelomalacia. However and despite the following speculation, ADM remains somewhat idiopathic.

The blood supply to the spinal cord has been described in Chapter 9. To summarize, the major blood supply is from the ventral spinal artery, which, in turn, is fed by vessels that enter the vertebral canal at each segment in conjunction with the nerve roots. It has been documented in both man and dogs that these segmental radicular arteries do not all develop or contribute blood supply to the ventral spinal artery equally. Particularly in the thoracolumbar region, it is well known that there can be great disparity between segmental artery diameters, and that often one vessel predominates over the others. This artery is termed the arteria radicularis magna (great radicular artery). In humans, the eponym "artery of Adamkiewicz" is used. It is further known that this artery is critical and that it supplies many segments cranially and caudally that are otherwise insufficiently supplied by the smaller radicular arteries at those levels. This is termed a "desegmented pattern" [10, 12, 34, 35]. It is so critical that many physician neurosurgeons will order angiograms prior to attempting vertebral or vascular surgery in the thoracolumbar region so as to know which radicular artery is serving as the main blood supply to the spinal cord (and to avoid compromising it) [36]. Traumatic, degenerative or iatrogenic compromise of the great radicular artery in humans is known to result in a widespread area of spinal cord ischemia and necrosis extending many segments superior and inferior to the entry point of the artery. This is termed the anterior spinal (cord) syndrome in humans, and it bears a striking similarity to the pathologic changes seen in dogs with ADM [37]. The segments of the spinal cord that lie between the great radicular artery in the thoracolumbar region and similar high-flow radicular arteries in the cervical spinal cord are termed "watershed" areas, and those segments are clearly more vulnerable to vascular injury of the type seen in the secondary phenomenon of acute SCI, and the more widespread destruction associated with ADM.

The vascular anatomy of the canine spinal cord has been studied, and a great radicular vessel has been identified, usually at L5 or L6, most often on the left side, but sometimes on the right or bilaterally [34, 35]. A veterinary neuropathologist has observed this artery entering at L4 and then seen it "recourse" caudally to L5 or L6 [38]. Moreover, it has been found in dogs that there is not always a radicular artery entering the vertebral canal bilaterally at every level between T10–T11 and L5–L6. Some dogs have unilateral or even bilateral deficiencies, with some dogs having as many as seven spinal cord segments being dependent on as few as two to four radicular arteries [34]. What this suggests is

that some dogs may be particularly vulnerable, especially if their great radicular artery supply enters more cranially, such as near the thoracolumbar junction, rather than at the more caudal lumbar area. In such a scenario, one could envision a combination of a dog with this particular vascular anomaly suffering from an acute IVDH, and thus being prone to ADM. Because it requires the unique combination of a thoracolumbar zone major radicular artery and a colocated disc herniation, it might explain the very low incidence of ADM in dogs with IVDH.

The observation of ADM "skipping" segments is consternating but could plausibly be explained if an uncompromised small intercostal artery could supply adequate blood flow to one or two segments between those that are not receiving blood flow from the ventral spinal artery.

Acknowledgment

The authors would like to acknowledge the conceptual and factual input to the material in this chapter from their late colleague Dr. Damon (Skip) Averill.

References

1. Olby N, Levine J, Harris T, Munana K, Skeen T, Sharp N. Long-term functional outcome of dogs with severe injuries of the thoracolumbar spinal cord: 87 cases (1996–2001). J Am Vet Med Assoc. 2003 Mar 15;222(6):762–9.
2. Das GD. Perspectives in anatomy and pathology of paraplegia in experimental animals. Brain Res Bull. 1989;22(1):7–32.
3. Griffiths IR. Some aspects of the pathology and pathogenesis of the myelopathy caused by disc protrusions in the dog. J Neurol Neurosurg Psychiatry. 1972 Jun;35(3):403–13.
4. McGrath JT. Neurologic Examination of the Dog. Philadelphia: Lea & Febiger; 1960.
5. Griffiths IR. The extensive myelopathy of intervertebral disc protrusions in dogs ("the ascending syndrome"). J Small Anim Pract. 1972;13(8):425–37.
6. Gage ED. Clinical recognition of progressive hemorrhagic myelomalacia in the dog. Southwest Vet. 1974;27:227–9.
7. Laitinen OM, Puerto DA. Surgical decompression in dogs with thoracolumbar intervertebral disc disease and loss of deep pain perception: a retrospective study of 46 cases. Acta Vet Scand. 2005;46(2):79.

8. Platt SR, McConnell J, Bestbier M. Magnetic resonance imaging characteristics of ascending hemorrhagic myelomalacia in a dog. Vet Radiol Ultrasound. 2006;47(1):78–82.

9. Okada M, Kitagawa M, Ito D, Itou T, Kanayama K, Sakai T. Magnetic resonance imaging features and clinical signs associated with presumptive and confirmed progressive myelomalacia in dogs: 12 cases (1997–2008). J Am Vet Med Assoc. 2010;237(10):1160–5.

10. de Lahunta A. Veterinary Neuroanatomy and Clinical Neurology. 2nd ed. Philadelphia: WB Saunders; 1983.

11. Oliver JE, Hoerlein BF. Veterinary Neurology. Philadelphia: WB Saunders; 1987.

12. Thacher C. Neuroanatomic and pathophysiologic aspects of intervertebral disc disease in the dog. Probl Vet Med. 1989;1(3):337.

13. Braund KG. Intervertebral Disc Disease. In: Bojrab MJ, editor. Disease Mechanisms in Small Animal Surgery. Philadelphia: Lea and Febiger; 1993. p. 966.

14. Oliver JE, Lorenz MD. Handbook of Veterinary Neurology. 2nd ed. Philadelphia: WB Saunders; 1993.

15. Wheeler SJ, Sharp NJH. Small Animal Spinal Disorders. London: Mosby-Wolfe; 1994.

16. Summers BA, Cummings JF, de Lahunta A. Veterinary Neuropathology. St. Louis: Mosby; 1995.

17. Coates JR. Intervertebral disk disease. Vet Clin North Am Small Anim Pract. 2000 Jan;30(1):77–110, vi.

18. Scott HW, McKee WM. Laminectomy for 34 dogs with thoracolumbar intervertebral disc disease and loss of deep pain perception. J Small Anim Pract. 1999 Sep;40(9):417–22.

19. Lu D, Lamb CR, Targett MP. Results of myelography in seven dogs with myelomalacia. Vet Radiol Ultrasound. 2002;43(4):326–30.

20. Laitinen OM, Puerto DA. Surgical decompression in dogs with thoracolumbar intervertebral disc disease and loss of deep pain perception: a retrospective study of 46 cases. Acta Vet Scand. 2005;46(1–2):79–85.

21. de Lahunta A. Unpublished observations.

22. Berg RJ, Rucker NC. Pathophysiology and medical management of acute spinal cord injury. Comp Cont Educ Pract Vet. 1985;7(8):646–652.

23. de la Torre JC. Spinal cord injury. Review of basic and applied research. Spine (Phila Pa 1976). 1981 Jul–Aug;6(4):315–35.

24. Demopoulos HB, Flamm ES, Pietronigro DD, Seligman ML. The free radical pathology and the microcirculation in the major central nervous system disorders. Acta Physiol Scand Suppl. 1980;492:91–119.

25. Griffiths IR. Some aspects of the pathogenesis and diagnosis of lumbar disc protrusion in the dog. J Small Anim Pract. 1972;13(8):439–47.

26. Griffiths IR. Spinal cord injuries: a pathological study of naturally occurring lesions in the dog and cat. J Comp Pathol. 1978;88(2):303–15.

27. Griffiths IR, Burns N, Crawford AR. Early vascular changes in the spinal grey matter following impact injury. Acta Neuropathol. 1978;41(1):33–9.

28. Griffiths IR, McCulloch M, Crawford RA. Ultrastructural appearances of the spinal microvasculature between 12 hours and 5 days after impact injury. Acta Neuropath. 1978;43(3):205–11.

29. Hall ED, Wolf DL. A pharmacological analysis of the pathophysiological mechanisms of posttraumatic spinal cord ischemia. J Neurosurg. 1986;64(6):951–61.

30. Janssen L, Hansebout RR. Pathogenesis of spinal cord injury and newer treatments. A review. Spine (Phila Pa 1976). 1989 Jan;14(1):23–32.

31. Jellinger K, Hansebout RR. Pathology of Spinal Cord Trauma. In: Errico TJ, Bauer RD, Waugh T, editors. Spinal Trauma. Philadelphia: JB Lippincott; 1989. pp. 455–95.

32. Tarlov IM, Klinger H. Spinal cord compression studies II. Time limits for recovery after acute compression in dogs. AMA Arch Neurol Psychiatry. 1954;71(3):271–90.

33. Tarlov IM. Spinal cord compression studies III. Time limits for recovery after gradual compression in dogs. AMA Arch Neurol Psychiatry. 1954;71(5):588–97.

34. Parker AJ. Distribution of spinal branches of the thoracolumbar segmental arteries in dogs. Am J Vet Res. 1973;34(10):1351–3.

35. Caulkins SE, Purinton PT, Oliver JE. Arterial supply to the spinal cord of dogs and cats. Am J Vet Res. 1989;50(3):425–30.

36. Benjamin MV, Ransohoff J. Thoracic Disc Disease. In: Rothman RH, Simeone FA, editors. The Spine. 2nd ed. Philadelphia: WB Saunders; 1982. p. 503.

37. Sliwa JA, Maclean IC. Ischemic myelopathy: a review of spinal vasculature and related clinical syndromes. Arch Phys Med Rehabil. 1992 Apr;73(4):365–72.

38. Averill D. Unpublished material. 2006.

13 Traumatic Disc Extrusions

Luisa De Risio, William B. Thomas, and James M. Fingeroth

Pathophysiology

Traumatic disc extrusions (TDE) may occur when an otherwise healthy intervertebral disc is subjected to excessive force such as during vigorous exercise (such as running and jumping) or trauma. A sudden increase in intradiscal pressure can cause rapid projection of hydrated nucleus pulposus (NP) toward the spinal cord through a tear in the annulus fibrosus. This results in spinal cord contusion and may or may not result in persistent spinal cord compression. The term *acute noncompressive nucleus pulposus extrusion (ANNPE)* has been proposed to indicate when the extruded NP contuses the spinal cord and then dissipates within the epidural space, causing minimal to no spinal cord compression [1]. Other terms to indicate this condition include traumatic disc prolapse, dorso-lateral intervertebral disc "explosion," and high-velocity–low-volume disc extrusion [2–4]. Some authors have also used the term Hansen type III intervertebral disc disease [5]. However, Hansen's terminology only included two types, and type III extrusions were originally described by Funquist

as extension of disc material "like a carpet over several vertebrae" [6]. Most recently, the term TDE has been used to indicate extrusion of either degenerated or nondegenerated intervertebral disc material following trauma to the spinal region [7].

ANNPE has been reported in several canine breeds and in a few cats [1–9]. Compressive hydrated nucleus pulposus extrusion (HNPE) has been reported in dogs and has been mainly characterized by ventral midline spinal cord compression [10]. Rarely, TDE can result in laceration of the dura mater and in some cases penetration of the spinal cord parenchyma [11–20]. Subarachnoid–pleural fistula has been reported in one dog following TDE at T11–T12, resulting in dura mater laceration and separation of the hypaxial muscle fascial planes and the parietal pleura [21].

TDE can also occur in association with vertebral fracture/luxation. In the authors' experience, this is infrequent in dogs and cats, and neurologic deficits are usually due to bony displacement or hematoma. However, in human patients, TDE has been reported in up to 40% of all fracture dislocations of the cervical spine [22–24].

Advances in Intervertebral Disc Disease in Dogs and Cats, First Edition. Edited by James M. Fingeroth and William B. Thomas.
© 2015 ACVS Foundation. Published 2015 by John Wiley & Sons, Inc.

Clinical presentation

The clinical presentation of dogs and cats with ANNPE is characterized by peracute onset of myelopathy that is nonprogressive after the first 24 h. Lateralization of neurological deficits has been reported in 62% of dogs and in two of the three cats reported [1, 8, 9]. Discomfort and hyperalgesia during palpation of the affected spinal segments have been described in 57% of dogs [1]. This is the most helpful clinical finding to differentiate ANNPE from fibrocartilaginous embolic myelopathy (see Chapter 9), although occasionally animals with fibrocartilaginous embolic myelopathy may have spinal pain or discomfort upon palpation in the first 24–48 h after onset. Male dogs seem to be affected more commonly with TDE than females. Median age at diagnosis in dogs has been reported as 6.7 years [1]. The T3–L3 spinal cord segments and in particular the T12–T13, T13–L1, and L1–L2 intervertebral disc spaces are most commonly affected [1, 25]. A transient decrease in magnitude of the flexor withdrawal reflex in the pelvic limbs has been reported in half of dogs with thoracolumbar ANNPE examined within hours to a few days after onset of signs and is probably due spinal shock [1].

The age at disease onset in the three cats reported with ANNPE was 16 months, 2 years, and 5 years, respectively [4, 8, 9]. Two cats were female and one was male. Breeds included domestic short and long haired and Siamese. Affected spinal cord segments were C2–C3, C3–C4, and L5–L6, respectively [4, 8, 9].

The clinical presentation of the cat and few dogs reported with TDE resulting in dura mater laceration and penetration of the spinal cord parenchyma was similar to the one described for ANNPE [11–20]. The thoracolumbar junction is most commonly affected, although cervical intervertebral discs can be affected [11–20].

To date, compressive HNPE has been reported in the cervical spine of 10 dogs [10]. In all but 1 of these 10 dogs, the onset of neurological signs was not associated with any type of physical activity (running, jumping, or playing) or traumatic event (road traffic accident). In the remaining dog, the onset of clinical signs appeared while running, without any witnessed traumatic event. All dogs had acute (<24 h) symmetric nonambulatory tetraparesis or tetraplegia. Respiratory dysfunction

was observed in 33% of dogs. The median age at diagnosis was 9 years (range, 8 to 13 years). Most dogs were nonchondrodystrophic and male. The most commonly affected IVD space was C4–C5 followed by C3–C4 [10]. The authors have observed compressive HNPE in the cervical and thoracolumbar spine of dogs following trauma or strenuous exercise.

In one study on 31 dogs with TDE [7], including dogs with intervertebral disc degeneration, 9 dogs (21%) had concurrent spinal cord compression and the remaining 22 (71%) had no spinal cord compression. Mean age was 6.3 years (range, 6 months to 15 years) and mean body weight was 14.2 kg (range, 2.5–32 kg). The most common sites for TDE (compressive and noncompressive) were the cervical and the thoracolumbar (T12–L4) regions of the spinal column. In addition to TDE, 7 of 9 dogs with spinal cord compression and 7 of 22 dogs without spinal cord compression had evidence of generalized IVD degeneration. Dogs with TDE and spinal cord compression were significantly older and more likely to be chondrodystrophic and have generalized IVD degeneration than were dogs with traumatic IVD extrusion without spinal cord compression. Body weight and initial neurologic grade did not differ significantly between dogs with and without spinal cord compression [7].

Diagnosis

The antemortem diagnosis of TDE is based on clinical features (acute onset of nonprogressive myelopathy following trauma or strenuous exercise) and MRI. The MRI findings of ANNPE include a focal area of T2 hyperintensity within the spinal cord overlying a narrowed intervertebral disc space, with absent or minimal spinal cord compression. There is decreased volume and signal intensity of the affected NP on T2-weighted images. Extraneous material or signal change may be evident in the epidural space dorsally [1, 25] (Figure 13.1). These MRI findings can help to differentiate ANNPE from fibrocartilaginous embolic myelopathy (see Chapter 9) and to identify penetration of NP material within the spinal cord [16, 17].

Myelography or CT myelography of dogs with dural lacerations may show extradural leakage of iodinated contrast medium or focal accumulation

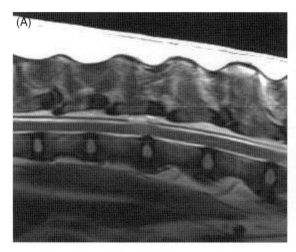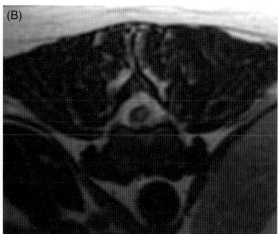

Figure 13.1   MRI of a dog with noncompressive traumatic disc extrusion (Source: Luisa De Risio ©). A 9-year-old neutered male Labrador suffered peracute left pelvic limb monoparesis while playing with a ball. When correcting for overshooting the ball, his left pelvic limb appeared to slide beneath him and he yelped. From that time, he was unable to use his left pelvic limb. Neurologic examination revealed severe paresis of the left pelvic limb.(A) Sagittal T2-weighted fast spin echo (FSE) MRI. There is mild swelling and ill-defined intramedullary hyperintensity of the spinal cord overlying the T13–L1 intervertebral disc space. There is disruption of the epidural space dorsally to the spinal cord. The size of the T13–L1 intervertebral nucleus pulposus appears slightly smaller than the volume adjacent discs. (B) Transverse T2-weighted FSE MRI. The intramedullary hyperintensity is left sided and immediately dorsal to the disrupted dorsal annulus on transverse T2-weighted images There is disruption of the epidural space dorsally and laterally on the left side (Source: Luisa De Risio ©).

of contrast within the spinal cord [11–15, 18, 20]. Traction of the cervical spine may result in penetration of myelographic contrast medium through a defect in the dura and annulus [13]. MRI allows visualization of disc material herniated within the spinal cord parenchyma and associated spinal cord edema and/or hemorrhage, as well as narrowing of the underlying intervertebral disc space with decreased volume and signal intensity of the NP on T2-weighted images (Figure 13.2). A communicating tract extending from the intervertebral disc into the spinal cord parenchyma can sometimes be seen [16, 17].

A definitive diagnosis of ANNPE is only possible at postmortem examination. Visualization of the extruded gelatinous NP may be difficult when it dissipates in the epidural space. However, rupture of the annulus fibrosus and spinal cord contusion or necrosis can be detected macroscopically and/or histologically [3].

The MRI features of compressive HNPE include extradural compressive material immediately dorsal to a narrowed IVD space and isointense to hydrated NP with ill-defined dorsal annulus and reduced NP volume [10] (Figure 13.3). Histopathology of the

extradural compressive material is necessary to achieve definitive diagnosis.

Treatment

At present, there is no evidence of any beneficial pharmacological treatment for ANNPE, including the use of methylprednisolone sodium succinate or other types of corticosteroids [1]. However, no controlled clinical trial has been performed to investigate the value of these or other pharmacological treatments in dogs or cats with TDE. Currently, treatment for ANNPE mainly consists of analgesia and nonsteroidal anti-inflammatory medications as needed, exercise restriction for 4–6 weeks, and physical rehabilitation. Dogs with compressive HNPE have been managed conservatively or surgically depending on the severity of neurologic dysfunction and degree of spinal cord compression [10]. Advances in the treatment of secondary spinal cord injury (see Chapter 25) may also benefit dogs with TDE.

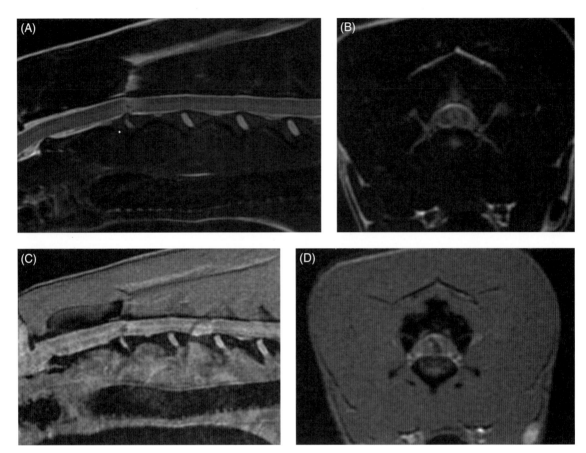

Figure 13.2 MRI of a dog with traumatic disc extrusion within the spinal cord parenchyma with associated intramedullary edema and hemorrhage (*Source*: Luisa De Risio ©). A 6-year-old female whippet presented with peracute onset nonambulatory tetraparesis after running into a wall. Cervical spinal hyperalgesia was detected on presentation 12 h after the trauma. (A) Sagittal T2-weigthed FSE MRI of the cervical spine. The C2–C3 intervertebral disc space is narrowed and the size and signal intensity of the nucleus pulposus is decreased, compared to adjacent intervertebral discs. There is an intramedullary focal hypointensity surrounded by ill-defined hyperintensity within the spinal cord overlying the C2–C3 intervertebral disc. (B) Transverse T2-weighted FSE image at the level of the C2–C3 intervertebral disc. As in A, there is an intramedullary focal hypointensity surrounded by ill-defined hyperintensity in the spinal cord overlying the C2–C3 intervertebral disc. (C) Sagittal T2* image of the cervical spine. The C2–C3 intervertebral disc space is narrowed, and there is intramedullary hypointensity within the overlying spinal cord. (D) Transverse T2* image at the level of the C2–C3 intervertebral disc. There is linear intramedullary hypointensity extending across the spinal cord overlying the C2–C3 intervertebral disc.

Outcome and prognosis

In the only published study of the outcome of ANNPE in 42 dogs, outcome was successful in 28 (67%) and unsuccessful in 14 (33%) [1]. Of the 14 dogs with an unsuccessful outcome, 10 had recovered nociception and ambulatory status but had persistent partial fecal and sometimes urinary incontinence. The intermittent fecal incontinence was not perceived as a major problem by the owners, similar to what has been reported for dogs with other types of acute thoracolumbar spinal cord injury [26]. The severity of neurologic deficits, extent of the intramedullary hyperintensity on sagittal and transverse T2-weighted MR images, and detection of intramedullary hypointensity on gradient echo images can help to predict outcome [1]. Maximal cross-sectional area of the intramedullary hyperintensity on transverse T2-weighted MR images has been reported as the most useful MRI variable to predict outcome [1].

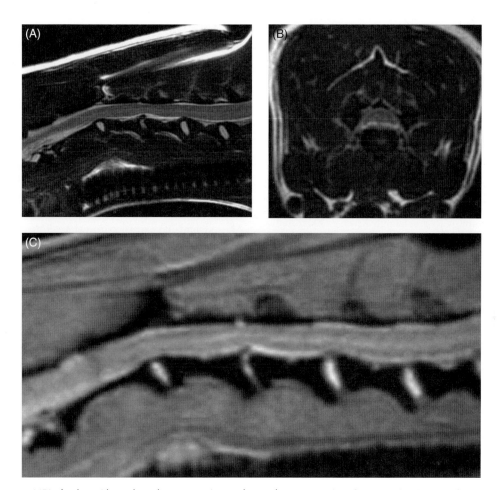

Figure 13.3   MRI of a dog with moderately compressive nucleus pulposus extrusion (Source: Luisa De Risio ©). A 9-year-and-5-month-old neutered male Yorkshire terrier–Jack Russell terrier cross was presented with a history of acute onset left pelvic limb paresis (during exercise) that progressed to nonambulatory tetraparesis over the following few hours.(A) Sagittal T2-weigthed FSE MRI of the cervical spine. There is extradural moderately compressive material isointense to hydrated nucleus pulposus dorsally to the C3–C4 intervertebral disc space and adjacent end plates. (B) Transverse T2-weighted FSE image. The extruded material lies symmetrically on the midline ventral to the spinal cord. The margin of the extruded material resembles a "seagull." (C) Sagittal T2* image of the cervical spine depicting the narrowed C3–C4 intervertebral disc space and the lack of mineralized material within the spinal canal (Luisa De Risio ©).

Of the three cats reported with ANNPE, two improved but had mild residual neurologic dysfunction and one fully recovered [4, 8, 9]. The majority of dogs with TDE resulting in dural laceration and penetration of the spinal cord parenchyma have been reported to have a favorable outcome following conservative management or surgery [11–13, 16, 18].

The majority of dogs (90%) with compressive HNPE had a favorable outcome and recovered ambulatory status within 2 weeks after onset [10]. In the study on 31 dogs with compressive and noncompressive TDE, including dogs with intervertebral disc degeneration, outcome was favorable except for dogs that had paraplegia and absence of deep pain sensation at initial examination [7]. Outcome, neurologic grade, and duration of hospitalization did not differ significantly between dogs with and without spinal cord compression [7].

References

1. De Risio L, Adams V, Dennis R, McConnell JF. 2009. Association of clinical and magnetic resonance imaging findings with outcome in dogs with presumptive acute noncompressive nucleus pulposus extrusion: 42 cases (2000–2007). *J Am Vet Med Assoc* 234:495–504.
2. Hansen HJ. 1952. A pathologic-anatomical study on disc degeneration in dog. *Acta Orthop Scand*, Charlotte, NC, 11:4–119.
3. Griffiths IR. 1970. A syndrome produced by dorso-lateral "explosions" of the cervical intervertebral discs. *Vet Rec* 87:737–741.
4. Lu D, Lamb CR, Wesselingh K, *et al.* 2002. Acute intervertebral disc extrusion in a cat: clinical and MRI findings. *J Feline Med Surg* 4:65–68.
5. Bagley RS. 2003. Spinal cord enigmas: fibrocartilaginous emboli, arachnoid cyst, and others, in *Proc 21st Annu Am Coll Vet Intern Med Forum*, Charlotte, NC, 10–11.
6. Funquist B. 1962. Thoraco-lumbar disk protrusion with severe cord compression in the dog. I. Clinical and patho-anatomic observations with special reference to the rate of development of the symptoms of motor loss. *Acta Vet Scand* 3:256–274.
7. Henke D, Gorgas D, Flegel T, Vanvelde M, Lang J, Doherr MG, Forterre F. 2013. Magnetic resonance imaging findings in dogs with traumatic intervertebral disk extrusion with and without spinal cord compression: 31 cases (2006–2010). *J Am Vet Med Assoc* 242:217–222.
8. Sanders S, Bagley RS, Tucker RL, Nelson NR. 1999. Radiographic diagnosis: Focal spinal cord malacia in a cat. *Vet Radiol Ultrasound* 40:122–125.
9. Chow K, Beatty JA, Voss K, Barrs VR. 2012. Probable lumbar acute non-compressive nucleus pulposus extrusion in a cat with acute onset paraparesis. *J Feline Med Surg* 14(10):764–767.
10. Beltran E, Dennis R, Doyle V, de Stefani A, Holloway A, De Risio L. 2012. Clinical and magnetic resonance imaging features of canine compressive cervical myelopathy with suspected hydrated nucleus pulposus extrusion. *J Small Anim Prac* 53:101–107.
11. Hay CW, Muir P. 2000. Tearing of the dura mater in three dogs. *Vet Rec* 146:279–282.
12. Yarrow TG, Jeffery ND. 2000. Dura mater laceration associated with acute paraplegia in three dogs. *Vet Rec* 146:138–139.
13. McKee WM, Downes CJ. 2008. Rupture of the dura mater in two dogs caused by the peracute extrusion of a cervical disc. *Vet Rec* 162:479–481.
14. Montavon PM, Weber U, Guscetti F, Sutter PF. 1990. What is your diagnosis? Swelling of spinal cord associated with dural tear between segments T13 and L1. *J Am Vet Med Assoc* 196:783–784.
15. Roush JK, Douglass JP, Hertzke D, Kennedy GA. 1992. Traumatic dural laceration in a racing greyhound. *Vet Radiol Ultrasound* 33:22–24.
16. Sanders SG, Bagley RS, Gavin PR. 2002. Intramedullary spinal cord damage associated with intervertebral disk material in a dog. *J Am Vet Med Assoc* 221:1594–1596.
17. MConnell JF, Garosi LS. 2004. Intramedullary intervertebral disk extrusion in a cat. *Vet Radiol Ultrasound* 45:327–330.
18. Kent M, Holmes S, Cohen E, Sakals S, Roach W, Platt S, Schatzberg S, Howerth E. 2011. Imaging diagnosis-CT myelography in a dog with intramedullary intervertebral disc herniation. *Vet Radiol Ultrasound* 52(2):185–187.
19. Kitagawa M, Okada M, Kanayama K, Sakai T. 2012. Identification of ventrolateral intramedullary intervertebral disc herniation in a dog. *J S Afr Vet Assoc* 83:4.
20. Meola SD, Swiderski JK, Randall EK, Kraft S, Palmer RH. 2007. What is your diagnosis? *J Vet Med Assoc* 230:1629–1630.
21. Packer RA, Frank PM, Chambers JN. 2004. Traumatic subarachnoid-pleural fistula in a dog. *Vet Radiol Ultrasound* 45:523–527.
22. Harrington JF, Likavec MJ, Smith AS. 1991. Disc herniation in cervical fracture subluxation. *Neurosurgery* 29:374–379.
23. Pratt ES, Green DA, Spengler DM. 1990. Herniated intervertebral discs associated with unstable spinal injuries. *Spine* 15:662–666.
24. Rizzolo SJ, Piazza MR, Cotler JM, Balderston RA, Schaefer D, Flanders A. 1991. Intervertebral disc injury complicating cervical spine trauma. *Spine* 16:S187–S189.
25. Chang Y, Dennis R, Platt SR, Penderis J. 2007. Magnetic resonance imaging features of traumatic intervertebral disc extrusion in dogs. *Vet Rec* 160:795–799.
26. Olby N, Levine J, Harris J, Munana K, Skeen T, Sharp N. 2003. Long-term functional outcome of dogs with severe injuries of the thoracolumbar spinal cord: 87 cases (1996–2001). *J Am Vet Med Assoc* 222:762–769.

14 "Discogenic" Pain (Signs Associated With Disc Degeneration But Without Herniation): Does It Occur?

James M. Fingeroth and James Melrose

Throughout this text, a distinction has been made between intervertebral disc *disease* (IVDD) and intervertebral disc *herniation* (IVDH). The main reason for this distinction is to differentiate clinical signs (pain and paresis) resulting from compressive lesions affecting the spinal cord and/or nerve roots (or well-innervated paradiscal structures such as the dorsal longitudinal ligament [1]), which are due to actual displacement of the disc, from clinical signs attributable to degenerative change in an intact, nonbulging intervertebral disc (IVD), leading to internal pain generation within this structure. A fair question to ask is whether patients can suffer symptoms of pain merely as a consequence of the degenerative processes that might be occurring in one or more IVDs [2].

A further complication that should be taken into account with regard to the generation of pain of discal origin is that, with the onset of age, the normal sequence of events in the IVD is for the disc cells to synthesize an altered form of aggrecan with smaller chondroitin sulfate (CS) side chains. Aggrecan is the major space-filling disc proteoglycan which conveys important weight-bearing properties to the nucleus pulposus (NP) [3]. Since there are no known mammalian chondroitinases (enzymes which degrade the CS side chains of aggrecan), this selective depolymerization process is the consequence of a change in how the aggrecan is biosynthesized by the disc cells and not due to a degradative event and is interpreted as an aging phenomenon. However, it still diminishes the biomechanical competence of the IVD as a weight-bearing structure. The consequence of this reduction in the hydrodynamic size and number of the CS chains attached to the aggrecan core protein is that the degree of hydration, which aggrecan can entrap in the NP, is reduced, leading to dehydration of this tissue with aging and a reduction in disc height. There may also be a compensatory increase in the synthesis of collagen which may lead to a further reduction in vertebral column flexibility. Axial loading to the vertebral column in these instances can lead to bulging of the annulus fibrosus (AF) since it is now required to take up a greater proportion of the compressive axial load. If annular nerve endings are indeed nociceptive, then this altered annular loading potentially can provide a mechanism for annular pain generation in an otherwise intact but aged

Advances in Intervertebral Disc Disease in Dogs and Cats, First Edition. Edited by James M. Fingeroth and William B. Thomas.
© 2015 ACVS Foundation. Published 2015 by John Wiley & Sons, Inc.

IVD. With aging, aggrecan can also undergo proteolytic degradation of its core protein through the action of matrix metalloproteinases, leading to fragmented forms of aggrecan devoid of their G1 N-terminal domains which formerly would have facilitated the interaction of aggrecan with hyaluronan to form massive macromolecular ternary complexes greater than 20 megadaltons in size [3]. In the healthy disc, these arrays are entrapped within the type II collagen network within the NP, and collectively, these provide hydrodynamic and viscoelastic weight-bearing properties to the NP of the composite disc structure. This fragmentation process constitutes part of the degradative events that occur in disc degeneration with normal aging. Traumatic overload of the biomechanically incompetent disc under such circumstances can lead to pathological failure of annular lamellae and extrusion of NP material into the vertebral canal. Such pathological change is therefore superimposed on normal age-related changes in disc composition and functional properties. A further consequence of the diminution of discal aggrecan with aging is that a significant fall in the intradiscal hydrostatic properties occurs, and this can promote ingrowth of nerves from the outer AF into the degenerate IVD. It remains controversial, however, as to whether these are nociceptive and contribute to discal pain generation. Age-related changes in disc composition are well documented in the chondrodystrophic canine breeds. Traumatic failure of discal components in the biomechanically compromised aged canine IVD may lead to extrusion of annular and nuclear material into the vertebral canal.

The anatomic basis for posing the existence of discogenic pain (i.e., pain resulting directly from degeneration within a contained disc that is not displaced or that creates any compressive lesion on neural tissues or other soft paradiscal tissue structures that are known to have pain receptors) requires that the disc itself possesses sensory nerve endings that transmit pain impulses to the brain. As discussed in Chapters 1 and 3, such a basis appears to exist in humans, where nerves penetrate as far as the inner AF [4–8].

Microscopic examination of canine discs reveals very sparse innervation, and such innervation appears to be confined to the outer layers of the annulus fibrosus [1, 9] or paradiscal structures. These may be affected when the normal disc undergoes degradative change in its extracellular matrix components, leading to annular remodeling, bulging, or failure. Annular bulging or annular tearing can lead to the so-called sciatic pain in man from localized pressure imposed on innervated paradiscal structures. This terminology is a misnomer given that the sciatic nerve is not actually impinged on in man, yet the term "sciatic low back pain" is a well-known term to the layman, and this incorrect terminology has persisted. Chemonucleolysis (see also Chapter 26) was an established treatment modality for lumbar disc disease in man for over 30 years following its introduction by Lyman Smith in 1963 [10–12]. The therapeutic basis of this treatment lay in its ability to reduce annular bulging, with a reduction in localized pressure on sensitized nerve endings providing a plausible explanation for pain alleviation. Anaphylaxis and medicolegal litigative issues however resulted in the procedure being withdrawn by the FDA. Chymopapain (chymodiactin) [13] and digestive proteinases from Antarctic krill [14] have both been evaluated for chemonucleolysis in the canine (see Chapter 26).

Discogenic pain is considered a real medical entity in man [6, 15–17]; however, it appears less likely to exist in the canine, given the very sparse innervation of the canine IVD.

The diagnosis and confirmation of discogenic pain is fraught with difficulty even in humans. Instances of symptomatic IVDs occur with no detectable change in the IVD evident using radiography or MRI and, conversely, the presence of radiographic or MRI abnormalities in IVDs of patients exhibiting no associated symptoms. Further, in some instances, the presence of extensively deranged IVDs has been confirmed at autopsy on individuals who had never complained of low back pain. Pain questionnaires, such as the Oswestry disability questionnaire, can however be useful in assessing the extent and duration of spinal pain in man. However, such interpretative findings cannot be collated in dogs other than as aberrations in their normal body behavior or other mannerisms subjectively detected by the owner or veterinarian.

One of the reasons that discogenic pain has been suggested by some as a cause for discomfort in dogs has been apparent failure of imaging studies to identify evidence of herniation in patients presenting with signs of vertebral column pain. However, it appears that this failure is attributable more to limitations with particular imaging modalities than an absence of demonstrable disc displacement. Starting with plain radiographs (see Chapter 16), it is well established that dogs can have IVDH and exhibit no radiographic signs (e.g., narrowed disc space, mineralization, etc.) as a consequence. Standard myelography too has some insensitivity for disc herniation. Small displacements of disc might result in little appreciable attenuation of the contrast columns and thus be misread as "negative." Moreover, lateralized disc displacements (foraminal discs) (see Chapters 16 and 30) may produce significant compression/attenuation of nerve roots, but as this is lateral to the vertebral canal proper, myelography may appear normal [18]. Interestingly, in dogs with suspected cervical disc herniation in which myelograms appear normal, the adjunctive use of obliqued radiographs (after clearance of the contrast agent from the subarachnoid space) may reveal evidence of mineralized disc material within the intervertebral foramen, an instance where the proper plain radiographic technique is superior to myelography [19].

The advent of cross-sectional imaging studies has sharply reduced the number of dogs with "negative" studies in cases where disc herniation is responsible for clinical signs. Computed tomography (CT), CT combined with myelography, and magnetic resonance imaging (MRI) are much less prone to false negatives (i.e., missing a macroscopic displacement of disc material) than plain radiography or standard myelography. For this reason, many fewer dogs today are suspected of having "discogenic" pain than before these more advanced modalities were widely available (Figure 14.1).

Because no imaging modality is 100% reliable, however, there are presumably still a few dogs that present with neck or back pain, where even MRI (the most sensitive imaging modality at present) does not disclose a macroscopic lesion. What is unknown is how many of these patients have false negative studies (i.e., there is, in fact, a disc displacement that was missed by the imaging or by the interpretation of the images) versus how many are found to have a specific cause for signs that is unrelated to disc disease/degeneration (e.g., where spinal fluid analysis reveals changes that suggest primary inflammation of the meninges or spinal cord parenchyma). Moreover, the clinical signs of neck or back pain that we as veterinarians use to deduce the *symptoms* being experienced by our patients (which they are unable to communicate subjectively) leave open the possibility that, for some of the patients we diagnose with neck or back pain, we are looking in the wrong place. All together, there will be very few, if any, cases where (a) we are absolutely sure the patient has neck or back pain, (b) we are absolutely

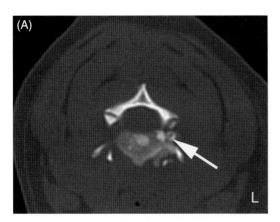
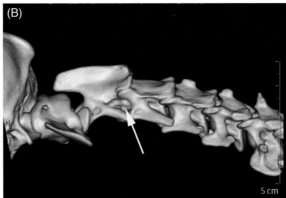

Figure 14.1   (A) Transverse CT image of a laterally herniated intervertebral disc (arrow) within the intervertebral foramen. The extruded disc causes nerve root compression (radiculopathy) but not spinal cord compression (i.e., no myelopathy) and would be undetectable with myelography. (B) Three-dimensional reconstruction from CT images of the cervical spine of a dog with severe neck pain. The arrow points to the lateral (foraminal) disc extrusion corresponding to the transverse image in (A). Absent such advanced imaging techniques, this dog might otherwise have been wrongly concluded to have been suffering from "discogenic pain."

sure that the imaging study is negative, and (c) we have ruled out all other causes for the clinical signs of pain we have identified. Only in those instances could we begin to consider the potential of "discogenic" pain, and even then, there may be a greater likelihood that we have missed a displacement lesion or other cause.

In conclusion, there is scant anatomic basis for diagnosing "discogenic" pain in dogs, and very few dogs with signs of neck or back pain related to disc disease will not have detectable signs of disc displacement. And in those few dogs that seem to defy this, we should be far more suspicious of our diagnostic accuracy than we should be of ascribing signs to discogenic pain. However, we should remain open to the possibility that, for some dogs, the degenerative process within a disc or discs may result in limited but significant impingement on the annulus or adjacent structures (e.g., dorsal longitudinal ligament) that possess nociceptive innervation and thus cause some degree of symptomatic discomfort.

References

1. Forsythe WB, Ghoshal NG. Innervation of the canine thoracolumbar vertebral column. Anat Rec. 1984 Jan;208(1):57–63.
2. Adams MA, Roughley PJ. What is intervertebral disc degeneration, and what causes it? Spine (Phila Pa 1976). 2006 Aug 15;31(18):2151–61.
3. Roughley PJ, Melching LI, Heathfield TF, Pearce RH, Mort JS. The structure and degradation of aggrecan in human intervertebral disc. Eur Spine J. 2006 Aug;15(Suppl 3):S326–32.
4. Bogduk N, Tynan W, Wilson AS. The nerve supply to the human lumbar intervertebral discs. J Anat. 1981 Jan;132(Pt 1):39–56.
5. Bogduk N, Windsor M, Inglis A. The innervation of the cervical intervertebral discs. Spine (Phila Pa 1976). 1988 Jan;13(1):2–8.
6. Coppes MH, Marani E, Thomeer RT, Oudega M, Groen GJ. Innervation of annulus fibrosis in low back pain. Lancet. 1990 Jul 21;336(8708):189–90.
7. Horackova L, Malinovsky L. Sensory innervation of the intervertebral joints in man. Folia Morphol (Praha). 1987;35(4):390–5.
8. Taylor JR, Twomey LT. Innervation of lumbar intervertebral discs. Med J Aust. 1979 Dec 29;2(13):701–2.
9. Willenegger S, Friess AE, Lang J, Stoffel MH. Immunohistochemical demonstration of lumbar intervertebral disc innervation in the dog. Anat Histol Embryol. 2005 Apr;34(2):123–8.
10. Simmons JW, Fraser RD. The rise and fall of chemonucleolysis. Arthrosc Endosc Spinal Surg. 2005;4: 351–8.
11. Simmons JW, Nordby EJ, Hadjipavlou AG. Chemonucleolysis: the state of the art. Eur Spine J. 2001 Jun;10(3):192–202.
12. Taylor TK, Ghosh P, Melrose J. Chemonucleolysis: a further look at a contentious issue. Med J Aust. 1990 Nov 19;153(10):575–8.
13. Melrose J, Taylor TK, Ghosh P, Holbert C, Macpherson C, Bellenger CR. Intervertebral disc reconstitution after chemonucleolysis with chymopapain is dependent on dosage. Spine (Phila Pa 1976). 1996 Jan 1;21(1):9–17.
14. Melrose J, Hall A, Macpherson C, Bellenger CR, Ghosh P. Evaluation of digestive proteinases from the Antarctic krill Euphasia superba as potential chemonucleolytic agents. In vitro and in vivo studies. Arch Orthop Trauma Surg. 1995;114(3):145–52.
15. Coppes MH, Marani E, Thomeer RT, Groen GJ. Innervation of "painful" lumbar discs. Spine (Phila Pa 1976). 1997 Oct 15;22(20):2342–9; discussion 9–50.
16. Freemont AJ, Peacock TE, Goupille P, Hoyland JA, O'Brien J, Jayson MI. Nerve ingrowth into diseased intervertebral disc in chronic back pain. Lancet. 1997 Jul 19;350(9072):178–81.
17. Freemont AJ, Watkins A, Le Maitre C, Baird P, Jeziorska M, Knight MT, et al. Nerve growth factor expression and innervation of the painful intervertebral disc. J Pathol. 2002 Jul;197(3):286–92.
18. Bagley RS, Tucker R, Harrington ML. Lateral and foraminal disk extrusion in dogs. Compend Contin Educ Pract Vet. 1996;18:795–805.
19. Felts JF, Prata RG. Cervical disk disease in the dog: Intraforaminal and lateral extrusions. J Am Anim Hosp Assoc. 1983;19:755–60.

15

Compressive and Contusive Spinal Cord Injury Secondary to Intervertebral Disc Displacement: A Clinical Perspective

James M. Fingeroth, Franck Forterre, and Jonathan M. Levine

When confronted with a patient with signs thought to be attributable to displacement of an intervertebral disc (IVD), one has to consider a range of prognostic and therapeutic possibilities. It can be helpful for clinicians to consider what is transpiring at the level of the spinal cord and how the interaction of the displaced disc with the spinal cord might influence the observed clinical signs and the utility/urgency of possible interventions.

For the purposes of simplification, we can consider *compressive spinal cord injury* (SCI) to represent spinal cord *deformation* and *shifting* from its normal position within the vertebral canal. *Contusive SCI*, on the other hand, is the actual *disruption of parenchyma* (neuronal cell bodies, axons, glial cells, myelin, and microvasculature) within the substance of the spinal cord. A simplified formula summarizes the primary (mechanical) events that occur in disc-associated SCI:

$$SCI = x \times compression + y \times contusion$$

where x and y are the relative contributions of mechanisms to SCI and $x + y = 100\%$.

While there is clearly going to be some overlap between these processes when an IVD displaces and contacts the spinal cord, it can be instructive to consider them as somewhat distinct entities for the purposes of clinical decision making. It is important to recognize that following compression or contusion, a series of secondary biochemical processes occurs including inflammation, oxidative stress, vascular events, and neurohormonal changes. Surgical intervention is best thought of as a means to relieve ongoing compressive SCI, which may in turn reduce the progression of these secondary mechanisms.

Seminal experimental studies by Tarlov and others demonstrated how slowly applied compression (such as inflation of an epidurally placed balloon catheter) would result in a predictable pattern of neurologic dysfunction and how, equally or more importantly, deflation of such catheters and thus "decompression" resulted in a predictable pattern of neurologic recovery [1]. We have long recognized this clinically, with many literature references establishing how paralyzed dogs will first recover normal nociception followed by recovery of motor function in the affected limbs

Advances in Intervertebral Disc Disease in Dogs and Cats, First Edition. Edited by James M. Fingeroth and William B. Thomas.
© 2015 ACVS Foundation. Published 2015 by John Wiley & Sons, Inc.

and finally fine motor skills and coordination [2, 3]. These experimental studies and clinical experience demonstrate that discomfort may be the first or only sign of disc displacement, followed by proprioceptive loss and ataxia, then paresis or paralysis, and finally loss of nociception.

The main deleterious effect of spinal cord compression (deformation/displacement) is **demyelination**, without transection of neurons or blood vessels [4]. Compression causes relative ischemia, and this ischemia, in turn, is responsible for the failure to maintain myelin coating on neurons [5, 6]. The axons and cell bodies themselves are more resistant to this relative level of ischemia, so are less affected.

While dwell time (the duration of compression) can be a factor in the severity of signs and the eventual development of intraparenchymal lesions beyond demyelination, we know that patients with even long-standing spinal cord compression, when it is slowly applied, can have complete and often rapid recovery once decompression is achieved [4, 7, 8]. Myelin serves as an "insulator" that helps speed electrical impulse conduction along the axon. After demyelination, conduction block might occur leading to paresis or even paralysis. Recovery occurs rapidly (within a few weeks) by restoration of continuous conduction prior to the return of saltatory conduction. This may be best illustrated in the clinical setting in animals with slow growing, extramedullary spinal cord tumors. In some cases, the spinal cord can be compressed down to a thin crescent, yet patients may have modest neurological deficits, and rapid improvement once the tumor has been excised. So, the take-home message is that **pure compression can be tolerated to an extraordinary degree by the spinal cord (especially when applied slowly), either producing minimal clinical signs (such as discomfort alone—usually due to nerve root compression/ischemia) or a predictable and gradual loss and then recovery of function.**

Contusive SCI, on the other hand, is internal disruption of the parenchyma *with or without* any associated compression. In addition to myelin disruption, there is actual compromise of the structural integrity of the spinal cord, including necrosis. Since the repair capabilities of the spinal cord are limited (see Chapter 25), such damage implies more severe neurological deficit and a slower, perhaps less complete recovery (or no recovery at all) *regardless of treatment.*

When discs displace, they can obviously cause a combination of compression and contusive SCI. Even with advanced imaging, we cannot know with precision the degree of each and thus will always have some uncertainty with respect to appropriate intervention. However, there are clues we can discern based on the history, clinical signs, and imaging studies that allow us to at least decide whether compression or contusion predominates, and thus help decide on a treatment strategy and prognosis. For example, it is intuitive and likely that a patient that develops signs gradually (over hours, days or longer) and, where those signs fit the pattern of initial discomfort followed by ataxia or proprioceptive loss and finally weakness, is much more likely to be suffering the effects of compression than parenchymal injury. Conversely, a patient that becomes suddenly paraplegic or tetraplegic within seconds or minutes may be more likely to have some degree of spinal cord contusion. The key tool for discrimination is spinal cord imaging (see Chapter 16) whereby the amount of compression (or lack thereof) can be ascertained, and that information is added to the clinical features (severity of deficits and onset of signs) to posit a mental construct of what is occurring at the level of the spinal cord. MR signal changes within the spinal cord (increased T2 signal) may be associated with contusion and have been shown to be a negative prognostic indicator in the setting of IVD herniation independent of physical examination based evaluation. Interestingly, no correlation between compressive indices and long-term outcome has been identified [9].

Clinicians must always bear in mind that **surgery for IVD herniation is, regardless of the nuances of particular technique, generally limited in therapeutic value to spinal cord decompression**. And, equally important, such decompression is only achieved when a deforming mass (disc, tumor, bone fragment, etc.) is effectively removed and the dural tube (with the enclosed spinal cord) is returned to its normal position and configuration. As noted in Chapters 9, 13, 28, and 33, there is minimal to no decompressive or other positive therapeutic effects to simple bone removal or durotomy when there is internal SCI. We cannot yet repair spinal cords with surgery. So, the basis for recommending surgery is the demonstration of spinal cord compression and the belief that the contusive component is not so severe as to preclude a beneficial effect from decompression. The latter is not always knowable (especially when clinical deficits are very severe, such as patients with apparent loss of nociception caudal to their lesion), but unless there is at least *some* degree of compression present, it is fair to conclude that surgery would not likely be helpful for a patient where imaging discloses no macroscopic extradural compressive lesion.

What determines the relative degrees of compression and contusion when a disc herniates?

The herniation of an IVD is governed by the Newtonian laws of physics. The herniated portion of the disc has mass, and it impacts the spinal cord with certain velocity. The kinetic energy delivered to the spinal cord can thus be defined as $\frac{1}{2}mV^2$, where m is the mass and V the velocity (or the force of the herniation can be defined as mA, mass times acceleration). We can further conclude that the greater the bolus of kinetic energy or force delivered to the spinal cord, the greater the risk for and degree of parenchymal injury [10, 11]. Therefore, when one considers the patient presented with signs attributable to suspected IVD herniation, one should consider the mass and velocity components of the equation, bearing in mind that the velocity component predominates because its value is *squared*.

The clinical implications of this concept are profound. For example, if one imagines a large mass of disc that herniates with close to zero velocity/acceleration, the resultant kinetic energy and force will also be close to zero. A patient so affected might be expected to have very modest signs (perhaps only some discomfort due to nerve root compression) and no other deficits despite severe spinal cord compression. This is exactly analogous to the prior examples of slowly applied compression from a balloon or tumor ("slowly" being the semantic equivalent of a low velocity). This concept is important to bear in mind as it demonstrates that **there may be no correlation between the size of the mass (i.e., degree of compression) and the severity of signs in dogs**. It is often seen in the clinical setting where patients with, say, severe and chronic neck pain are treated for prolonged times with conservative, nonsurgical methods because the clinician was under the misapprehension that such modest signs indicated that there was minimal compression to be

concerned about and thus no justification for considering imaging or surgery. This is also seen in thoracolumbar disc herniations where the patient is ambulatory and has minimal neurologic deficits, but imaging demonstrates marked spinal cord compression. Conversely, a minute fragment of disc (low mass) ejected at high velocity will deliver a huge bolus of energy and force to the spinal cord (perhaps resulting in focal myelomalacia), and yet there will be no compressive element for which surgery could play a role in treatment. These are so-called noncompressive discs described elsewhere (Chapters 4, 6, 9, and 13). Further, the degenerative state of the disc may also play a role in the pathophysiology of the lesion. It can be expected that a nondegenerated disc in which higher pressures are exerted will mainly lead to a severe contusion when extruding. Its high water content will also lead to its rapid distribution within the spinal canal without severe spinal cord compression. It is also apparent how two patients, presented with identical neurological examinations and deficits, can have very different outcomes regardless of treatment.

In conclusion, prognostication and therapeutic recommendations for patients with suspected IVD herniation can largely be based on a careful consideration of the onset of clinical signs, the severity of those signs, the degree of spinal cord compression (and bearing in mind that the latter can only be defined by imaging, and **not** based on the severity of signs), consideration of estimated mass and indirect signs indicating high velocity of the disc herniation (high T2 signal with minimal compression), and theoretical envisioning of the degree to which spinal cord compression vs. spinal cord contusion is contributing to the observed signs.

In recent studies, a supplementary epidural inflammatory role has been attributed to the herniated disc itself. This finding would modify the initial formula to

$$SCI = x \times compression + y \times contusion + z \times inflammation$$

where, x, y, and z are the percentile values of SCI and $x + y + z = 100\%$.

How far this finding may influence the decision-making process for therapy in dogs is actually unknown and has to be elucidated in the future.

References

1. Tarlov IM, Klinger H, Vitale S. Spinal cord compression studies. I. Experimental techniques to produce acute and gradual compression. AMA Arch Neurol Psychiatr. 1953 Dec;70(6):813–9.
2. Olby N, Levine J, Harris T, Munana K, Skeen T, Sharp N. Long-term functional outcome of dogs with severe injuries of the thoracolumbar spinal cord: 87 cases (1996–2001). J Am Vet Med Assoc. 2003 Mar 15;222(6):762–9.
3. Olby N, Harris T, Burr J, Munana K, Sharp N, Keene B. Recovery of pelvic limb function in dogs following acute intervertebral disc herniations. J Neurotrauma. 2004 Jan;21(1):49–59.
4. Delamarter RB, Sherman J, Carr JB. Pathophysiology of spinal cord injury. Recovery after immediate and delayed decompression. J Bone Joint Surg Am. 1995 Jul;77(7):1042–9.
5. Griffiths IR, Trench JG, Crawford RA. Spinal cord blood flow and conduction during experimental cord compression in normotensive and hypotensive dogs. J Neurosurg. 1979;50:353–63.
6. Malik Y, Spreng D, Konar M, Doherr MG, Jaggy A, Howard J, et al. Laser-Doppler measurements of spinal cord blood flow changes during hemilaminectomy in chondrodystrophic dogs with disk extrusion. Vet Surg. 2009 Jun;38(4):457–62.
7. Lonjon N, Kouyoumdjian P, Prieto M, Bauchet L, Haton H, Gaviria M, et al. Early functional outcomes and histological analysis after spinal cord compression injury in rats. J Neurosurg Spine. 2010 Jan;12(1):106–13.
8. Swartz KR, Scheff NN, Roberts KN, Fee DB. Exacerbation of spinal cord injury due to static compression occurring early after onset. J Neurosurg Spine. 2009;11:570–4.
9. Levine JM, Fosgate GT, Chen AV, Rushing R, Nghiem PP, Platt SR, et al. Magnetic resonance imaging in dogs with neurologic impairment due to acute thoracic and lumbar intervertebral disk herniation. J Vet Intern Med. 2009 Nov–Dec;23(6):1220–6.
10. Brasso DM, Beattie MS, Breshnahan JC. Graded histological and locomotor outcomes after spinal cord contusion using the NYU weight-drop device versus transection. Exp Neurol. 1996;139:244–56.
11. Rosenzweig ES, McDonald JW. Rodent models for treatment of spinal cord injury: research trends and progress toward useful repair. Curr Opin Neurol. 2004 Apr;17(2):121–31.

16 Advances in Imaging for Intervertebral Disc Disease

Patrick R. Gavin and Jonathan M. Levine

Introduction

As pointed out elsewhere in this text, diagnostic imaging is a necessary step for establishing the cause and options for treatment in all animals with clinical signs consistent with vertebral column pathology. In regard to imaging for suspected intervertebral disc herniation (IVDH), approaches vary depending on whether medical or surgical therapy is deemed most likely. It is critical for clinicians making imaging decisions to understand the limitations of various modalities. For example, radiography is a good, cost-effective screening tool. However, it is not adequate to diagnose IVDH definitively, does not provide sufficient information for planning decompressive surgery, and does not permit imaging of the actual spinal cord.

There are various imaging modalities employed for dogs and cats with suspected IVDH. These are reviewed in the following in their order of historical appearance and ascending order of preference. Reviewed elsewhere in this text is the subject of discography for direct imaging of the intervertebral discs (see Chapter 26).

Radiography

Conventional radiography became widely available in the 1950s and 1960s in the veterinary profession. During this time period, radiography was commonly used to definitively diagnose IVDH [1–3]. Currently, many clinicians use vertebral radiography as a means to help exclude diseases such as overt osseous neoplasia, vertebral fracture/luxation, and discospondylitis [4]. The sensitivity of radiographs for detecting vertebral fracture/luxation and discospondylitis approximates 75 and 80%, respectively [5, 6]. Vertebral radiography has relatively poor accuracy for identifying sites of surgical IVDH in the thoracic and even less so in the cervical vertebral column [7, 8]. Additionally, it does not permit the reliable differentiation of multisite IVDH from single-site lesions [9].

Careful attention to positioning and coned-down views to reduce parallax of the image in orthogonal projections facilitate the diagnosis of vertebral column diseases. Accurate positioning requires heavy sedation or general anesthesia.

Advances in Intervertebral Disc Disease in Dogs and Cats, First Edition. Edited by James M. Fingeroth and William B. Thomas.

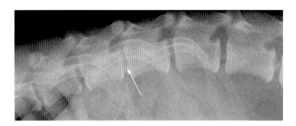

Figure 16.1 Lateral radiograph. Intervertebral disc narrowing at T12–T13. Arrow indicates the narrowed space. Any opacification of the intervertebral foramina is difficult to judge due to superimposition of the rib. It must be remembered that discs can herniate laterally and ventrally as well as dorsally and narrowed disc spaces cannot be used alone as a determinant of the cause for the animal's clinical signs.

Even with this effort, plain film radiography has been shown to be inaccurate and subject to marked interobserver variation. Radiography can demonstrate increased opacification of discs and in some cases can demonstrate opacified disc material superimposed within the vertebral canal (Figure 16.1). However, the spinal cord and spinal nerves cannot be visualized, thus making it impossible to conclude if there is actual disc herniation resulting in neural compression. While disc space narrowing and collapse of the diarthrodial joints can be identified in some instances, and might possibly be related to underlying IVDD at that level, this radiographic change can be spurious or misleading. Improper positioning can lead to artifactual "narrowing" of disc spaces, and there can be no certainty that any such lesion, even if real (i.e., correlated with disc degeneration at that level), corresponds to the lesion that is responsible for the current clinical signs in the patient that has prompted the imaging investigation in the first place. Hence, plain radiography is neither particularly sensitive nor specific when trying to confirm a diagnosis of disc disease or herniation, and generally cannot be relied on for surgical planning.

Myelography

In the 1970s, nonionic iodinated contrast agents were developed. These contrast agents facilitated the use of myelography in the dog. Prior to the nonionic contrast agents, iodinated lipid agents were used in human patients. Due to the small subarachnoid space in dogs and cats, these contrast agents were not useful in veterinary patients.

However, the water-soluble nonionic contrast agents were an improvement over plain film radiography [10].

Myelography requires general anesthesia and a degree of skill in the placement of the material within the subarachnoid space. While the atlanto-occipital region (cisterna magna or cerebellomedullary junction) is the easiest place to access the subarachnoid space, most radiologists favor the use of a low lumbar puncture at L5–L6. Cervical puncture requires gravity to distribute the contrast agent along the vertebral column, and swelling of the spinal cord can stop the advancement of the contrast agent before it can demonstrate the level of the actual lesion. A caudal lumbar injection allows pressure to be used to enhance the flow of the material cranially, although this can still be stymied by the presence of severe spinal cord swelling and/or extradural compression. In some instances where flow is blocked subarachnoid injections of contrast can be made both from the cervical end and lumbar end. However, when there is substantial spinal cord swelling, this may still fail to demonstrate the specific site of the lesion, and might only reveal a zone of several segments where contrast cannot be seen. Injection from both ends also increases the total dose of contrast, which could result in higher complication rates (such as seizures). In such instances, the radiologist and surgeon usually interpolate the approximate center of this zone and hypothesize that this is the likely level of disc herniation. Alternatively, discography could be used to try and determine the precise level of the herniation lesion (see Chapter 26) [11]. Another limitation with myelography, especially in those cases where the contrast does not opacify the subarachnoid space at the level of the lesion, is that it may not be possible to determine which side of the vertebral canal the disc material is predominantly lying on [12–14]. This hampers the surgeon from knowing with assurance which side to approach for hemilaminectomy (see Chapter 31). When there is such a multisegmental zone of absent contrast, it is also important to observe whether there is any evidence of contrast centrally, within the area where the spinal cord itself should be lying, and interpret the myelogram in light of clinical deficits, since some of these cases could represent a dog with widespread myelomalacia (see Chapter 12).

Another drawback to myelography occurs when the imager is having difficulty accessing the

L5–L6 subarachnoid space, either being unable to inject it at all or having only a portion of the contrast actually produce a myelogram, while the balance produces a nonuseful and confounding epidurogram. This sometimes prompts the imager to attempt lumbar puncture at a higher level (e.g., L4–L5 or even L3–L4), and this can result in significant spinal cord trauma and worsened neurologic deficits.

While the newer contrast agents offered a large improvement in safety and reduced toxicity, problems still exist with myelography, where the invasive nature of the procedure could result in spinal cord damage. Myelography is limited to the same orthogonal projections as radiographs (with some oblique views being helpful) [15], and myelography only demonstrates the subarachnoid space and not the spinal cord tissues themselves (Figures 16.2 and 16.3). Complications include seizures (especially with cervical injections) and poor studies due to epidural contamination with the contrast agent, failure to access the subarachnoid space, and the aforementioned problems associated with spinal cord swelling and failure of contrast to fill the area of the spinal cord lesion [16].

Computed tomography

Computed tomography (CT) started to become available to the veterinary profession in the 1980s and currently has widespread acceptance. CT offered improved visualization of tissues due to the ability to manipulate the contrast windows and levels. In chondrodystrophoid dogs, disc extrusions are often mineralized. Plain CT can detect this mineralized disc material as well as hemorrhage in the vertebral canal (Figures 16.4 and 16.5) [17]. It is common practice in some hospitals to perform CT on chondrodystrophoid dogs suspected of having an intervertebral disc extrusion [18]. In many cases, disc-associated spinal cord compressive lesions are readily identified. With the advent of helical scanning, the procedure can be extremely rapid. The study can be reconstructed in multiple planes, improving conspicuity [19]. However, nonmineralized disc

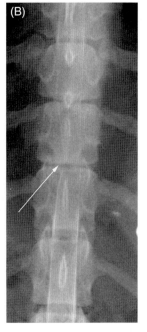

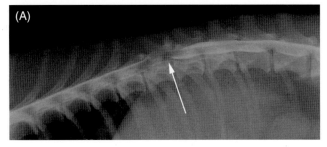

Figure 16.2   (A) Contrast myelogram. An extradural lesion is seen in the ventral vertebral canal displacing the ventral subarachnoid column and thinning the dorsal subarachnoid column. The arrow indicates the site at T11–T12. (B) Ventrodorsal view of the myelogram of the same patient. The narrowness of the intervertebral disc space on this ventrodorsal film can be seen to be more right sided.

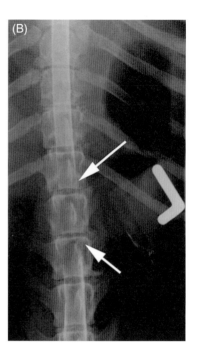

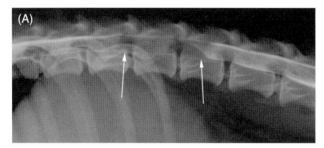

Figure 16.3 (A) Sagittal myelogram. (B) Ventrodorsal myelogram. Area of subarachnoid space that is thinned but no definitive extradural compression can be seen (between the white arrows). Thin columns go from caudal T13 to cranial L2 (arrows). Extradural compressions cannot be seen. The spinal cord is obviously not visible. Cause of the thin columns cannot be ascertained.

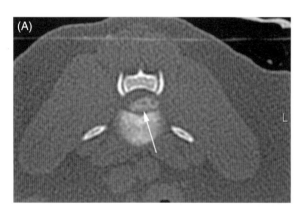
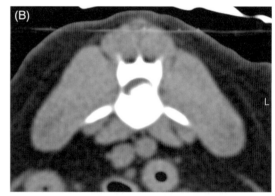

Figure 16.4 Transverse CT. (A) Bone window. (B) Soft tissue window. High-opacity material (arrow) can be seen in the ventral left vertebral canal (arrow) and compressing the spinal cord. Measuring the density of the material may help indicate the presence of mineralized material versus hemorrhage, but at times, there is overlap between the two tissue densities depending on the degree of mineralization.

extrusions may not be identified. The reported accuracy of noncontrast CT for identifying IVDH in the thoracolumbar vertebral column is roughly equivalent to myelography across several recent studies [18, 20, 21]. CT does appear to more accurately determine the side of disc-associated compression compared to myelography.

CT myelography

The combination of myelography and CT yields an improved diagnostic capability [22–25]. Change in the subarachnoid space can be seen in the absence of mineralized or hemorrhagic material within the vertebral canal. Nonopaque changes to

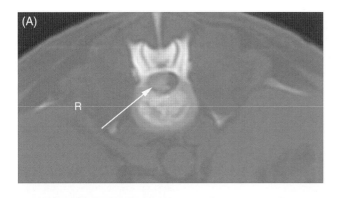

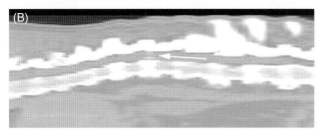

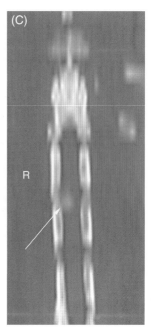

Figure 16.5 (A) CT showing opaque material in the right parasagittal vertebral canal causing spinal cord compression. Arrow points to the opaque material. (B) Sagittal reconstruction of CT in (A). Again, the arrow points to the compressive material. (C) Dorsal reconstruction showing the compressive material in the right vertebral canal (arrow). By using various images of this reconstruction, the location, in comparison to the last pair of ribs, is easily ascertained.

the epidural, dural, or intramedullary regions may be detected via myelography. It is common practice in many institutions that if the plain CT is nondiagnostic, then it will be followed by a CT myelogram. While there is improved conspicuity, the same toxic problems and other complications associated with myelography exist with CT myelography (Figure 16.6).

In an attempt to identify more paraspinal disease and vertebral disease, some hospitals augment CT myelography with injection of an intravenous contrast agent for improved visualization of paravertebral lesions and vertebral disorders [26].

Magnetic resonance imaging

Magnetic resonance imaging (MRI) became more available in the beginning of the twenty-first century. It is widely accepted that MRI has improved visualization of spinal disease [27–53]. The ability to see the intervertebral discs, vertebrae, vertebral canal, nerve roots, and spinal cord is unmatched by the other modalities.

Paravertebral tissues are readily visualized. A myelogram appearance can be obtained from manipulation of the imaging sequence and the subarachnoid columns can be readily displayed without the need for any injection into the subarachnoid space. Gadolinium-based paramagnetic contrast agents can be used in some cases to provide information about the vascularity of the spinal disease and to help distinguish intervertebral disc-induced lesions from other causes [54]. A recent study found MRI to be more sensitive than CT (98.5% vs. 88.6%, respectively) and more accurate for identifying the site of thoracolumbar IVDH in dogs [55].

On occasion, MRI cannot be used due to the presence of a pacemaker, vascular coil (such as those sometimes used for closure of a patent ductus arteriosus), or a magnetic material present within the tissues. Metallic agents that can cause problems include BBs and the wire associated with identification microchips [56]. While imaging patients with metal implants such as stainless steel orthopedic devices, BBs or microchips will cause no harm to the patient, it may create an artifact that prevents proper

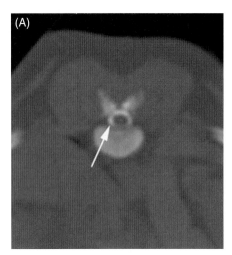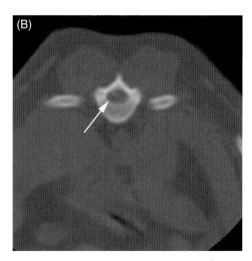

Figure 16.6   (A) Myelogram CT. The subarachnoid columns are normal. Arrow indicates normal subarachnoid column with iodine contrast. (B) There is loss of the columns and there appears to be material of low signal intensity in the ventral right spinal canal. There may be numerous causes for this, including tumors, non-mineralized disc material, hemorrhage, and other causes. The arrow points to the material in the ventral right spinal canal and the thinned displaced subarachnoid column.

visualization of the spine and spinal cord. The offending material can be removed, or at times just displaced with skin manipulation, to a satisfactory degree to allow imaging. Titanium implants are generally compatible with MRI and do not cause loss of signal artifact as seen with stainless steel implants.

Due to the time required for MRI, general anesthesia is needed for animal patients. However, the improved visualization of the tissues, improved safety, and decreased morbidity when compared to the other available modalities dictate that magnetic resonance is the clear preference for spinal imaging. If MRI is not available, then CT myelography, myelography, or radiography, as available, could be used with the aforementioned limitations. At this time, and in many locations, MRI is readily or increasingly available and should preferentially be utilized for spinal imaging whenever possible.

The magnetic resonance sequences are numerous and there is no single method applicable in each case. Various protocols can be devised for different patient subsets, and based on the magnet strength of the machine being used. For the typical chondrodystrophic or small-breed patient with an acute thoracolumbar myelopathy, the imaging may consist of the MR myelogram, T2-weighted images in the sagittal and transverse planes, and a T1 or other

coronal (dorsal plane) images for correct vertebral count [57, 58]. Such a study can be done in 20 min or less with the proper magnet and a skilled MR technologist (Figure 16.7) [59]. In other cases where the differential diagnosis beyond IVDH is much broader initially, sequences would include MR myelograms, T2-weighted images, short-tau inversion recovery (STIR) sequences, and possibly T1-weighted images before and after intravenous gadolinium contrast agent administration (Figure 16.8) [60, 61]. One complication to MR is the need to limit the field of view to a specific zone. In patients where the neurolocalization is no more specific than "T3–L3 segments" (see Chapter 10), this might require two separate studies (depending on the size of the patient) in order to image the entire area of interest. This can result in longer anesthetic times and higher costs. This potential problem is only exacerbated when there is concern or suspicion for both cervical and (thoraco)lumbar lesions, and the entire vertebral column needs to be evaluated.

MR myelograms are heavily T2 weighted to allow the visualization of only fluid. These can be acquired in numerous ways, either as one thick slab or as multiple slices, and then reconstructed using a maximum intensity projection (MIP). In either case, a volume image is obtained. T2-weighted images are generally preferable

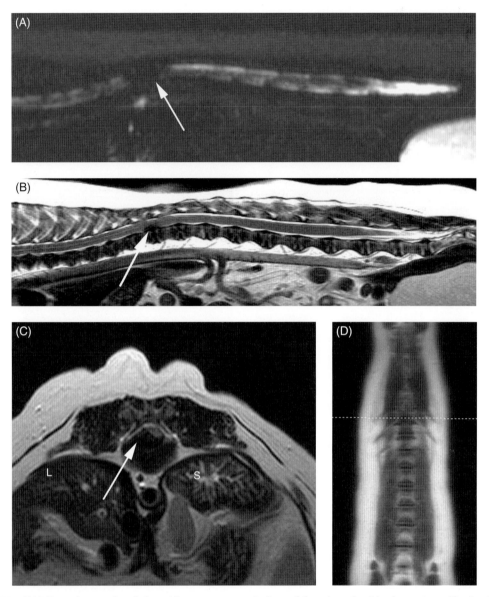

Figure 16.7   (A) MR myelogram. Small dog with acute paraparesis. Loss of the subarachnoid columns is readily visualized on the MR myelogram. This procedure takes less than 1 min to obtain. (B) T2 sagittal there appears to be a disc extrusion at T11–12, assuming a normal 7 lumbar vertebrae. The material is more right-sided on (C), T2 transverse, with the material in the ventral and right parasagittal spinal canal causing marked compression of the spinal cord. Arrow points to the low signal intense extruded disc material. (D) It is a dorsal plane scout image. The line is the site of the previous transverse image of (C). This confirmed that the disc extrusion is at T11–12.

over T1-weighted images for the detection of spinal cord disease in small animal patients. The increased intensity of the subarachnoid fluid on T2-weighting facilitates diagnosis [62]. T1-weighted images may provide better visualization of the vertebrae and on occasion, better visualization of the abnormality, but it is uncommon for T1-weighting to increase conspicuity. Contrast agents may be helpful in some cases, but in most cases of IVDH, contrast agents are not needed and may only cause confusion in the diagnosis.

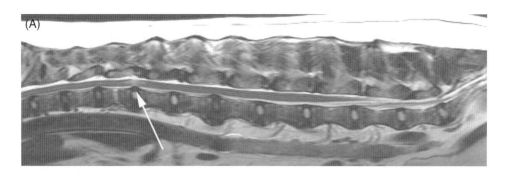

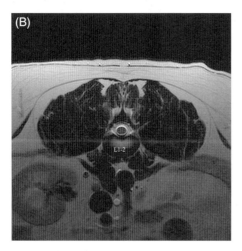

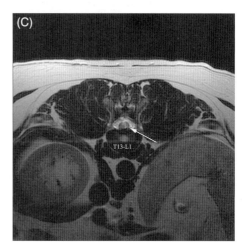

Figure 16.8   (A) Dog has suffered an acute paraparesis. Dog is nonpainful now. Arrow points to elevation of the annulus at T13-L1, assuming a normal seven lumbar vertebrae. There is increased signal intensity to the spinal cord immediately above this site. (B) The disc space caudal to this at L1-2 appears normal. Notice the large amount of nucleus pulposus present above the label. (C) T13-L1 disc space—notice the small amount of nucleus pulposus. Arrow points to an increased signal intensity to the spinal cord that is intramedullary. Also notice the epidural space has an amorphous material, presumably hemorrhage. This is a classic appearance of a noncompressive disc extrusion.

A T2* sequence may help in the detection and confirmation of hemorrhage [63]. Some favor the use of a fluid attenuation and inversion recovery (FLAIR) sequence for the confirmation that the abnormality seen on T2- and T1-weighted images are consistent with cerebrospinal fluid and not another disease process. Use of MR myelograms removes the necessity for FLAIR sequences (Figure 16.9).

Conclusion

There has been a major shift in the imaging of intervertebral disc disease with ever-increasing improvement in the diagnosis, which is leading to improved therapies and clinical outcomes. MRI is the only technique that allows direct visualization of the spinal cord while still imaging the subarachnoid and epidural spaces, the vertebrae, and the intervertebral discs. CT and CT myelography have been a large improvement over plain radiography and myelography [64]. Both MRI and CT reduce the risk of incorrectly identifying the side of disc herniation in cases that are not strictly midline, and this is especially valuable to surgeons who typically prefer a unilateral (hemilaminectomy or pediculectomy) approach to the vertebral canal. Only MRI visualizes the noncompressive disc extrusions with associated spinal cord contusions (see Chapters 9, 13, and 15), and only MRI can distinguish IVDH from spinal cord infarction (fibrocartilaginous embolism; see Chapter 9). Hence, this modality must be considered the gold standard at the present time [64].

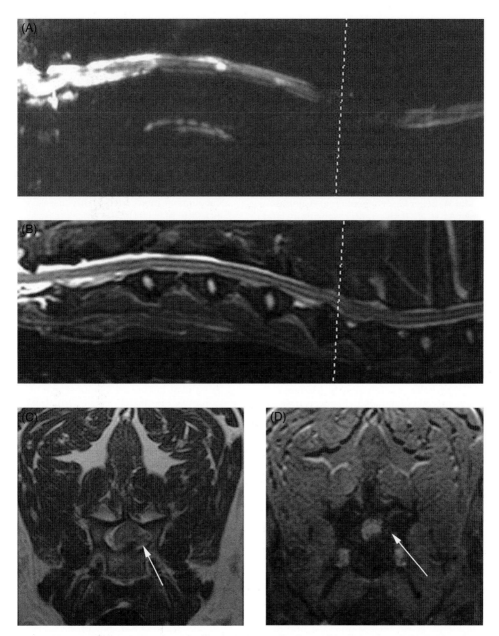

Figure 16.9   (A) MR myelogram of the cervical spine. Notice that there is loss of the subarachnoid columns in the caudal cervical region. (B) T2-weighted sagittal sequence. There is desiccation of the intervertebral discs at C5–C6 and C6–C7. The line indicates the site of the transverse images of (C) and (D). (C) T2 transverse image. There is material present in the left parasagittal vertebral canal that is similar in signal intensity to the spinal cord. (D) Gradient echo sequence, sensitive for magnetic inhomogeneities. The very low-signal intense material in the same area as seen on (C) is indicative of hemorrhage. This gradient echo sequence can be used to distinguish hemorrhage from other extradural material.

References

1. Hoerlein BF. Intervertebral disc protrusions in the dog. III. Radiological diagnosis. Am J Vet Res. 1953 Apr;14(51):275–86.
2. Lee R. Interpretation of radiographs: inter-vertebral disc lesions in the dog. J Small Anim Pract. 1973 Feb;14(2):111–2.
3. Lewis RE. Roentgen signs of the spine. Vet Clin North Am. 1974 Nov;4(4):647–61.
4. Bennett D, Carmichael S, Griffiths IR. Discospondylitis in the dog. J Small Anim Pract. 1981 Aug;22(8): 539–47.
5. Kinns J, Mai W, Seiler G, Zwingenberger A, Johnson V, Caceres A, et al. Radiographic sensitivity and negative predictive value for acute canine spinal trauma. Vet Radiol Ultrasound. 2006 Oct–Nov;47(6):563–70.
6. Carrera I, Sullivan M, McConnell F, Goncalves R. Magnetic resonance imaging features of discospondylitis in dogs. Vet Radiol Ultrasound. 2011 Mar–Apr;52(2):125–31.
7. Somerville ME, Anderson SM, Gill PJ, Kantrowitz BJ, Stowater JL. Accuracy of localization of cervical intervertebral disk extrusion or protrusion using survey radiography in dogs. J Am Anim Hosp Assoc. 2001 Nov–Dec;37(6):563–72.
8. Lamb CR, Nicholls A, Targett M, Mannion P. Accuracy of survey radiographic diagnosis of intervertebral disc protrusion in dogs. Vet Radiol Ultrasound. 2002 May–Jun;43(3):222–8.
9. Burk R. Problems in the radiographic interpretation of intervertebral disc disease in the dog. Probl Vet Med. 1988;1(3):381–401.
10. Morgan JP, Suter PF, Holliday TA. Myelography with water-soluble contrast medium. Radiographic interpretation of disc herniation in dogs. Acta Radiol Suppl. 1972;319:217–30.
11. Kahanovitz N, Arnoczky SP, Sissons HA, Steiner GC, Schwarez P. The effect of discography on the canine intervertebral disc. Spine (Phila Pa 1976). 1986 Jan–Feb;11(1):26–7.
12. Bos AS, Brisson BA, Holmberg DL, Nykamp SG. Use of the ventrodorsal myelographic view to predict lateralization of extruded disk material in small-breed dogs with thoracolumbar intervertebral disk extrusion: 104 cases (2004–2005). J Am Vet Med Assoc. 2007 Jun 15;230(12):1860–5.
13. Gibbons SE, Macias C, De Stefani A, Pinchbeck GL, McKee WM. The value of oblique versus ventrodorsal myelographic views for lesion lateralisation in canine thoracolumbar disc disease. J Small Anim Pract. 2006 Nov;47(11):658–62.
14. Schulz KS, Walker M, Moon M, Waldron D, Slater M, McDonald DE. Correlation of clinical, radiographic, and surgical localization of intervertebral disc extrusion in small-breed dogs: a prospective study of 50 cases. Vet Surg. 1998 Mar–Apr;27(2):105–11.
15. Tanaka H, Nakayama M, Takase K. Usefulness of myelography with multiple views in diagnosis of circumferential location of disc material in dogs with thoracolumbar intervertebral disc herniation. J Vet Med Sci. 2004 Jul;66(7):827–33.
16. Lexmaulova L, Zatloukal J, Proks P, Dvorak M, Srnec R, Rauser P, et al. Incidence of seizures associated with iopamidol or iomeprol myelography in dogs with intervertebral disk disease: 161 cases (2000–2002). J Vet Emerg Crit Care (San Antonio). 2009 Dec;19(6):611–6.
17. Lim C, Kweon OK, Choi MC, Choi J, Yoon J. Computed tomographic characteristics of acute thoracolumbar intervertebral disc disease in dogs. J Vet Sci. 2010 Mar;11(1):73–9.
18. Hecht S, Thomas WB, Marioni-Henry K, Echandi RL, Matthews AR, Adams WH. Myelography vs. computed tomography in the evaluation of acute thoracolumbar intervertebral disk extrusion in chondrodystrophic dogs. Vet Radiol Ultrasound. 2009 Jul–Aug;50(4):353–9.
19. King JB, Jones JC, Rossmeisl JH, Harper TA, Lanz OI, Werre SR. Effect of multi-planar CT image reformatting on surgeon diagnostic performance for localizing thoracolumbar disc extrusions in dogs. J Vet Sci. 2009;10(3):225–32.
20. Olby NJ, Munana KR, Sharp NJ, Thrall DE. The computed tomographic appearance of acute thoracolumbar intervertebral disc herniations in dogs. Vet Radiol Ultrasound. 2000 Sep–Oct;41(5):396–402.
21. Kuroki K, Vitale CL, Essman SC, Pithua P, Coates JR. Computed tomographic and histological findings of Hansen type I intervertebral disc herniation in dogs. Vet Comp Orthop Traumatol. 2013;26(5):379–84.
22. Kent M, Holmes S, Cohen E, Sakals S, Roach W, Platt S, et al. Imaging diagnosis-CT myelography in a dog with intramedullary intervertebral disc herniation. Vet Radiol Ultrasound. 2011 Mar–Apr;52(2):185–7.
23. Hara Y, Tagawa M, Ejima H, Orima H, Fujita M. Usefulness of computed tomography after myelography for surgery on dogs with cervical intervertebral disc protrusion. J Vet Med Sci. 1994 Aug;56(4): 791–4.
24. Jones JC, Inzana KD, Rossmeisl JH, Bergman RL, Wells T, Butler K. CT myelography of the thoracolumbar spine in 8 dogs with degenerative myelopathy. J Vet Sci. 2005 Dec;6(4):341–8.
25. Shimizu J, Yamada K, Mochida K, Kako T, Muroya N, Teratani Y, et al. Comparison of the diagnosis of intervertebral disc herniation in dogs by CT before and after contrast enhancement of the subarachnoid space. Vet Rec. 2009 Aug 15;165(7):200–2.
26. Schroeder R, Pelsue DH, Park RD, Gasso D, Bruecker KA. Contrast-enhanced CT for localizing compressive thoracolumbar intervertebral disc extrusion. J Am Anim Hosp Assoc. 2011 May–Jun;47(3):203–9.
27. Adamiak Z, Pomianowski A, Zhalniarovich Y, Kwiatkowska M, Jaskolska M, Bochenska A.

A comparison of magnetic resonance imaging sequences in evaluating pathological changes in the canine spinal cord. Pol J Vet Sci. 2011;14(3):481–4.

28. Amort KH, Ondreka N, Rudorf H, Stock KF, Distl O, Tellhelm B, et al. MR-imaging of lumbosacral intervertebral disc degeneration in clinically sound German shepherd dogs compared to other breeds. Vet Radiol Ultrasound. 2012 May–Jun;53(3):289–95.

29. Beltran E, Dennis R, Doyle V, de Stefani A, Holloway A, de Risio L. Clinical and magnetic resonance imaging features of canine compressive cervical myelopathy with suspected hydrated nucleus pulposus extrusion. J Small Anim Pract. 2012 Feb;53(2):101–7.

30. Bergknut N, Grinwis G, Pickee E, Auriemma E, Lagerstedt AS, Hagman R, et al. Reliability of macroscopic grading of intervertebral disk degeneration in dogs by use of the Thompson system and comparison with low-field magnetic resonance imaging findings. Am J Vet Res. 2011;72(7):899–904.

31. Besalti O, Pekcan Z, Sirin YS, Erbas G. Magnetic resonance imaging findings in dogs with thoracolumbar intervertebral disk disease: 69 cases (1997–2005). J Am Vet Med Assoc. 2006 Mar 15;228(6):902–8.

32. Chambers JN, Selcer BA, Sullivan SA, Coates JR. Diagnosis of lateralized lumbosacral disk herniation with magnetic resonance imaging. J Am Anim Hosp Assoc. 1997 Jul–Aug;33(4):296–9.

33. Chang Y, Dennis R, Platt SR, Penderis J. Magnetic resonance imaging of traumatic intervertebral disc extension in dogs. Vet Rec. 2007;160(23):795–9.

34. De Decker S, Gielen IMVL, Duchateau L, Polis I, Van Bree HJJ, Van Ham LML. Agreement and repeatability of linear vertebral body and canal measurements using computed tomography (CT) and low field magnetic resonance imaging (MRI). Vet Surg. 2010;39(1):28–34.

35. de Haan JJ, Shelton SB, Ackerman N. Magnetic resonance imaging in the diagnosis of degenerative lumbosacral stenosis in four dogs. Vet Surg. 1993 Jan–Feb;22(1):1–4.

36. De Risio L, Platt SR. Fibrocartilaginous embolic myelopathy in small animals. Vet Clin North Am Small Anim Pract. 2010 Sep;40(5):859–69.

37. Freeman AC, Platt SR, Kent M, Howerth E, Holmes SP. Magnetic resonance imaging enhancement of intervertebral disc disease in 30 dogs following chemical fat saturation. J Small Anim Pract. 2012 Feb;53(2):120–5.

38. Freeman P. Sacrococcygeal intervertebral disc extrusion in a dachshund. Vet Rec. 2010;167(16):618–9.

39. Forterre F, Gorgas D, Dickomeit M, Jaggy A, Lang J, Spreng D. Incidence of spinal compressive lesions in chondrodystrophic dogs with abnormal recovery after hemilaminectomy for treatment of thoracolumbar disc disease: a prospective magnetic resonance imaging study. Vet Surg. 2010 Feb;39(2):165–72.

40. Gambino J. What is your diagnosis? J Am Vet Med Assoc. 2010;236(11):1177–8.

41. Gendron K, Doherr MG, Gavin PR, Lang J. Magnetic resonance imaging characterization of vertebral endplate changes in the dog. Vet Radiol Ultrasound. 2012;53(1):50–6.

42. Gonzalo-Orden JM, Altonaga JR, Orden MA, Gonzalo JM. Magnetic resonance, computed tomographic and radiologic findings in a dog with discospondylitis. Vet Radiol Ultrasound. 2000 Mar–Apr;41(2):142–4.

43. Grunenfelder FI, Weishaupt D, Green R, Steffen F. Magnetic resonance imaging findings in spinal cord infarction in three small breed dogs. Vet Radiol Ultrasound. 2005 Mar–Apr;46(2):91–6.

44. Ito D, Matsunaga S, Jeffery ND, Sasaki N, Nishimura R, Mochizuki M, et al. Prognostic value of magnetic resonance imaging in dogs with paraplegia caused by thoracolumbar intervertebral disk extrusion: 77 cases (2000–2003). J Am Vet Med Assoc. 2005 Nov 1;227(9):1454–60.

45. Konar M, Lang J, Fluhmann G, Forterre F. Ventral intraspinal cysts associated with the intervertebral disc: magnetic resonance imaging observations in seven dogs. Vet Surg. 2008 Jan;37(1):94–101.

46. Kraft SL, Mussman JM, Smith T, Biller DS, Hoskinson JJ. Magnetic resonance imaging of presumptive lumbosacral discospondylitis in a dog. Vet Radiol Ultrasound. 1998 Jan–Feb;39(1):9–13.

47. Lawson CM, Reichle JK, McKlveen T, Smith MO. Imaging findings in dogs with caudal intervertebral disc herniation. Vet Radiol Ultrasound. 2011 Sep–Oct;52(5):487–91.

48. Lowrie M, Carrera I, Trevail T, Wessmann A. What is your diagnosis? Hansen type 1 intervertebral disk disease. J Am Vet Med Assoc. 2009 Oct 1;235(7):823–4.

49. Mateo I, Lorenzo V, Foradada L, Munoz A. Clinical, pathologic, and magnetic resonance imaging characteristics of canine disc extrusion accompanied by epidural hemorrhage or inflammation. Vet Radiol Ultrasound. 2011 Jan–Feb;52(1):17–24.

50. Nakamoto Y, Ozawa T, Katakabe K, Nishiya K, Yasuda N, Mashita T, et al. Fibrocartilaginous embolism of the spinal cord diagnosed by characteristic clinical findings and magnetic resonance imaging in 26 dogs. J Vet Med Sci. 2009 Feb;71(2):171–6.

51. Penning VA, Benigni L, Steeves E, Cappello R. Imaging diagnosis—degenerative intraspinal cyst associated with an intervertebral disc. Vet Radiol Ultrasound. 2007 Sep–Oct;48(5):424–7.

52. Platt SR, McConnell JF, Bestbier M. Magnetic resonance imaging characteristics of ascending hemorrhagic myelomalacia in a dog. Vet Radiol Ultrasound. 2006 Jan–Feb;47(1):78–82.

53. Seiler G, Hani H, Scheidegger J, Busato A, Lang J. Staging of lumbar intervertebral disc degeneration in nonchondrodystrophic dogs using low-field magnetic resonance imaging. Vet Radiol Ultrasound. 2003 Mar–Apr;44(2):179–84.

54. An HS, Nguyen C, Haughton VM, Ho KC, Hasegawa T. Gadolinium-enhancement characteristics of magnetic resonance imaging in distinguishing herniated intervertebral disc versus scar in dogs. Spine (Phila Pa 1976). 1994 Sep 15;19(18):2089–94; discussion 95.

55. Cooper JJ, Young BD, Griffin JFt, Fosgate GT, Levine JM. Comparison between noncontrast computed tomography and magnetic resonance imaging for detection and characterization of thoracolumbar myelopathy caused by intervertebral disk herniation in dogs. Vet Radiol Ultrasound. 2013 Oct 9;55: 182–90.

56. Freer SR, Scrivani PV. Postoperative susceptibility artifact during magnetic resonance imaging of the vertebral column in two dogs and a cat. Vet Radiol Ultrasound. 2008 Jan–Feb;49(1):30–4.

57. Guillem Gallach R, Suran J, Caceres AV, Reetz JA, Brown DC, Mai W. Reliability of T2-weighted sagittal magnetic resonance images for determining the location of compressive disk herniation in dogs. Vet Radiol Ultrasound. 2011 Sep–Oct;52(5):479–86.

58. Levine JM, Fosgate GT, Chen AV, Rushing R, Nghiem PP, Platt SR, et al. Magnetic resonance imaging in dogs with neurologic impairment due to acute thoracic and lumbar intervertebral disk herniation. J Vet Intern Med. 2009 Nov–Dec;23(6):1220–6.

59. Yamada K, Nakagawa M, Kato T, Shigeno S, Hirose T, Miyahara K, et al. Application of short-time magnetic resonance examination for intervertebral disc diseases in dogs. J Vet Med Sci. 2001 Jan;63(1):51–4.

60. Naude SH, Lambrechts NE, Wagner WM, Thompson PN. Association of preoperative magnetic resonance imaging findings with surgical features in Dachshunds with thoracolumbar intervertebral disk extrusion. J Am Vet Med Assoc. 2008 Mar 1;232(5):702–8.

61. Suran JN, Durham A, Mai W, Seiler GS. Contrast enhancement of extradural compressive material on magnetic resonance imaging. Vet Radiol Ultrasound. 2011 Jan–Feb;52(1):10–6.

62. Mankin JM, Hecht S, Thomas WB. Agreement between T2 and haste sequences in the evaluation of thoracolumbar intervertebral disc disease in dogs. Vet Radiol Ultrasound. 2012 Mar–Apr;53(2):162–6.

63. Tidwell AS, Specht A, Blaeser L, Kent M. Magnetic resonance imaging features of extradural hematomas associated with intervertebral disc herniation in a dog. Vet Radiol Ultrasound. 2002 Jul–Aug; 43(4):319–24.

64. Robertson I, Thrall DE. Imaging dogs with suspected disc herniation: pros and cons of myelography, computed tomography, and magnetic resonance. Vet Radiol Ultrasound. 2011 Mar–Apr;52(1 Suppl 1): S81–4.

17 The Role of Nonimaging-Based Diagnostic Studies for Intervertebral Disc Herniation

Gwendolyn J. Levine

Introduction

Imaging modalities are the cornerstone of intervertebral disc herniation (IVDH) diagnosis, and advanced imaging techniques, such as magnetic resonance imaging (MRI), have supplanted the necessity of ancillary diagnostics such as cerebrospinal fluid (CSF) and electrophysiology in the opinion of some practitioners. CSF analysis remains an important tool to diagnose diseases mimicking IVDH, especially in cases where imaging findings are equivocal. CSF analysis is also gaining recent attention in veterinary medicine as a source of prognostic information in the evaluation of patients with IVDH. Electromyography (EMG) and somatosensory evoked potentials (SSEPs) have been used in the research setting to quantify functional recovery following spinal cord injury (SCI); their role in the clinical management of IVDH has been more limited.

CSF analysis: Typical findings in IVDH

CSF analysis has the most utility in alerting the clinician to the presence of an inflammatory disease (e.g., granulomatous meningoencephalomyelitis) in cases where imaging results are equivocal or nondiagnostic. Dogs afflicted with myelitis or meningoencephalomyelitis may have their condition exacerbated by the injection of myelographic contrast into the thecal space; therefore, the nucleated cell count of the fluid as well as the microprotein concentration should be determined prior to contrast administration. Most investigators view MRI as superior to myelography or computed tomography for detecting IVDH and differentiating it from diseases that may have similar clinical signs.

Between 26 and 82% of CSF samples acquired from dogs with IVDH have parameters outside of accepted reference ranges (Table 17.1) [1–4]. The most common abnormality observed in patients

Advances in Intervertebral Disc Disease in Dogs and Cats, First Edition. Edited by James M. Fingeroth and William B. Thomas.
© 2015 ACVS Foundation. Published 2015 by John Wiley & Sons, Inc.

Table 17.1   Cerebrospinal fluid (CSF) characteristics in dogs with intervertebral disc herniation (IVDH)

Site	No. of animals	Acquisition location	% Abnormal	Protein range, mg/dl	NC/µl range	Cytology	Ref
C	111	Lumbar	82% (85/104) protein increased 23% (26/111) NC increased	10–306 (median, 60)	0–54 (median, 2)	Lymphocytic (11/26) Neutrophilic (8/26)	[6]
C	25	CM	44% (11/25)	Median, 21	0–12 (median, 2)	Mononuclear	[1]
TL	312	Lumbar	66% (152/232) protein increased 61% (190/312) NC increased	3–1920 (median, 57)	0–428 (median, 8)	Lymphocytic (78/190) Neutrophilic (60/190)	[6]
TL	54	CM	54% (29/54) NC increased 16% (4/25) increased protein	0–228.5 (median, 4.2)	0–104 (median, 6)	Neutrophils most common cell type (60%)	[4]
TL	54	CM	51% (28/54) protein increased 31% (17/54) NC increased	12–110 (median, 28)	0–245 (median, 3)	Neutrophilic (12/17) Mixed (4/17)	[5]
TL	35	CM	26% (9/35)	10–42 (mean, 19)	0–11 (mean, 2)	N/A	[5]

with IVDH is albuminocytologic dissociation. This occurs when there is an elevation in CSF microprotein concentration without a corresponding pleocytosis (elevated cell count) and may indicate leakage of protein through the blood/spinal cord/CSF barrier.

The least common finding in analysis of the CSF from IVDH dogs is that of a pleocytosis (23–61% of assessed samples). Reports vary widely in the literature regarding what type of pleocytosis is the most common. Some authors found that mixed cell pleocytoses are the most common, while others state that neutrophilic pleocytosis is the most often diagnosed [3, 5]. Still other researchers state that lymphocytic pleocytosis occurs with the highest frequency [2]. Even eosinophilic pleocytosis has been reported with IVDH, although thus far it has not been seen with great frequency in any case series [6].

The wide variation in pleocytosis findings may be explained by several factors. The site of CSF collection (lumbar vs. cisternal) may affect the cell population, especially as blood contamination is most common in lumbar taps and contamination of CSF with peripheral blood would lead to an increase in neutrophil percentage. Cisternal CSF is more commonly abnormal in dogs with cervical IVDH, while lumbar CSF is more commonly abnormal in dogs with thoracolumbar IVDH. The duration of time between SCI onset and CSF acquisition may also affect the cell population. While neutrophils are the most common cell type to arrive first following SCI, they are replaced by increased numbers of macrophages and lymphocytes after 24–48 h [2, 7]. So CSF acquired at a late time point from the initial injury may have more lymphocytes or macrophages than neutrophils, and a mixed pleocytosis may occur during this cell population switch. Injury severity may also affect the cell populations present in CSF; in one study, higher macrophage percentage was associated with severe injury and poor functional outcome [4].

CSF biomarkers: Novel biomarkers may provide important prognostic information

While CSF analysis may not provide a definitive diagnosis of IVDH, researchers are evaluating substances found in CSF that may provide prognostic information for affected dogs. The first step in this process is detecting the protein of interest in the CSF of dogs with IVDH, and the next step is determining whether the concentration of that protein differs from that found in normal dogs, varies depending on the severity of injury, or is a predictor of outcome in injured dogs.

Substances that have been detected in CSF include matrix metalloproteinase 9 (MMP9), myelin basic protein (MBP), creatine kinase (CK), cartilage oligomeric matrix protein (COMP), and beta-2 microglobulin (B2m). MMP9 is a gelatinase that degrades extracellular matrix, facilitates innate inflammatory responses, and may result in neuronal apoptosis. Expression of MMP9 occurs shortly after SCI and has been correlated to behavioral and histologically severe injury in rodent models. In one report, dogs with acute IVDH and those with paraplegia were more likely to have detectable levels of MMP9 compared to nonparaplegic dogs; another report suggested that CSF MMP9 activity is correlated with poor long-term outcome in dogs with IVDH [3, 8]. MBP release into the CSF is associated with demyelination in a variety of neurological diseases. In animals with SCI, it may play a direct role in secondary mechanisms. In one report [5] on dogs with thoracolumbar IVDH, animals that were nonambulatory at a 6-week follow-up had higher cisternal CSF MBP concentrations than control dogs; a cutoff of greater than 3 ng/ml MBP had a sensitivity of 78% and a specificity of 76% to predict unsuccessful outcome in dogs with thoracolumbar IVDH. High activity (>20 IU/ml) of CK has been associated with poor prognosis in dogs with IVDH, especially those lacking nociception and having elevated MBP [9]. COMP has been shown to promote the early association of collagen molecules, support matrix interactions, and facilitate normal chondrocyte behavior [10]. In dogs with IVDH, COMP was detected at higher levels in lumbar CSF compared to cisternal CSF, indicating that it accumulates caudal to the site of injury. B2m is a protein that is bound to the surface of nucleated cells and is normally shed during cell membrane turnover [11]. While B2m was elevated in dogs with IVDH compared to controls, concentrations were not as high as those observed in dogs with inflammatory diseases.

Electrophysiology

Electrophysiologic testing can be used to evaluate spinal cord function in dogs with IVDH. SSEPs have been the most widely employed technique and are performed by stimulating sensory nerve fibers in the pelvic limb. This stimulus generates action potentials within the ascending sensory tracts of the spinal cord and brain that can be recorded as far-field potentials at sites somewhat distant to the central nervous system parenchyma. Recorded spinal SSEPs have been hypothesized to originate from the dorsal columns or dorsolateral fasciculus, whereas cortical SSEPs arise from electrical events in cortical neurons, synapses, or axons [12, 13]. Dogs with anatomic or functional spinal cord transection have absent SSEPs cranial to the lesion; injury potentials (large positive spikes) may be recorded at the lesion site. In animals with incomplete lesions or those that are recovering, SSEPs can be recorded cranial to the lesion but may be reduced in amplitude or have delays in latency. These changes are believed to occur due to axonal loss and/or demyelination within the spinal cord parenchyma [14].

Standard electrophysiologic techniques such as EMG and peripheral nerve conduction studies do not directly evaluate spinal cord tracts and have not been rigorously assessed in dogs with IVDH. Abnormal spontaneous activity on EMG of limb musculature may be present if there is denervation due to gray matter loss following SCI. However, abnormal spontaneous activities can occur with peripheral axonal injuries or direct muscle trauma and are variable in their magnitude and timing after SCI. Additionally, standard veterinary EMG studies (which are performed when muscle is not being volitionally activated) provide no information concerning white matter spinal cord tracts. In animal models of SCI and humans with SCI, EMG can be used during kinematic gait studies to assess patterns of muscle activation during recovery. Motor nerve conduction studies have been used in humans with SCI to evaluate peripheral nervous system changes in the setting of chronic injury.

It must be remembered that SSEPs and other electrophysiologic studies do not allow clinicians to determine the underlying etiology responsible for SCI. Rather, evoked potentials like SSEPs are measures of the physiologic integrity of the central nervous system parenchyma. The role of EMG in dogs with IVDH is unknown and for the time being would seem to be limited to the research setting, where it could be used to assess muscle activation during walking.

Conclusions

Despite the rapid advances in neuroimaging over the last decade in veterinary medicine, CSF analysis remains a vital diagnostic test in animals with spinal cord disease. Although CSF analysis cannot be used to diagnose IVDH, understanding typical CSF patterns can be helpful when neuroimaging is equivocal or if another disease process is suspected. Electrophysiology will likely continue to play a minor role in the assessment of veterinary patients with SCI in the clinical setting. Like CSF, results are not etiology specific. However, electrophysiology can provide information concerning the functional status of the central nervous system.

References

1. Thomson CE, Kornegay JN, Stevens JB. Analysis of cerebrospinal fluid from the cerebellomedullary and lumbar cisterns of dogs with focal neurologic disease: 145 cases (1985–1987). J Am Vet Med Assoc. 1990 Jun 1;196(11):1841–4.
2. Windsor RC, Vernau KM, Sturges BK, Kass PH, Vernau W. Lumbar cerebrospinal fluid in dogs with type I intervertebral disc herniation. J Vet Intern Med. 2008 Jul–Aug;22(4):954–60.
3. Levine JM, Ruaux CG, Bergman RL, Coates JR, Steiner JM, Williams DA. Matrix metalloproteinase-9 activity in the cerebrospinal fluid and serum of dogs with acute spinal cord trauma from intervertebral disk disease. Am J Vet Res. 2006 Feb;67(2): 283–7.
4. Srugo I, Aroch I, Christopher MM, Chai O, Goralnik L, Bdolah-Abram T, et al. Association of cerebrospinal fluid analysis findings with clinical signs and outcome

in acute nonambulatory thoracolumbar disc disease in dogs. J Vet Intern Med /. 2011 Jul–Aug;25(4):846–55.
5. Levine GJ, Levine JM, Witsberger TH, Kerwin SC, Russell KE, Suchodolski J, et al. Cerebrospinal fluid myelin basic protein as a prognostic biomarker in dogs with thoracolumbar intervertebral disk herniation. J Vet Intern Med. 2010 Jul–Aug;24(4):890–6.
6. Windsor RC, Sturges BK, Vernau KM, Vernau W. Cerebrospinal fluid eosinophilia in dogs. J Vet Intern Med. 2009 Mar–Apr;23(2):275–81.
7. Levine JM, Levine GJ, Porter BF, Topp K, Noble-Haeusslein LJ. Naturally occurring disk herniation in dogs: an opportunity for pre-clinical spinal cord injury research. J Neurotrauma. 2011 Apr;28(4): 675–88.
8. Nagano S, Kim SH, Tokunaga S, Arai K, Fujiki M, Misumi K. Matrix metalloprotease-9 activity in the cerebrospinal fluid and spinal injury severity in dogs with intervertebral disc herniation. Res Vet Sci. 2011 Dec;91(3):482–5.
9. Witsberger TW, Levine JM, Slater MR, Kerwin SC, Russell KE, Levine GJ, et al. Cerebrospinal fluid biomarkers and neurologic outcome in dogs with acute intervertebral disc herniation. J Am Vet Med Assoc. 2012;240(5):555–62.
10. Tokunaga S, Yamanokuchi K, Yabuki A, Fujiki M, Misumi K. Cartilage oligomeric matrix protein in canine spinal cord appears in the cerebrospinal fluid associated with intervertebral disc herniation. Spine (Phila Pa 1976). 2010 Jan 1;35(1):4–9.
11. Munana KR, Saito M, Hoshi F. Beta-2-microglobulin levels in the cerebrospinal fluid of normal dogs and dogs with neurological disease. Vet Clin Pathol. 2007 Jun;36(2):173–8.
12. Poncelet L, Michaux C, Balligand M. Study of spinal cord evoked injury potential by use of computer modeling and in dogs with naturally acquired thoracolumbar spinal cord compression. Am J Vet Res. 1998;59:300–6.
13. Shores A, Redding RW, Knecht CD. Spinal-evoked potentials in dogs with acute compressive thoracolumbar spinal cord disease. Am J Vet Res. 1987;48: 1525–30.
14. Borgens RB, Toombs JP, Breur GJ, Widmer WR, Waters D. An imposed oscillatory electrical field improves the recovery of function in neurologically complete paraplegic dogs. J Neurotraum. 1999;16: 639–57.

18 Recurrent Intervertebral Disc Herniation

Brigitte A. Brisson

Recurrent intervertebral disc (IVD) herniation was recognized as early as 1970 with Funkquist reporting that recurrent signs of disc herniation were at least as frequent in patients that had undergone a laminectomy alone as in patients that had been treated conservatively [1]. More recently, publications have focused on early and late recurrence in dogs treated conservatively or with decompressive surgery as well as on lack of postoperative improvement and the presence of residual disc material following surgical decompression. Fenestration of the affected herniated disc space at the time of decompressive surgery has since been recommended by several authors to prevent further extrusion of disc material through the ruptured annulus fibrosus (AF) in the early postoperative period [1–6]. A recent study that performed repeat thoracolumbar (TL) magnetic resonance imaging (MRI) immediately and 6 weeks postoperatively confirmed recurrent disc herniation at the same site in 6 of 10 patients that did not undergo fenestration of the affected disc space at the time of surgical decompression, compared to none of the 9 patients

that had the disc space fenestrated at the time of first surgery [3]. Three of these six patients displayed clinical signs (pain and/or paresis) compatible with the recurrent herniation noted on MRI, while the others were subclinical for the recurrent extrusion. This study has since been supported by others that document early recurrent disc extrusion with advanced imaging and repeat surgery following an initial hemilaminectomy [5, 7]. These reports do not support the previous claims suggesting that recurrent herniated disc material would likely move spontaneously outside of the canal through the laminectomy site and not cause clinical deterioration. It is however possible that the previously made laminectomy offers some relief from spinal cord or nerve root compression which could explain why some dogs documented as having recurrent herniated material did not develop neurological deficits or any signs at all in one study [3]. Similarly, dogs with residual disc material identified immediately following hemilaminectomy were found to achieve functional recovery regardless of the amount of residual disc material identified,

Advances in Intervertebral Disc Disease in Dogs and Cats, First Edition. Edited by James M. Fingeroth and William B. Thomas.
© 2015 ACVS Foundation. Published 2015 by John Wiley & Sons, Inc.

suggesting that complete decompression by removal of all herniated disc material may not be necessary [8].

The effect of fat grafts or gelatin sponges, which are used by some surgeons to cover the laminectomy site prior to closure, is unknown. It is unclear whether or not the presence of a fat graft could prevent early recurrent extruded disc material from spontaneously moving away from the spinal cord, thus increasing the risk of postoperative clinical deterioration [5] (see Chapter 34). The effect of early postoperative rehabilitation on recurrent disc herniation is also unknown. Several recent publications describing early recurrence of disc extrusion at the site of surgery included dogs that received underwater treadmill therapy within 2–3 days of surgery and were reported to develop early signs of recurrent disc extrusion confirmed with imaging and/or surgery [3, 7, 9].

The overall conclusion is that decompression alone does not prevent any remaining nucleus pulposus from extruding through the damaged AF in the postoperative period and that fenestration of the affected disc space should be performed when possible to reduce the risk of early recurrent herniation [3, 5, 10]. Although early recurrence has been reported to occur in spite of disc fenestration [5], other studies have shown that fenestration of the affected disc space prevented early recurrence in all reported cases [3, 10].

Early recurrence

Early recurrence reportedly occurs within 4–6 weeks of surgery and is most commonly associated with recurrent nuclear extrusion at the site of initial IVD extrusion [3, 11, 12]. Differential diagnoses for early postoperative deterioration or failure to improve postoperatively include iatrogenic trauma, failure to remove the compressive mass at surgery, continued or second disc herniation, hemorrhage, infection, spinal instability, and myelomalacia [5, 7–9, 13]. Although the potential for early recurrence should be considered in patients showing deterioration after initial postoperative improvement, an early recurrence rate of only 2% over a 4-year period was reported in a recent study [7], which is consistent with the rate of 1% over 15 years previously reported in another study [11]. Lack of improvement after decompressive surgery has generally been associated with the disease process itself (primary and secondary spinal cord injury) or with the presence of residual disc material within the vertebral canal. The presence of residual disc material after surgery is thought to be influenced by the surgeon's ability to evacuate disc material [9, 11]. In a study that reviewed 178 postoperative cases of TL IVD herniation, 10 dogs (5.8%) had clinical deterioration within 1–10 days of surgery, some for residual disc at the site of initial surgery and others because the initial surgery was performed at a site immediately adjacent to the affected disc space resulting in only partial removal of the extruded disc material [9]. Of the 10 dogs in the study, 8 underwent a second surgery to remove residual disc material and recovered uneventfully. In contrast, a recent study found residual disc material in 100% of 40 dogs when assessed by computed tomography (CT) immediately following hemilaminectomy [8]. In contrast to the previously mentioned studies, residual disc material was not surgeon dependent in this study and was not associated with failure to achieve a functional recovery [8]. Similarly, a study evaluating residual disc material by comparing pre- and postoperative MRI found residual material in 10 of 10 dogs following hemilaminectomy and 4 of 9 dogs following mini-hemilaminectomy for an extruded TL disc [14]. This suggests that the presence of residual material is possible with various surgical techniques [14]. Since clinical recovery is the most important postoperative factor, repeat diagnostic imaging should be performed when feasible in any patient that fails to improve or deteriorates postoperatively [7, 9, 11].

Imaging options for early recurrent lesions are the same as for first-time lesions. Of course, CT and MRI have the advantage of providing more detail and improving lesion localization with regard to the previous surgical site. This is especially important when CT or MRI was used at the time of initial imaging in order to assess the amount of disc material that was actually removed during surgical decompression or whether or not disc material might have been displaced to the contralateral side of the vertebral canal. Previously reported cases where details of imaging were provided confirmed that although the recurrent lesion can be located on the contralateral side of the initial surgical site, it is more frequently located on the same side as the previous laminectomy

[3, 5, 7, 9]. Differentiating disc material from hemorrhage can be challenging postoperatively and in one study was suspected to be the reason why some dogs were found to have a residual disc percentage higher than 100% compared to preoperatively using CT [8]. MRI may be better suited to differentiate between disc material and hemorrhage [14, 15]. Postoperative susceptibility artifacts seen on MRI can also lead to misinterpretation of the images or preclude image interpretation altogether [16]. Suspected causes for postoperative susceptibility artifacts include microscopic metal fragments from the burr, suction tip, or other instruments; hemorrhage; or paramagnetic suture material [16]. These microscopic paramagnetic substances are typically not visible radiographically or on CT [16].

All IVDs are subject to degeneration, and chondrodystrophic breeds have been reported to develop on average of 2.5 IVD herniations per dog [17, 18]. Fenestration of IVDs adjacent to the surgical lesion has been advocated as a prophylactic measure to prevent future disc herniation from these other sites [1, 19–29]. Recurrence rates of 0–24.4% with prophylactic fenestration [19, 20, 24, 25, 28, 30] and 2.67–41.7% without prophylactic fenestration [1, 2, 11, 20, 28, 31–33] have been reported. The most recent retrospective studies report unconfirmed recurrence rates of 19.2% without prophylactic fenestration [34] and confirmed recurrence rates of 4.4% in a population of dogs that frequently underwent prophylactic fenestration [6]. The latter study also revealed that 15.8% of dog owners reached by telephone follow-up reported that their dog developed signs compatible with recurrent IVD herniation and that 44% of these dogs were euthanized elsewhere for suspected recurrence [6].

More recently, a prospective study randomized 207 small-breed dogs undergoing surgical decompression for TL IVD extrusion to either receive single-site fenestration at the site of decompression ($n = 103$) or multiple-site prophylactic fenestration of all disc spaces between T11 and L4 ($n = 104$) and followed dogs for signs of recurrence for a median time of 3.4 years [10]. The surgically confirmed recurrence rate for new disc lesions (at a site other than the original level of decompression) in this study was 12.7% with a significantly lower recurrence rate for dogs in the multiple-site fenestration group (7.45%) compared

to dogs in the single-site fenestration group (17.89%) [10]. This study revealed that dogs that did not receive prophylactic fenestration of additional disc spaces beyond the surgically decompressed disc space were 2.7 times more likely to undergo surgery for a second disc extrusion than those that did. In addition, only dogs from the single-site fenestration group developed more than one recurrence in this study [10]. Finally, the most recent retrospective study available followed 662 chondrodystrophic dogs that recovered from hemilaminectomy and prophylactic disc fenestration of at least 3 TL IVD spaces and showed a 2.3% rate of recurrence confirmed by a second surgery [12]. In addition, 10% of dogs in this study developed signs of recurrence that were managed conservatively, so the unconfirmed rate of recurrence in this study could have been as high as 12.3% [12]. Although this study only included dogs that received prophylactic fenestration, it revealed that nonfenestrated discs were 26.2 times more likely than fenestrated discs to be the cause of a surgically confirmed second disc extrusion [12]. This is higher than the rate of 5.86 times previously reported in a smaller study [6]. Similarly to what has been published in small dogs, the rate of recurrent IVD herniation for large-breed dogs has been reported at 11–12% [35, 36].

Although in some studies dachshunds were more likely to develop recurrent TL IVD herniation compared with other breeds [6, 11], this was not confirmed by other studies [10, 12, 34]. Age was not found to be associated with recurrence in some studies [11, 34], while it was in a larger prospective study [10]. Other factors such as sex, body weight, lesion location, neurological grade, and decompressive surgical technique were not associated with an increased risk of recurrence [6, 10, 11, 34]. In contrast, radiographic evidence of TL disc mineralization at the time of first surgery has been associated with recurrent TL IVD herniation in dogs [10, 34] whereby the risk of recurrence increased by 1.4 times for each opacified disc [34].

Late recurrence

Late recurrent TL IVD herniation occurs at a mean time of 8 to 14 months after the first surgery and typically develops within 36 months of the first event [6, 10, 11, 24, 33, 34]. Recurrences have however been reported as late as 71 months after surgery [6, 10, 12, 34]. Recurrences occur at a new disc space in 88–100% of cases [6, 10–12, 33], and more than 70% of recurrences occur in a region that could have been prophylactically fenestrated at the first surgery [10, 11]. Most recurrences occur at a site immediately adjacent to or one disc space away from the first lesion or from a fenestrated disc space, suggesting that disc herniation and fenestration may have a biomechanical effect on adjacent disc spaces [6, 10–12, 34]. This finding is supported by the fact that the AF has been shown to be an important stabilizing structure and that fenestration significantly contributes to vertebral instability in both the TL and cervical portions of the spine [37, 38]. The incidence of recurrence at L4–L5 and L5–L6 in dogs prophylactically fenestrated between T11–T12 and L3–L4 is reportedly 45.5–57.1%[6, 10]; this is considered high because the reported rate of naturally occurring disc herniation at these disc spaces is between 3.7 and 7% [6, 17, 26, 31]. It is however important to reiterate that although recurrence appears to occur most frequently at a disc space adjacent to or one space away from a previously herniated or fenestrated disc space, fenestration itself does not "provoke" or increase the risk of further herniation and has been shown to reduce the overall rate of recurrence [5, 6, 10].

Late recurrent cases have been shown to present earlier and with less severe neurologic deficits, presumably because the owners are more attentive to the dog's neurological signs [11]. Imaging studies focused on patients that develop signs of late recurrence are yet to be published. However, similar to what was shown in first-time disc herniation [15], MRI was shown to be superior to myelography to localize the extruded disc material circumferentially within the vertebral canal and also to identify the previous site and side of surgery in dogs with recurrent signs of disc herniation after the first decompressive surgery [39]. The prognosis for functional recovery after repeat surgery for recurrent TL IVD extrusion appears to be identical to that of first-time extrusion [10–12, 40].

Conclusions

In summary, early and late recurrences of IVD herniation are clinically relevant entities that deserve consideration when managing patients with IVD herniation. Owners should be aware that recurrence is possible after an initial event and that this may necessitate repeat imaging and surgery in the future. Further, owners should be advised that the prognosis for recurrent herniation appears to be as good for a second or third event and does not warrant euthanasia.

References

1. Funkquist B. Decompressive laminectomy in thoraco-lumbar disc protrusion with paraplegia in the dog. J Small Anim Pract. 1970;11(7):445–51.
2. Scott HW. Hemilaminectomy for the treatment of thoracolumbar disc disease in the dog: a follow-up study of 40 cases. J Small Anim Pract. 1997 Nov; 38(11):488–94.
3. Forterre F, Konar M, Spreng D, Jaggy A, Lang J. Influence of intervertebral disc fenestration at the herniation site in association with hemilaminectomy on recurrence in chondrodystrophic dogs with thoracolumbar disc disease: a prospective MRI study. Vet Surg. 2008;37(4):399–405.
4. Fingeroth JM. Fenestration. Pros and cons. Probl Vet Med. 1989;1:445–66.
5. Stigen Ø, Ottesen N, Jäderlund KH. Early recurrence of thoracolumbar intervertebral disc extrusion after surgical decompression: a report of three cases. Acta Vet Scand. 2010;52(1):10.
6. Brisson BA, Moffatt SL, Swayne SL, Parent JM. Recurrence of thoracolumbar intervertebral disk extrusion in chondrodystrophic dogs after surgical decompression with or without prophylactic fenestration: 265 cases (1995–1999). J Am Vet Med Assoc. 2004 Jun 1;224(11):1808–14.
7. Hettlich BF, Kerwin SC, Levine JM. Early reherniation of disk material in eleven dogs with surgically treated thoracolumbar intervertebral disk extrusion. Vet Surg. 2012 Feb;41(2):215–20.
8. Roach WJ, Thomas M, Weh JM, Bleedorn J, Wells K. Residual herniated disc material following hemilaminectomy in chondrodystrophic dogs with thoracolumbar intervertebral disc disease. Vet Comp Orthop Traumatol. 2012;25(2):109–15.
9. Forterre F, Gorgas D, Dickomeit M, Jaggy A, Lang J, Spreng D. Incidence of spinal compressive lesions in chondrodystrophic dogs with abnormal recovery after hemilaminectomy for treatment of thoracolumbar disc disease: a prospective magnetic resonance imaging study. Vet Surg. 2010 Feb;39(2):165–72.
10. Brisson BA, Holmberg DL, Parent J, Sears WC, Wick SE. Comparison of the effect of single-site and multiple-site disk fenestration on the rate of recurrence of thoracolumbar intervertebral disk herniation in dogs. J Am Vet Med Assoc. 2011 Jun 15;238(12):1593–600.

11. Dhupa S, Glickman N, Waters DJ. Reoperative neurosurgery in dogs with thoracolumbar disc disease. Vet Surg. 1999;28(6):421–8.

12. Aikawa T, Fujita H, Shibata M, Takahashi T. Recurrent thoracolumbar intervertebral disc extrusion after hemilaminectomy and concomitant prophylactic fenestration in 662 chondrodystrophic dogs. Vet Surg. 2012 Apr 41(3):381–90.

13. Arthurs G. Spinal instability resulting from bilateral mini-hemilaminectomy and pediculectomy. Vet Comp Orthop Traumatol. 2009;22(5):422–6.

14. Huska JL, Gaitero L, Brisson BA, Nykamp S, Thomason J, Sears WC. Presence of residual material following mini-hemilaminectomy in dogs with thoracolumbar intervertebral disc extrusion. Can Vet J. in press.

15. Bos AS, Brisson BA, Nykamp SG, Poma R, Foster RA. Accuracy, intermethod agreement, and interreviewer agreement for use of magnetic resonance imaging and myelography in small-breed dogs with naturally occurring first-time intervertebral disk extrusion. J Am Vet Med Assoc. 2012;240(8):969–77.

16. Freer SR, Scrivani PV. Postoperative susceptibility artifact during magnetic resonance imaging of the vertebral column in two dogs and a cat. Vet Radiol Ultrasound. 2008 Jan–Feb;49(1):30–4.

17. Hansen H-J. A pathologic-anatomical interpretation of disc degeneration in dogs. Acta Orthop. 1951; 20(4):280–93.

18. Hansen HJ. A pathologic-anatomical study on disc degeneration in dog, with special reference to the so-called enchondrosis intervertebralis. Acta Orthop Scand Suppl. 1952;11:1–117.

19. Black A. Lateral spinal decompression in the dog: a review of 39 cases. J Small Anim Pract. 1988;29(9): 581–8.

20. Davies J, Sharp N. A comparison of conservative treatment and fenestration for thoracolumbar intervertebral disc disease in the dog. J Small Anim Pract. 1983;24(12):721–9.

21. Olsson S-E. Observations concerning disc fenestration in dogs. Acta Orthop. 1951;20(4):349–56.

22. Olsson SE. Surgical treatment with special reference to the value of disc fenestration. Acta Orthop Scand Suppl. 1951;8:51–70.

23. Hoerlein B. The status of the various intervertebral disc surgeries for the dog in 1978. J Am Anim Hosp Assoc. 1978;14:563–70.

24. Funkquist B. Investigations of the therapeutic and prophylactic effects of disc evacuation in cases of thoraco-lumbar herniated discs in dogs. Acta Vet Scand. 1978;19(3):441–57.

25. Butterworth SJ, Denny HR. Follow-up study of 100 cases with thoracolumbar disc protrusions treated by lateral fenestration. J Small Anim Pract. 1991;32:443–7.

26. Gage ED. Incidence of clinical disk disease. J Am Anim Hosp Assoc. 1975;11:135–8.

27. Braund K, Taylor T, Ghosh P, Sherwood A. Lateral spinal decompression in the dog. J Small Anim Pract. 1976;17(9):583–92.

28. Levine S, Caywood D. Recurrence of neurological deficits in dogs treated for thoracolumbar disk disease. J Am Anim Hosp Assoc. 1984;20.

29. McKee WM. A comparison of hemilaminectomy (with concomitant disk fenestration) and dorsal laminectomy for the treatment of thoracolumbar disk protrusion in dogs. Vet Rec. 1992;130:296–300.

30. Knapp D, Pope E, Hewett J, Bojrab M. A retrospective study of thoracolumbar disk fenestration in dogs using a ventral approach: 160 cases (1976 to 1986). J Am Anim Hosp Assoc. 1990;26(5):543–9.

31. Brown NO, Helphrey ML, Prata RG. Thoracolumbar disk disease in the dog: a retrospective analysis of 187 cases. J Am Anim Hosp Assoc. 1977;13:665–72.

32. Prata RG. Neurosurgical treatment of thoracolumbar disks: the rationale and value of laminectomy with concomitant disk removal. J Am Anim Hosp Assoc. 1981;17:17–26.

33. Necas A. Clinical aspects of surgical treatment of thoracolumbar disc disease in dogs. A retrospective study of 300 cases. Acta Vet Brno. 1999;68:121–30.

34. Mayhew PD, McLear RC, Ziemer LS, Culp WT, Russell KN, Shofer FS, et al. Risk factors for recurrence of clinical signs associated with thoracolumbar intervertebral disk herniation in dogs: 229 cases (1994–2000). J Am Vet Med Assoc. 2004;225(8):1231–6.

35. Cudia SP, Duval JM. Thoracolumbar intervertebral disk disease in large, nonchondrodystrophic dogs: a retrospective study. J Am Anim Hosp Assoc. 1997 Sep–Oct;33(5):456–60.

36. Macias C, McKee WM, May C, Innes JF. Thoracolumbar disc disease in large dogs: a study of 99 cases. J Small Anim Pract. 2002 Oct;43(10):439–46.

37. Hill TP, Lubbe AM, Guthrie AJ. Lumbar spine stability following hemilaminectomy, pediculectomy, and fenestration. Vet Comp Orthop Traumatol. 2000;13:165–71.

38. Fauber AE, Wade JA, Lipka AE, McCabe GP, Aper RL. Effect of width of disk fenestration and a ventral slot on biomechanics of the canine C5-C6 vertebral motion unit. Am J Vet Res. 2006 Nov;67(11):1844–8.

39. Reynolds D, Brisson BA, Nykamp SG. Agreement between magnetic resonance imaging, myelography, and surgery for detecting recurrent, thoracolumbar intervertebral disc extrusion. Vet Comp Orthop Traumatol. 2013;26(1):12–8.

40. Ruddle TL, Allen DA, Schertel ER, Wilson MD, Barnhart ER, Lineberger JA, et al. Outcome and prognostic factors in non-ambulatory Hansen type Ii ntervertebral disc extrusions: 308 cases. Vet Comp Orthop Traumatol. 2006;19:29–34.

19 When Should Dogs Be Referred for Imaging and Surgery?

James M. Fingeroth and William B. Thomas

Clinicians are frequently confronted with patients in which intervertebral disc herniation (IVDH) is considered the working diagnosis. Elsewhere in this text, we have addressed the need for caution in assuming that all dogs that presented with neck pain, back pain, or paresis and ataxia do so because of disc-related disease. We have also touched on (see Chapters 13, 15, and 28) the reasons why there might be a poor correlation between severity of signs and the role that surgery could play in treating those signs. We will expand on that discussion here. The challenge for clinicians is to combine all the information available and recommend treatment that is neither too conservative nor overly aggressive.

There are two key concepts that should always be borne in mind when making clinical decisions for dogs and patients with suspected IVDH. First, surgery is only sensible when there is spinal cord compression. As has been demonstrated in other chapters there is a very questionable and probably insignificant value to operations that provide access to the vertebral canal and dural tube/spinal cord, but do not remove a compressive mass. Second, one can neither assume that mild signs

(such as discomfort without other deficits) imply minimal spinal cord/nerve root compression, nor the converse that severe signs (tetra or paraplegia) indicate that there must be a significant compressive lesion present.

Hence, the clinician uses both inductive and deductive reasoning to decide if a patient might have a compressive lesion for which surgery could be helpful and must further decide when surgery should be considered rather than nonsurgical management. A helpful mental tool in this regard is the construction of a time–sign graph (Figure 19.1). The signs plotted might represent the severity of either discomfort or paresis or both. First, one must consider the historical onset of signs: Did they develop gradually, over days, or longer or were they acute/peracute in onset? Since their initial recognition, how have these signs progressed? Have they stayed the same? Improved? Worsened? If medical intervention was initiated, how has that intervention impacted on the plotted trend? As one considers the onset and progression of signs over time, one can then mentally extrapolate the data to suggest what will transpire over the ensuing time periods. It is from this extrapolation that one can

Advances in Intervertebral Disc Disease in Dogs and Cats, First Edition. Edited by James M. Fingeroth and William B. Thomas.
© 2015 ACVS Foundation. Published 2015 by John Wiley & Sons, Inc.

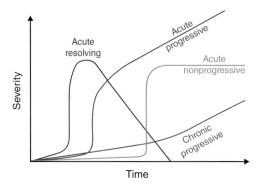

Figure 19.1   Time–sign graph. Clinical decision making can be aided by the mental construct of a graph that establishes the onset, severity, and rapidity of progression of clinical signs or deficits. Response (or lack thereof) to medical interventions can be incorporated in the graph. In general, patients at risk for permanent paralysis (correlated with severity of deficits and rapidity of progression), progression of deficits despite appropriate nonsurgical interventions, and failure to improve (even if signs are limited to discomfort alone or mild neurologic deficits) are considered candidates for referral for possible surgical intervention. The urgency of such referral is based on extrapolation of the time–sign graph generated for that patient into the subsequent hours or days, assuming previous trends are maintained.

make decisions regarding continuation of medical-only treatment versus referral for possible surgery. In any instance, a trend that suggests either a failure to improve with current treatment and more time or worsening of signs in spite of current treatment would warrant a shift in therapeutic intervention. Moreover, and especially in regard to patients with severe paresis, the goal should always be to intervene aggressively to prevent progression to a state where deep pain perception distal to the lesion is diminished or lost, since (as discussed in Chapter 11) the loss of deep pain is associated with a poorer chance for recovery.

It should be noted that severity of signs at any given time is not as useful in making decisions as is consideration of those signs in the context of onset, progression and response to therapy. Two patients might present with identical signs, but if one reached that point of impairment over a period of days, and the other was normal just a few hours before, it suggests that the latter may have the more emergent condition. It also implies that severity of signs alone is not the only determinant of a need for advanced imaging and surgery. If two patients are presented with, say, signs of

severe neck pain but the onset in one occurred just today while the other has been suffering and medically treated for 3 weeks, it is entirely appropriate to consider more aggressive treatment for the latter even though there may yet be no signs of paresis or other neurologic deficits. It is here that we again must remind ourselves that it is quite possible for dogs with signs of discomfort alone to have marked compression of their spinal cords and/or nerve roots, and thus, they are more likely to be benefited from decompressive surgery than from continued medical management [1–3].

Should I take plain radiographs of patients in which I suspect have IVDH?

This is a common question and one without a simple or definitive answer. However, we can look at some of the pros and cons of plain radiographs, and how the results of such radiography might impinge on treatment recommendations.

As noted in Chapter 16, radiographs provide useful clues regarding the presence and site of IVDH. However, as also demonstrated in that chapter, there are many possible artifacts and red herrings that may be seen as well, even when radiographs are done with optimal positioning and technique. There may also be signs of disc degeneration that can occur without corresponding disc herniation (and vice versa), rendering information derived from plain radiographs generally insufficient for a surgeon to base his or her operative planning on. Therefore, the first take-home message is that plain radiographs provided by an attending clinician to a neurosurgeon will, with very rare exception, not obviate the need for subsequent imaging studies. So there should be no motivation for a clinician to obtain plain radiographs as part of a basic database that he or she feels might be helpful to or needed by the neurosurgeon.

As with almost any use of radiography, the essential question any clinician should ask is, "How will the results of this imaging alter my diagnostic or treatment strategy for this patient?" As already stated, it is rare for even the best of radiographs to be definitive for making the diagnosis of IVDH. So, if your differential diagnosis list is headed by IVDH, and you consider alternatives to be very unlikely, there is almost no value to having plain radiographs in that circumstance. Your treatment decisions are based on the time–sign graph or similar assessment of the urgency of the case and whether nonsurgical management is or is not appropriate at this time. Hence, if the working diagnosis is IVDH but based on the progression and severity of signs (or the client's stated intention not to pursue surgery no matter what) you are not currently considering referral for surgery, there is no advantage in having radiographs that may or may not indicate disc disease or even disc herniation. Knowing that there is a narrowed disc space at, say, T13–L1 versus L2–L3 will have no impact on treatment planning or efficacy. And considering the added cost for radiography and morbidity involved (either restraining an anxious patient or those in pain or anesthetizing the patient), it might be considered detrimental to pursue plain radiographs.

That all said, we do have to remember that a putative diagnosis of IVDH is just that, and so an argument can be made for using radiographs to screen for the presence of nondisc-related lesions. These can include fractures/luxations (although, in most cases, the history will indicate if external trauma should be considered in the differential diagnosis), discospondylitis (Chapter 20), and vertebral or disc neoplasia (Chapter 21). However, the sensitivity for each of these alternate diagnoses via plain radiography is less than 100%, so negative plain radiographs (especially if obtained with less than optimal positioning, technique, or orthogonal views) cannot rule out any diagnosis. Many patients may also have developmental/anomalous lesions such as hemivertebrae, block vertebrae, butterfly vertebrae, extra or missing vertebrae, or degenerative lesions such as spondylosis deformans, diffuse idiopathic skeletal hyperostosis (DISH), or mineralized discs that may have no relation to current signs of discomfort and/or paresis. So the value of plain radiographs to rule in or rule out alternative diagnoses to IVDH, just as with trying to prove IVDH via plain radiography, is questionable. However, if referral for advanced imaging/surgery entails a great distance or other major logistical hurdle for the client, it can be logically argued that plain radiographs for screening, even in the face of possible false negatives and false positives, should be considered, since a definitive finding of pathology other then IVDH might alter the plans for referral.

As a general rule, however, the foregoing should at least sway clinicians from a "knee-jerk" policy of diagnosing a patient with neck or back disease, assuming it to be IVDH, and automatically taking radiographs. If a patient is to be classified a surgical candidate, that classification is based on the differential diagnosis (could there be a compressive lesion affecting the spinal cord and/or nerve roots, be it disc or something else?), the consideration of severity of signs, progression over time, anticipated progression/course without surgery, and the desire to avoid loss of deep pain. Client willingness to pursue referral for possible surgery and response to any medical intervention already initiated are also important considerations. Once the clinical decision is made to recommend referral for surgery, it is only then that imaging studies need to be performed. There are virtually no instances where the results of radiography in the primary clinician's facility or emergency clinic will or should instigate a recommendation for surgery if no such recommendation was being considered before those radiographs were obtained. And if referral for surgery is deemed warranted, any surgical intervention will be predicated on an advanced imaging modality (Chapter 16), making radiographs prior to referral essentially useless, except for the screening motive addressed earlier in instances where the referral might be a logistical hardship for the client.

Examples

Consider how this information is applied in the following case examples.

A 5-year-old dachshund presented with a 24h duration of thoracolumbar pain and no neurologic deficits. Based on the signalment and other clinical features, IVDH is the most likely diagnosis. Considering the short and nonprogressive course of mild clinical signs, the initial treatment of choice is nonsurgical therapy. Radiographs are likely to be either normal or show signs of IVDD, neither of which will change the initial treatment recommendations.

A 5-year-old dachshund presented with a 24h duration of neck pain with no neurologic deficits. Conservative therapy for presumed IVDH is started, consisting of strict crate rest and analgesics. Three weeks later, the dog is still substantially in pain with no neurologic deficits. Because the signs are persisting despite appropriate conservative therapy, referral for imaging and potential surgery is indicated. Results of plain radiographs are very unlikely to change this recommendation and advanced imaging such as computed tomography, magnetic resonance imaging or myelography will be necessary for definitive diagnosis and surgical planning. Although this patient does not have neurologic deficits, refractory pain can be just as detrimental to quality of life as paresis or paralysis so surgery is justified.

A 4-year-old male pointer presented with a recent onset of thoracolumbar pain and fever. While IVDH is a potential diagnostic consideration, the signalment is not typical for IVDH, and the fever increases the index of suspicion of alternative diagnoses, such as discospondylitis. In this case, spinal radiographs are indicated.

A 5-year-old dachshund presented with a sudden onset of back pain and paraplegia. Neurologic examination shows paraplegia with intact spinal reflexes and absent deep pain perception in the pelvic limbs. There is focal pain at the thoracolumbar junction and a loss of the cutaneous trunci reflex caudal to L1. The clinical features are highly suggestive of acute IVDH. Immediate referral for imaging and surgery is indicated in an effort to relieve any spinal cord compression before there is irreversible damage to the spinal cord. There is no need for plain radiographs because results are very unlikely to change recommendations and surgery will require advanced imaging anyway.

A 5-year-old dachshund started showing signs of thoracolumbar pain 5 days ago. Three days before presentation, the client noticed swaying, scuffing, and staggering in the pelvic limbs, which progressively worsened to the point that the patient is unable to walk. Neurologic examination shows nonambulatory paraparesis with intact spinal reflexes and clear evidence of superficial pain perception. Referral for potential surgery is recommended based on the progression and severity of the neurologic deficits. In this patient, the need for surgery is not emergent as it was in the previous case because of the slower progression of signs

and presence of some motor function. However, referral should be pursued relatively soon before the neurologic status deteriorates further.

A 5-year-old dachshund presented with a 2-day duration of paraparesis progressing to paraplegia. Neurologic examination shows complete loss of voluntary movement in the pelvic limbs with normal spinal reflexes and intact pain perception. Due to the severity of the neurologic deficits, urgent referral is indicated. A potential mistake in these patients is to treat conservatively, periodically assess deep pain perception, and only refer if deep pain perception is lost. However, the prognosis for neurologic recovery decreases to approximately 50% once deep pain perception is lost, compared to approximately 95% if surgery is performed when pain perception is still intact [4–8].

Conclusions

Referral to a surgeon is based on the severity of signs, the historical progression of those signs, and the extrapolated progression of signs, with consideration of the efficacy (or lack thereof) of prior or current medical interventions.

Loss of deep pain or anticipated loss of deep pain is an emergency situation and always warrants referral to determine if there is an operable lesion.

It is improper to limit referrals only to patients with paraplegia or tetraplegia, or to delay referral of such patients until such time as deep pain is diminished. If a patient still has some function (e.g., voluntary motor function) but the history suggests rapid and ongoing deterioration or a failure to respond to medical therapy, the goal should be to intervene surgically (if appropriate) before signs worsen.

Intractable discomfort, even in the absence of any other neurologic deficits, warrants referral just as much as signs of paresis, since patients so affected may have IVDH and profound compressive lesions that might more quickly and completely be resolved than with ongoing medical therapy.

Plain radiographs are of limited and often dubious value in patients likely to be suffering from IVDH. One needs to first establish a neuroanatomic diagnosis ("where is the lesion?") and then a differential diagnosis and finally decide whether radiographs might alter the treatment choices or decision to refer for possible surgery based on the aforementioned. Clinicians should be able to discuss a tentative diagnosis of IVDH with their clients without the crutch of displaying a radiograph of that particular patient, especially since it is quite common for the lesion pointed out by the initial clinician to the client to end up NOT being the one actually causing the patient's signs.

Such lesions as narrowed disc spaces, disc mineralization, and spondylosis may indicate disc degeneration, but neither prove disc herniation has occurred nor that any such herniation causing the patient's signs corresponds to the lesion seen on plain radiographs. Radiographic signs of disc degeneration are common and quite expected in chondrodystrophoid dogs (with or without clinical signs), and so their findings in a clinically affected patient are as likely to be red herrings as they are to be the actual location of the lesion. And even if the lesion seen corresponds to the site where herniation and spinal cord/nerve root compression are occurring, the decision whether to refer for surgery is not altered by this knowledge (just as the converse is true, the absence of plain radiographic lesions should not dissuade referral).

References

1. Morgan P, Parent J, Holmberg D. Cervical pain secondary to intervertebral disc disease in dogs; radiographic findings and surgical implications. Prog Vet Neurol. 1993;4:76–80.

2. Sukhiani HR, Parent JM, Atilola MA, Holmberg DL. Intervertebral disk disease in dogs with signs of back pain alone: 25 cases (1986–1993). J Am Vet Med Assoc. 1996 Oct 1;209(7):1275–9.

3. Fry TR, Johnson AL, Hungerford L, Toombs J. Surgical treatment of cervical disc herniations in ambulatory dogs: ventral decompression vs. fenestration, 111 cases (1980–1988). Prog Vet Neurol. 1991;2:165–73.

4. Ruddle TL, Allen DA, Schertel ER, Barnhart MD, Wilson ER, Lineberger JA, et al. Outcome and prognostic factors in non-ambulatory Hansen Type I intervertebral disc extrusions: 308 cases. Vet Comp Orthop Traumatol. 2006;19(1):29–34.

5. Amsellum PM, Toombs JP, Laverty PH, Breur GJ. Loss of deep pain sensation following thoracolumbar intervertebral disk herniation in dogs: treatment and prognosis. Compend Contin Educ Pract Vet. 2003;24:266–74.

6. Ferreira AJ, Correia JH, Jaggy A. Thoracolumbar disc disease in 71 paraplegic dogs: influence of rate of onset and duration of clinical signs on treatment results. J Small Anim Pract. 2002 Apr;43(4):158–63.

7. Brisson BA, Moffatt SL, Swayne SL, Parent JM. Recurrence of thoracolumbar intervertebral disk extrusion in chondrodystrophic dogs after surgical decompression with or without prophylactic fenestration: 265 cases (1995–1999). J Am Vet Med Assoc. 2004 Jun 1;224(11):1808–14.

8. Gambardelli PC. Dorsal decompressive laminectomy for treatment of thoracolumbar disc disease in dogs: A retrospective study of 98 cases. Vet Surg. 1980;9:24–26.

20 Discospondylitis and Related Spinal Infections in the Dog and Cat

Sharon Kerwin

Introduction

Spinal infection in dogs and cats may involve the vertebral body[1, 2], vertebral physes [3, 4], intervertebral disc, epidural space [5], or paravertebral soft tissues [6]. Spinal infection is being increasingly recognized as imaging techniques become more sophisticated and available [7].

Definitions

Vertebral physitis is infection centered on the vertebral physis, with no initial involvement of the disc space. It is generally identified in dogs less than 2 years of age and typically observed in the lumbar vertebrae [4]. **Spondylitis or vertebral osteomyelitis** refers to infection of the vertebral bone and occurs most frequently as a result of direct inoculation of pathogens. **Discitis** refers to infection of the intervertebral disc only. **Discospondylitis** (which has also in some literature been termed "intradiscal osteomyelitis") refers to an infection of the cartilaginous end plates with secondary involvement of the disc [8]. There is no such entity as "discospondylosis" (a term occasionally referred to by veterinarians), and spondylosis deformans is not at all the same thing as discospondylitis, although patients with discospondylitis might consequently develop spondylosis at the affected level(s) (see also Chapter 8).

Spinal epidural empyema (abscess) is a suppurative, septic process within the epidural space of the vertebral canal, with accumulation of purulent, septic material [5, 9]. **Paraspinal infection** refers to infection of the muscles surrounding the spine (longus colli, iliopsoas, epaxial muscles) and may arise from osteomyelitis, discospondylitis, or direct inoculation [6].

Pathophysiology

The source of spinal infection may be autogenous or iatrogenic. The majority of cases are thought to result from hematogenous spread of infection from a distant site. Infection may become

Advances in Intervertebral Disc Disease in Dogs and Cats, First Edition. Edited by James M. Fingeroth and William B. Thomas.
© 2015 ACVS Foundation. Published 2015 by John Wiley & Sons, Inc.

established in the highly vascular, slow flowing metaphyseal and epiphyseal capillary beds with rapid extension into the disc. In humans, it is thought that infection may begin in the anterior longitudinal ligament, which extends along the ventral surface of the spine and serves as the periosteum [10]. As our ability to image cases earlier improves, we may be able to more accurately describe the initial location of infection and subsequent progression [11].

Iatrogenic discospondylitis of the lumbosacral disc has been reported after epidural injection [12, 13]. In both reported cases, intestinal perforation, possibly associated with the use of an excessively long 3.5 inch spinal needle, was theorized as a potential source of infection, based on isolation of enteric organisms (*E. coli*, *Enterococcus* spp.). Interestingly, both cases were adult German shepherd dogs.

Iatrogenic discospondylitis has also been reported after fenestration carried out during surgery to treat intervertebral disc herniation [14, 15]. In one report, documenting two cases of iatrogenic methicillin-resistant *Staphylococcus aureus* infection, high-dose steroids were theorized as a possible risk factor [14].

Spinal infection may also occur after migration of foreign bodies [16] or abnormal migration of parasites [17, 18]. In hunting dogs, grass awns are thought to be inhaled, penetrate the lungs into the pleural cavity and then forced between the pleural layers in a caudal direction by respiratory movements. The foreign bodies then migrate along the attachment of the diaphragm and into the sublumbar musculature and infect the L2 to L4 vertebra, where the crura of the diaphragm attach. Commensal organisms in the mucous membrane may colonize the plant material. An oral route of migration through the esophagus or caudal duodenal flexure in the dog has also been proposed [16]. Although most foreign bodies associated with infection around the spine lodge in the musculature, the plant material may also lodge directly within the vertebral body [19].

History and clinical signs

Clinical signs of spinal infection in dogs can include spinal pain, fever, lameness, anorexia, weight loss, abdominal pain, and neurologic deficits ranging from mild ataxia and paresis to nonambulatory paraplegia with absence of deep nociception. Neurologic deficits are only seen in about half of presenting cases [15]. In cases of exogenous spinal infection (e.g., foreign bodies), fistulous tracts may be present [16]. Although pain on palpation of the affected vertebral column is often present, it may not be detected in stoic dogs. Although presentation can be peracute [20], clinical signs may wax and wane, and the history may be vague and can span over a period of years [19].

Spinal infection is much less commonly reported in cats than in dogs. Signs may include lameness, reluctance to ambulate, spinal pain, paresis, or paralysis. A history of trauma, in particular bite wounds adjacent to the spinal column, may be present [21].

Risk factors

Male dogs were twice as likely as females to be affected in one large study, and urinary tract infections were the most commonly diagnosed concurrent disease. Great danes, boxers, rottweilers, English bulldogs, German shepherd dogs, and Doberman pinschers appeared to be at higher risk than mixed breed dogs [15]. In the United States, discospondylitis appears to be more prevalent in the southern region of the country.

Imaging

Radiographs

Initial radiographic changes of **vertebral physitis** are a lucent widening of the caudal vertebral physis accompanied by hazy loss of definition of the metaphyseal and epiphyseal margins of the physis. This later gives way to increasing sclerosis in the surrounding cancellous bone, collapse of the physis, and remodeling of the ventrocaudal aspect of the affected vertebra, with preservation of the caudal end plate and absence of disc space narrowing [4].

Discospondylitis is first characterized by symmetric loss of definition of the vertebral end plates of the affected disc space with progressive lucency and loss of bone from the subchondral bone plate or may be first observed as a collapse of the intervertebral disc space alone [8]. Radiographic changes have been reported to lag behind clinical signs by several weeks in dogs [14] and 2–8 weeks in humans [10]. Progressive lysis and sclerosis of both end plates and vertebral bodies, leading to extensive remodeling and partial collapse of the disc space, occur over time, with ventral spondylosis and eventual ankylosis of the space [8].

Vertebral osteomyelitis, with sparing of the disc space and end plates, has been described in the dog as osteolytic and osteoproliferative changes including intense periosteal reaction of the vertebral bodies [2].

Myelography

Myelography may be useful in combination with radiographs for diagnosis of space-occupying extradural lesions, determining the degree of spinal cord compression, and assessing vertebral instability in association with spinal infections but is being supplanted by advanced imaging in many practices [5, 18, 22].

Computed tomography

Computed tomography (CT) is a very effective tool for diagnosing osteomyelitis of bone as it has the ability to detect bone changes earlier than conventional radiography, and the cross sectional anatomy is helpful for surgical planning. Combination CT with myelography has been used to diagnose epidural empyema in the dog. The additional use of intravenous contrast medium aids detection of enhancing lesions both in the epidural space and within the surrounding soft tissues. Multiple areas of punctate osteolysis may be present in the end plates surrounding involved disc space in discospondylitis [21, 23, 24]. Although CT documentation in small animals has been reported in several types of spinal infections in dogs and cats, a case series describing sensitivity and specificity both for diagnosis and for monitoring treatment has not been reported.

Magnetic resonance imaging

Magnetic resonance imaging (MRI) is considered the most sensitive and specific imaging modality for inflammatory and infectious disease of the human spine and was reported for the diagnosis of discospondylitis in the dog as early as 1998 [25], as well as for the diagnosis of canine paraspinal infections [6, 16]. Carrera et al. [7] reported MRI findings in 13 dogs with confirmed (culture positive, presumed hematogenous origin) discospondylitis. There was always involvement of two adjacent vertebral end plates and the associated disc. The involved end plates and adjacent marrow were hypointense on T1-weighted imaging, and all dogs also had contrast enhancement of end plates and paravertebral soft tissues after administration of paramagnetic contrast agents. The end plates and involved marrow were hyperintense on short tau inversion recovery (STIR) images (generally used to eliminate fat from the image), and the affected intervertebral discs were hyperintense in T2-weighted and STIR images. The intervertebral discs exhibited contrast enhancement in 15 of 17 (88%) of affected sites. End plate erosion could be observed in 15 sites, but was not observable either on MRI or plain radiography in two sites. Epidural extension could be seen on contrast at 15 sites and all affected dogs had neurologic signs [7].

Harris et al. reported the MRI findings in 23 dogs with discospondylitis; an infectious organism was identified in 18 of 23 dogs [26]. Vertebral end plate irregularity and erosion were observed in most cases. The most common findings on T2-weighted images were hyperintensity of the disc space, multifocal hyperintensity of the vertebral end plates, and isointensity to hyperintensity of paravertebral soft tissue. On T1-weighted imaging after contrast administration, there was frequent and heterogeneous enhancement of the disc and vertebral end plates. Of the 23 dogs, 17 had one or more sites of compression of the spinal cord or cauda equina, and both the severity of compression and the number of sites of compression correlated to the severity of the neurologic deficits [26].

It is important to consider other potential causes of signal changes of vertebral end plates and adjacent subchondral bone in MRI of dogs. A recent study reviewed spinal MRI of 75 dogs acquired over a 7-year period [27]. Diagnostic categories included reactive end plate changes (10 dogs, 13%), discospondylitis (29 dogs, 38%), vertebral osteochondrosis (7 dogs, 9%), intravertebral disc herniation (Schmorl's nodes in 4 dogs), and fatty infiltration (26 dogs, 34%). MRI criteria for discospondylitis in this study included paravertebral STIR hyperintensity or contrast enhancement, T2- and STIR-hyperintense and T1-hypointense signal from end plates, contrast enhancement of end plates, possible contrast enhancement of the disc space, end plate erosion, and collapse of the intervertebral space. Reactive end plate changes were characterized by T2 and STIR hyperintensity and T1 end plate hypointensity, with or without end plate enhancement. Osteochondrosis was diagnosed when a defect was observed on the dorsal edge of an end plate, with or without a matching bone fragment, with disc-isointense material filling the gap. Fatty replacement was significantly more common in small breeds, and the lumbosacral joint was a predilected site for end plate lesions, except for fatty deposits. Limitations of the study included lack of histologic confirmation and use of a low-field MRI, which implies that changes reported may not apply to high-field MRI. Causes for reactive end plate changes are unknown but may be related to disc injury [27].

MRI is also helpful in identifying paraspinal infections of the thoracolumbar spine. T2-hyperintense soft tissues, abscessation, mild inherent T1 hyperintensity of muscle, and abscesses along with postcontrast enhancement have been reported. In one study evaluating 22 dogs and 2 cats with paraspinal infection, lumbar vertebrae periosteal reactions were identified in 19/23 patients on MRI as compared with 15/17 patients with radiography. MRI permitted the extent of changes associated with paraspinal infection to be characterized and allowed the location, number, and any communication of sinus tracts to be documented [6].

Ultrasound

Ultrasound of paraspinal infection, either related to foreign bodies such as grass awns or of unknown cause, can be a helpful adjunct in lesion characterization and in monitoring response to treatment. Ultrasonography can demonstrate an increase in diameter of muscle as compared to normal and identify abscesses, which have an unstructured hypoechoic appearance with anechoic areas with possibly hyperechoic areas associated with the

foreign material and in some cases surrounded by an anechoic area [16]. In addition, ultrasound guided aspiration of lesions can provide material for culture and can also be utilized for drainage [6]. Ultrasonography has also been used to describe the intraoperative appearance of various spinal cord conditions, including discospondylitis and associated empyema, allowing the surgeon to more accurately extend the bony resection to more completely decompress or access the lesion [28].

Scintigraphy

Skeletal scintigraphy (bone scan), using intravenous injection of technetium-labeled diphosphonates, is a sensitive technique to detect early skeletal remodeling and to evaluate the activity of bony lesions. The 99mTc-MDP is incorporated into bone mineral and accurately reflects the status of bone remodeling as well as tissue perfusion [29]. Scintigraphy has been useful in identifying occult spinal or paraspinal infection in several case reports [1, 3, 16].

Identifying the organism

Once lesions consistent with spinal infection have been identified on imaging, the next important step in case management is to identify the underlying organism. A high level of suspicion is necessary to identify spinal infection in the early stages, and accurate identification of the underlying cause (where possible) and actual infective organism, is essential to prevent spread of the infection and avoid structural compromise of the vertebral bodies resulting in kyphosis, pathologic fracture and neurological deterioration. The wide variety of reported causative organisms, including aerobic and anaerobic bacteria as well as an increasing variety of fungi, combined with increasingly resistant strains of common bacteria, make empirical antibiotic treatment often unrewarding. The "gold standard" for diagnosis is surgically obtained biopsy and culture. However, the invasive nature and expense of surgery may not be financially or clinically feasible for all clients. Particularly in dogs and cats without neurologic compromise, other methods of organism identification may be used. Because urinary or reproductive tract infections are the most commonly reported concurrent conditions, it is sometimes possible to isolate the offending organism from the urine (success in about 29% of cases in one study) [15]. Blood culture can also be useful and was positive in 34% of cases in that same study. Common isolates include *Staphylococcus* spp., *Streptococcus*, and *E. coli*, but many others have been reported including *Pseudomonas aeruginosa*, *Enterococcus*, *Bordetella*, and *Pasteurella* [2, 30, 31].

Depending on the signalment, geographic location, and history, infectious disease titers may be helpful. In several studies, *Brucella canis* was identified as one of the most common causative organisms. A rapid slide agglutination test (RSAT), tube agglutination test (TAT), or ELISA can be useful screening tests, as they are highly sensitive, and a negative test is generally sufficient evidence that infection is not present. A positive screening test for *B. canis* should be confirmed by an agar gel immunodiffusion test (AGID) [32].

Aspergillus infection should be considered when the dog affected by discospondylitis is a German shepherd or German shepherd mix, although other breeds can be affected by this organism as well [33]. Although serologic testing can be performed, results are not as accurate as for *Brucella canis* [34]. Although it is unusual, spinal infection can lead to pleural or peritoneal effusion, and aspiration, cytology, and culture of that effusion may be used to diagnose the causative agent [35].

A definitive diagnosis of the causative agent can sometimes be made by percutaneous aspiration of the disc [36], and fluoroscopy-guided aspiration is the gold standard for diagnosis in humans [10]. Microbial culture of samples obtained by surgical biopsy, although more invasive, have a higher success rate. It should be kept in mind that in some cases, polymicrobial infections are present and that blood and urine cultures may not reveal the same organism as that identified from that directly sampled from the lesion [15].

Treatment

Treatment with antimicrobial drugs is recommended on the basis of results of microbial culture and susceptibility testing. Cage rest, particularly in dogs that may be at risk for pathologic fracture or kyphosis based on imaging, may be helpful, although appropriate duration of rest has not been reported for the dog and cat. Although *Staphylococcus intermedius* is one of the most common isolates of all types of spinal infection in the dog, increasing resistance means that empiric administration of a first-generation cephalosporin drug alone may not be effective in controlling the infection [37, 38]. If an organism is not identified on initial testing or if the animal is not responding to treatment, additional, repeat, or more aggressive testing is indicated, including surgical biopsy and culture if possible.

There is not a standard duration of treatment recommended in the veterinary literature for satisfactory resolution of spinal infection. However, if there is bony involvement, the clinician should treat as for any osteomyelitis. In humans with spondylodiscitis, 6 weeks of intravenous antibiotics are recommended, with follow-up oral antibiotics for an additional 3–6 months in many cases, with clearance of the infection monitored using erythrocyte sedimentation rate (ESR) and C-reactive protein testing [10].

In one study in dogs, a mean of 53 weeks of antimicrobial administration was reported. Lack of identification of the causative organism, inability to provide long-term intravenous antibiotics, client compliance, and relapse all likely play a role in the apparent need for much longer-term antimicrobial therapy than is typically seen for other types of osteomyelitis [8, 15].

Dogs with brucellosis should be considered potentially infected for life, and owners should be warned by the veterinarian about zoonotic transmission as well as being referred to their physician for testing and treatment if exposed. *Brucella canis* infection has recently been reported in two immunocompromised humans and in an outbreak involving two families with small children who interacted with infected dogs [39–41]. If owners choose treatment for their dogs, they should be counseled to neuter the pet to reduce shedding of organisms into the environment, and to wear impermeable gloves to clean up any urine and feces. Combination antibiotic therapy (e.g., doxycycline and enrofloxacin) should be considered, and serologic testing should be repeated every 4–6 months [32].

Little is known regarding the use of imaging to guide the decision to stop antimicrobial drug therapy, with no reports of using CT, MRI, or scintigraphy as follow-up tools in dogs or cats with spinal infection and only one report regarding radiographic findings during recovery from discospondylitis [8]. Until further evidence becomes available, a combination of clinical signs (e.g., complete resolution of vertebral column pain on deep palpation) and absence of radiographic evidence of active disease are recommended. Markers of radiographic quiescence include absence of a lytic focus, smoothing and then loss of the sclerotic margins formed around the lytic focus, or replacement by bridging of the involved vertebrae [15].

Surgical decompression is indicated when there is evidence of significant spinal cord compression, as in empyema [5, 24], or evidence of vertebral column instability and neurologic compromise [20]. Surgery may also allow the application of local antibiotic therapy, including gentamicin-impregnated bone cement, gentamicin-impregnated resorbable collagen sponge, or local injection of cefazolin in conjunction with fluoroscopy-guided percutaneous discectomy [20, 42, 43]. Surgery has also been reported to remove a bony sequestrum to facilitate resolution of vertebral physitis [3] and to decompress paraspinal abscess [6].

Summary

Spinal infections are becoming increasingly recognized in small animals, and early diagnosis is more likely to lead to clinical resolution with less risk of vertebral column instability. Diagnosis and treatment can be challenging, with a wide variety of clinical presentations. The clinician should be aggressive regarding both recommendation for diagnostic imaging and also obtaining appropriate samples from the infected site in the spine for microbial culture, particularly in animals with neurologic compromise or who are not responding to initial treatment, even when blood or urine cultures yielded positive results. Treatment should not be withdrawn prematurely, as relapse is common in cases where discontinuation of treatment was based solely on perception of improved clinical signs.

References

1. Rabillard M, Souchu L, Niebauer GW, Gauthier O. Haematogenous osteomyelitis: clinical presentation and outcome in three dogs. Vet Comp Orthop Traumatol. 2011;24(2):146–50.
2. Csebi P, Jakab C, Janosi K, Sellyei B, Ipolyt T, Szabo Z, et al. Vertebral osteomyelitis and meningomyelitis caused by pasteurella canis in a dog-clinicopathological case report. Acta Vet Hung. 2010;58(4):413–21.
3. Walker M, Platt SR, Graham JP, Clemmons RM. Vertebral physitis with epiphyseal sequestration and a portosystemic shunt in a Pekingese dog. J Small Anim Pract. 1999;40:525–8.
4. Jimenez MM, O'Callaghan MW. Vertebral physitis: a radiographic diagnosis to be separated from discospondylitis. Vet Radiol Ultrasound. 1995;36(3): 188–95.
5. Lavely JA, Vernau KM, Vernau W, Herrgesell EJ, LeCouteur RA. Spinal epidural empyema in seven dogs. Vet Surg. 2006 Feb;35(2):176–85.
6. Holloway A, Dennis R, McConnell F, Herrtage M. Magnetic resonance imaging features of paraspinal infection in the dog and cat. Vet Radiol Ultrasound. 2009 May–Jun;50(3):285–91.
7. Carrera I, Sullivan M, McConnell F, Goncalves R. Magnetic resonance imaging features of discospondylitis in dogs. Vet Radiol Ultrasound. 2011 Mar–Apr;52(2):125–31.
8. Shamir MH, Tavor N, Aizenberg T. Radiographic findings during recovery from discospondylitis. Vet Radiol Ultrasound. 2001 Nov–Dec;42(6):496–503.
9. Cherrone KL, Eich CS, Bonzynski JJ. Suspected paraspinal abscess and spinal epidural empyema in a dog. J Am Anim Hosp Assoc. 2002 Mar–Apr; 38(2):149–51.
10. Lehovsky J. Pyogenic vertebral osteomyelitis/disc infection. Baillieres Best Pract Res Clin Rheumatol. 1999 Mar;13(1):59–75.
11. Dunbar JA, Sandoe JA, Rao AS, Crimmins DW, Baig W, Rankine JJ. The MRI appearances of early vertebral osteomyelitis and discitis. Clin Radiol. 2010 Dec;65(12):974–81.
12. MacFarlane PD, Iff I. Discospondylitis in a dog after attempted extradural injection. Vet Anaesth Analg. 2011 May;38(3):272–3.
13. Remedios AM, Wagner R, Caulkett NA, Duke T. Epidural abscess and discospondylitis in a dog after administration of a lumbosacral epidural analgesic. Can Vet J. 1996 Feb;37(2):106–7.
14. Schwartz M, Boettcher IC, Kramer S, Tipold A. Two dogs with iatrogenic discospondylitis caused by meticillin-resistant Staphylococcus aureus. J Small Anim Pract. 2009 Apr;50(4):201–5.
15. Burkert BA, Kerwin SC, Hosgood GL, Pechman RD, Fontenelle JP. Signalment and clinical features of diskospondylitis in dogs: 513 cases (1980–2001). J Am Vet Med Assoc. 2005 Jul 15;227(2):268–75.

16. Frendin J, Funkquist B, Hansson K, Lonnemark M, Carlsten J. Diagnostic imaging of foreign body reactions in dogs with diffuse back pain. J Small Anim Pract. 1999;40:278–85.

17. Du Plessis CJ, Keller N, Millward IR. Aberrant extra-dural spinal migration of Spirocerca lupi: four dogs. J Small Anim Prac. 2007 May;48(5):275–8.

18. Maritato KC, Colon JA, Ryan KA. What is your diagnosis? J Am Vet Med Assoc. 2007;230(6):821–22.

19. Sutton A, May C, Coughlan A. Spinal osteomyelitis and epidural empyema in a dog due to migrating conifer material. Vet Rec. 2010;166:693–4.

20. Cabassu J, Moissonnier P. Surgical treatment of a vertebral fracture associated with a haematogenous osteomyelitis in a dog. Vet Comp Orthop Traumatol. 2007;20(3):227–30.

21. Packer RA, Coates JR, Cook CR, Lattimer JC, O'Brien DP. Sublumbar abscess and diskospondylitis in a cat. Vet Radiol Ultrasound. 2005 Sep–Oct;46(5):396–9.

22. Davis MJ, Dewey CW, Walker MA, Kerwin SC, Moon ML, Kortz GD, et al. Contrast radiographic findings in canine bacterial discospondylitis: a multicenter, retrospective study of 27 cases. J Am Anim Hosp Assoc. 2000;36:81–5.

23. Nykamp SG, Steffey MA, Scrivani PV, Schatzberg SJ. Computed tomographic appearance of epidural empyema in a dog. Can Vet J. 2003 Sep;44(9):729–31.

24. Granger N, Hidalgo A, Leperlier D, Gnirs K, Thibaud JL, Delisle F, et al. Successful treatment of cervical spinal epidural empyema secondary to grass awn migration in a cat. J Feline Med Surg. 2007 Aug;9(4):340–5.

25. Kraft SL, Mussman JM, Smith T, Biller DS, Hoskinson JJ. Magnetic resonance imaging of presumptive lumbosacral discospondylitis in a dog. Vet Radiol Ultrasound. 1998 Jan–Feb;39(1):9–13.

26. Harris JM, Chen AV, Tucker RL, Mattoon JS. Clinical features and magnetic resonance imaging characteristics of diskospondylitis in dogs: 23 cases (1997–2010). J Am Vet Med Assoc. 2013 Feb 1;242(3):359–65.

27. Gendron K, Doherr MG, Gavin P, Lang J. Magnetic resonance imaging characterization of vertebral endplate changes in the dog. Vet Radiol Ultrasound. 2011 Oct 12;53:50–6.

28. Nanai B, Lyman R, Bichsel PS. Use of intraoperative ultrasonography in canine spinal cord lesions. Vet Radiol Ultrasound. 2007 May–Jun;48(3):254–61.

29. Samoy Y, Van Ryssen B, Van Caelenberg A, Gielen I, Van Vynckt D, Van Bree H, et al. Single-phase bone scintigraphy in dogs with obscure lameness. J Small Anim Pract. 2008 Sep;49(9):444–50.

30. Adamo PF, Cherubini GB. Discospondylitis associated with three unreported bacteria in the dog. J Small Anim Pract. 2001;42:352–5.

31. Cherubini GB, Cappello R, Lu D, Targett M, Wessmann A, Mantis P. MRI findings in a dog with discospondylitis caused by Bordetella species. J Small Anim Pract. 2004 Aug;45(8):417–20.

32. Makloski CL. Canine brucellosis management. Vet Clin North Am Small Anim Pract. 2011 Nov;41(6):1209–19.

33. Zhang S, Corapi W, Quist E, Griffin S, Zhang M. Aspergillus versicolor, a new causative agent of canine disseminated aspergillosis. J Clin Microbiol. 2012 Jan;50(1):187–91.

34. Billen F, Peeters D, Peters IR, Helps CR, Huynen P, De Mol P, et al. Comparison of the value of measurement of serum galactomannan and Aspergillus-specific antibodies in the diagnosis of canine sino-nasal aspergillosis. Vet Microbiol. 2009 Feb 2;133(4):358–65.

35. Quance-Fitch FJ, Schachter S, Christopher MM. Pleural effusion in a dog with discospondylitis. Vet Clin Pathol. 2002;31(2):69–71.

36. Fischer A, Mahaffey MB, Oliver JE. Fluoroscopically guided percutaneous disk aspiration in 10 dogs with diskospondylitis. J Vet Intern Med. 1997;11:284–7.

37. Fitzgerald JR. The Staphylococcus intermedius group of bacterial pathogens: species re-classification, pathogenesis and the emergence of meticillin resistance. Vet Dermatol. 2009 Oct;20(5–6):490–5.

38. Guardabassi L, Loeber ME, Jacobson A. Transmission of multiple antimicrobial-resistant Staphylococcus intermedius between dogs affected by deep pyoderma and their owners. Vet Microbiol. 2004 Jan 14; 98(1):23–7.

39. Lucero NE, Corazza R, Almuzara MN, Reynes E, Escobar GI, Boeri E, et al. Human Brucella canis outbreak linked to infection in dogs. Epidemiol Infect. 2010 Feb;138(2):280–5.

40. Lucero NE, Maldonado PI, Kaufman S, Escobar GI, Boeri E, Jacob NR. Brucella canis causing infection in an HIV-infected patient. Vector Borne Zoonotic Dis. 2010 Jun;10(5):527–9.

41. Lawaczeck E, Toporek J, Cwikla J, Mathison BA. Brucella canis in a HIV-infected patient. Zoonoses Public Health. 2011 Mar;58(2):150–2.

42. Renwick AI, Dennis R, Gemmill TJ. Treatment of lumbosacral discospondylitis by surgical stabilisation and application of a gentamicin-impregnated collagen sponge. Vet Comp Orthop Traumatol. 2010;23(4):266–72.

43. Kinzel S, Koch J, Buecker A, Krombach G, Stopinski T, Afify M, et al. Treatment of 10 dogs with discospondylitis by fluoroscopy-guided percutaneous discectomy. Vet Rec. 2005 Jan 15;156(3):78–81.

21 Neoplasias Mimicking Intervertebral Disc Herniation

Gwendolyn J. Levine

Introduction

Tumors originating from the vertebral bodies or epidural space are relatively uncommon in veterinary medicine, while neoplasia developing from the intervertebral disc itself has not been reported. Tumors arising from vertebrae or within the epidural space may mimic intervertebral disc herniation (IVDH) on currently available imaging and will be discussed in this chapter.

Patients afflicted with neoplasia of the vertebral column or structures within the epidural space may have similar clinical signs compared to those with IVDH. Often the course is progressive in dogs with these neoplasms, with clinical signs reported from months to years prior to presentation. Some animals with vertebral neoplasia may have acute onset dysfunction or rapid deterioration after a slowly progressive course of disease due to pathologic fracture, vascular events, or rapid tumor growth. Animals with vertebral neoplasms mimicking IVDH will exhibit levels of neurologic dysfunction ranging from paraspinal hyperesthesia only to paralysis with no deep pain perception. Patients with neoplasia may or may not exhibit pain on palpation of the affected area of the vertebral column. Occasionally, paraneoplastic symptoms may be present, such as polyuria and polydipsia secondary to humoral hypercalcemia of malignancy as a result of lymphoma, or seizures due to hyperviscosity syndrome arising from markedly elevated protein concentrations in the blood from multiple myeloma.

Neoplasia sharing embryonic origin within the intervertebral disc: Chordoma

Although no chordomas in the veterinary literature have been reported to arise from the intervertebral disc itself, these tumors share a common origin with the nucleus pulposus [1]. The nucleus pulposus is the surviving structure of the embryologic notochord in the adult animal. Chordomas are thought to arise from notochordal

Advances in Intervertebral Disc Disease in Dogs and Cats, First Edition. Edited by James M. Fingeroth and William B. Thomas.
© 2015 ACVS Foundation. Published 2015 by John Wiley & Sons, Inc.

rests or remnants outside of the nucleus pulposus. These tumors are rare in dogs, with fewer than 10 cases reported in the veterinary literature since 1933 [1–7].

In humans, chordomas are most commonly found at the extreme cranial and caudal ends of the vertebral column [8]. In dogs, locations range from the skin over the parietal bone on the skull [4], intramedullary or extradural masses in the cervical spinal cord [3, 7], to the lumbar and coccygeal vertebrae [5]. A chordoma was also reported to arise within the meninges adjacent to the cerebellar fossa, while another was found between the trachea and ventral muscles of the vertebral column, ventral to C1 [4, 7].

Although a male sex predilection was initially reported in dogs [4], the sample size available in peer-reviewed literature is too small to make such a generalization, as females have also been described with this neoplasm. Breeds ranging from Shetland Sheepdogs to Labrador retrievers have been affected, with no two reports sharing a common breed thus far.

In humans, the imaging features of chordoma often include vertebral body lysis, infiltration of the intervertebral disc space, and extradural compression of neuroparenchyma [8]. There are limited data in veterinary medicine concerning the radiographic, computed tomographic, and magnetic resonance imaging (MRI) appearance of chordoma. In dogs, chordomas can appear very similar to herniated disc material on radiographs (if located within the vertebral canal) and will occasionally contain multifocal areas of mineralization [9]. In two dogs, computed tomography suggested the presence of soft tissue dense masses with areas of mineralization that were either extradural or intramedullary; bony lysis was not identified [7, 9]. In one dog with chordoma, MRI revealed a T2 hyperintense lesion within the spinal cord parenchyma; the lesion was initially interpreted as spinal cord contusion secondary to disc herniation or neoplasia [3].

In human patients, chordomas are characterized by local invasiveness, aggressive regrowth at the site of resection, and late metastasis [8]. In the veterinary literature, there has been a single paper describing regrowth following incomplete surgical resection and no reports of metastasis [4].

Neoplasms mimicking IVDH: Tumors of the surrounding vertebrae

These neoplasms originate in the vertebral column and can extend into the epidural space, mimicking the appearance of a disc extrusion or protrusion. Reported vertebral tumors include osteosarcoma, chondrosarcoma, myeloma, fibrosarcoma, and hemangiosarcoma. These tumors often compromise the structural integrity of the vertebral body, resulting in pathologic fracture and severe neurologic dysfunction.

Osteosarcoma is the most common tumor of bone in the dog [10]. It arises from malignant primitive bone cells, which produce osteoid, and is most commonly seen in the appendicular skeleton of dogs. Approximately 25% of osteosarcomas are found in the axial skeleton [11]. Of these, only 15% originate in the vertebral column, and osteosarcoma is the most common extradural spinal neoplasm. In one report, 46% of dogs presenting with axial osteosarcoma had documented metastatic disease [10]. While large-breed dogs account for a majority of cases of osteosarcoma, small-breed dogs have a relatively higher incidence of axial compared to appendicular osteosarcoma [12]. Affected vertebrae do not have a consistent or specific radiographic or other imaging appearance. Biopsy with cytology and/ or histopathologic examination is recommended for diagnosis of this tumor.

Chondrosarcoma is the next most common primary bone tumor and approximately 61% originate in flat bones as opposed to the appendicular skeleton [13]. These tumors are slow growing, and metastasize slowly; therefore, if complete resection is possible, patients have long median survival times.

Plasma cell tumors are uncommon in dogs, and account for less than 4% of all vertebral neoplasms [14]. These tumors may present as solitary plasmacytomas or as multiple myeloma. In multiple myeloma, there is multifocal involvement of the bone marrow, often with presence of an intact or fragmented immunoglobulin in the peripheral blood, light chain (Bence Jones) proteinuria, and osteolytic lesions. The spleen and liver may also be infiltrated by neoplastic plasma cells. A strong male predilection was noted in a paper describing vertebral plasma cell tumors in eight dogs [14].

In that same report, lumbar location was exquisitely common and survival time in dogs receiving treatment ranged from 4 to 65 months.

Fibrosarcoma is a relatively uncommon primary tumor of bone, and the vertebral body is an uncommonly affected location. A report of 20 vertebral tumors contained six dogs with either primary or metastatic fibrosarcoma of the vertebral body [15]. No breed or sex predilection was evident. Many of these dogs were treated with surgery and had survival times ranging from 15 to 600 days.

Primary hemangiosarcomas of bone are an uncommon primary bone tumor, and occur in very low frequency in the vertebral column. These tumors arise from neoplastic endothelial cells, and are composed of myriad, large, disorganized vascular structures lined by plump endothelial cells. A breed predisposition for this tumor in this location has not been identified, which is likely a factor of how few cases have been reported. Hemangiosarcomas are highly malignant and rapidly metastasize.

Neoplasms mimicking disc displacement: Tumors of the epidural space

These neoplasms can be limited to the epidural space, resembling herniated disc material, or they may extend into the spinal cord itself, increasing the clinical suspicion of a neoplastic process on advanced imaging. Approximately 50% of reported spinal tumors in dogs are located within the epidural space [16]. Osteosarcoma and hemangiosarcoma can be found in this location without vertebral involvement (see previous discussion).

Nerve sheath tumors are the most common type of spinal tumor according to one source and may be extradural, intradural/extramedullary, or intramedullary [16]. The majority of nerve sheath tumors occur in the cervical region. Often, these tumors arise in the peripheral nerves and invade proximal structures including the spinal cord. They are most easily detected on MRI. Rarely, intervertebral disc material can herniate out of the intervertebral foramen, resembling a thickened nerve root (Figure 21.1). As extruded disc material within the intervertebral foramen and nerve sheath tumor may enhance on T1-weighted MRI,

differentiation of these etiologies can be difficult in some cases [17].

Lymphoma arising within the epidural space is relatively uncommon in dogs [16]. It has been rarely reported, and no breed, sex, or vertebral column location predilections have been determined. Limited data are available concerning MRI appearance, and survival data have been suggested to be poor.

Lipomas and myelolipomas have been reported in the epidural space. Myelolipomas are uncommon tumors composed of hematopoietic precursor cells and neoplastic adipocytes [18]. These tumors are more commonly found in the spleen, liver, and adrenal glands. Myelolipomas appear to have mixed signal intensity on MRI due to their composition of marrow elements and fat [18]. These tumors can be relatively nonaggressive without evidence of regrowth if complete surgical resection is achieved. Considering their epidural location and the variable signal characteristics reported in IVDH, it seems conceivable that these neoplasms could be mistaken for IVDH based on imaging.

Although meningiomas most commonly arise rostral to the foramen magnum, they can occur in the meninges of the vertebral column. Meningiomas are often seen in an intradural/extramedullary location; however, they have been reported in strictly extradural locations [19]. In dogs, approximately 70% of meningiomas occur within the cervical region [19]. Most affected animals are middle aged, and no clear gender predilection has been identified. On MRI, spinal meningiomas are typically well-marginated, broad-based lesions that are typically hyperintense on T2-weighted images, mildly hyperintense on T1-weighted images, and strongly contrast enhanced on T1-weighted images following the administration of gadolinium [19]. In a case series of 10 dogs, mean survival following surgical excision alone was 19 months [19].

Conclusion

Various neoplasms of the vertebral body and epidural space may mimic IVDH. The advent of high field MRI has significantly reduced the possibility of misclassifying tumors originating within vertebrae as IVDH. Sequences such as short tau inversion recovery (STIR) and T2 with chemical

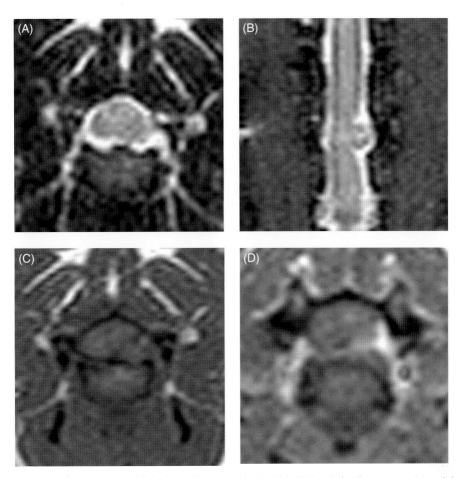

Figure 21.1   MR images from a 5-year-old dachshund suspected of IVDH. STIR-weighted transverse (A) and dorsal (B) images centered at the C5–C6 vertebral articulation show an isointense mass-like lesion located within the left ventrolateral epidural space and intervertebral foramen. On precontrast T1-weighted transverse images (C), the lesion was isointense to spinal cord parenchyma. Postcontrast T1-weighted transverse images (D) identified uniform, strong contrast enhancement of the majority of the lesion. At the time of evaluation, proximal nerve sheath tumor and lateralized disc extrusion were considered most likely. Histopathology confirmed the presence of disc extrusion adhered to the C6 spinal nerve and ventral nerve root.

fat saturation are exquisitely sensitive for destructive lesions within bone, which will appear hyperintense on these particular weightings. At centers using myelography to diagnose IVDH, misclassification may be possible as radiographic evidence of bone destruction is not always obvious.

Even with the advent of high field MRI, tumors and other lesions that are extradural and do not involve the vertebrae themselves may be challenging to differentiate from IVDH (Figure 21.2). In these cases, strong consideration should be given toward surgical exploration and biopsy or extradural compressive material.

References

1. Spoden JE, Bumsted RM, Warner ED. Chondroid chordoma. Case report and literature review. Ann Otol Rhinol Laryngol. 1980 May–Jun;89(3 Pt 1):279–85.
2. Ball V, Auger L. Les chordomas su tumeurs de la dorsale chez l'homme et les animaux. Rev Vet Zootech. 1933;85:185–95.
3. Gruber A, Kneissl S, Vidoni B, Url A. Cervical spinal chordoma with chondromatous component in a dog. Vet Pathol. 2008 Sep;45(5):650–3.
4. Jabara AG, Jubb KV. A case of a probable chordoma in a dog. Aust Vet J. 1971 Aug;47(8):394–7.

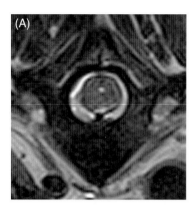
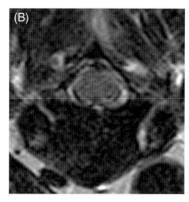
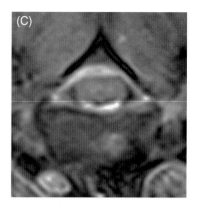

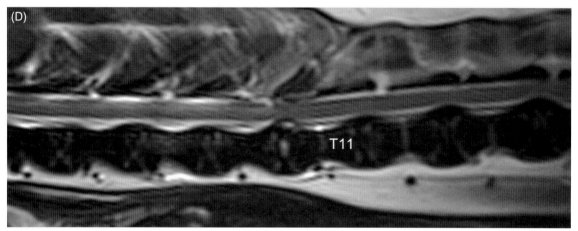

Figure 21.2 MR images from a 6-year-old dachshund suspected of IVDH. Transverse T2-weighted images clearly demonstrate the presence of normal epidural fat and spinal cord shape cranial to the lesion (A) and marked dorsolateral compression of the spinal cord at the T10–T11 vertebral articulation. On T2-weighted images, the compressive material is of mixed signal intensity. On T1-weighted postcontrast images (C) at the level of T10–T11, there is uniform, strong contrast enhancement of the entire lesion. A sagittal T2-weighted image (D) suggests the presence of hypo- and hyperintense material intimately associated with dorsal annulus of the T10–T11 intervertebral disc. At the time of evaluation, intervertebral disc extrusion was deemed most likely with secondary consideration given to neoplasia mimicking disc extrusion. Histopathology confirmed the presence of sterile, epidural steatitis, which may represent an immune-mediated disease process.

5. Munday JS, Brown CA, Weiss R. Coccygeal chordoma in a dog. J Vet. Diag Invest. 2003 May;15(3):285–8.
6. Saliba AM, Neto ZL, Greechi R, Mariano M, Martin BW, Migliano MF. Chordoma in two dogs. Arq Inst Biol S Paulo. 1967;34:45–50.
7. Woo GH, Bak EJ, Lee YW, Nakayama H, Sasaki N, Doi K. Cervical chondroid chordoma in a Shetland sheep dog. J Comp Pathol. 2008 May;138(4):218–23.
8. Sciubba DM, Chi JH, Rhines LD, Gokaslan ZL. Chordoma of the spinal column. Neurosurg Clin N Am. 2008;19:5–15.
9. Pease AP, Berry CR, Mott JP, Peck JN, Mays MB, Hinton D. Radiographic, computed tomographic and histopathologic appearance of a presumed spinal chordoma in a dog. Vet Radiol Ultrasound. 2002 Jul–Aug;43(4):338–42.
10. Dickerson ME, Page RL, LaDue TA, Hauck ML, Thrall DE, Stebbins ME, et al. Retrospective analysis of axial skeleton osteosarcoma in 22 large-breed dogs. J Vet Intern Med. 2001 Mar–Apr;15(2):120–4.
11. Knecht CD, Priester WA. Musculoskeletal tumors in dogs. J Am Vet Med Assoc. 1978;172:72–4.
12. Cooley DM, Waters DJ. Skeletal neoplasms of small dogs: a retrospective study and literature review. J Am Anim Hosp Assoc. 1997;33:11–23.
13. Popovitch CA, Weinstein MJ, Goldschmidt MH, Shofer FS. Chondrosarcoma: a retrospective study of 97 dogs (1987–1990). J Am Anim Hosp Assoc. 1994;30:81–5.
14. Rusbridge C, Wheeler SJ, Lamb CR, Page RL, Carmichael S, Brearley MJ, et al. Vertebral plasma cell tumors in 8 dogs. J Vet Intern Med. 1999 Mar–Apr; 13(2):126–33.

15. Dernell WS, Van Vechten BJ, Straw RC, LaRue SM, Powers BE, Withrow SJ. Outcome following treatment of vertebral tumors in 20 dogs (1986–1995). J Am Anim Hosp Assoc. 2000 May–Jun;36(3):245–51.

16. Levy MS, Kapatkin AS, Patnaik AK, Mauldin GN, Mauldin GE. Spinal tumors in 37 dogs: clinical outcome and long-term survival (1987–1994). J Am Anim Hosp Assoc. 1997 Jul–Aug;33(4):307–12.

17. Suran JN, Durham A, Mai W, Seiler GS. Contrast enhancement of extradural compressive material on magnetic resonance imaging. Vet Radiol Ultrasound. 2011 Jan–Feb;52(1):10–16.

18. Ueno H, Miyake T, Kobayashi Y, Yamada K, Uzuka Y. Epidural spinal myelolipoma in a dog. J Am Anim Hosp Assoc. 2007 Mar–Apr;43(2):132–5.

19. Petersen SA, Sturges BK, Dickinson PJ, Pollard RE, Kass PH, Kent M, et al. Canine intraspinal meningiomas: imaging features, histopathologic classification, and long-term outcome in 34 dogs. J Vet Intern Med. 2008 Jul–Aug;22(4):946–53.

22 Client Communications When Confronted with a Patient with Suspected Intervertebral Disc Herniation

James M. Fingeroth and William B. Thomas

Veterinarians confronted with a patient exhibiting signs of discomfort and/or neurologic deficits, and in whom spinal cord disease is suspected as the cause, properly include intervertebral disc disease (IVDD) in their differential diagnoses. Elsewhere in this book, the difference between IVDD and intervertebral disc herniation (IVDH) has been addressed, as has the concept of "discogenic" pain not associated with actual disc displacement. When speaking with clients the attending clinician should bear these distinctions in mind since having the correct concept of what is really transpiring in the patient can influence what information we convey to clients, and the sense of urgency we need to express. The focus of this chapter is not so much about what actions the attending veterinarian should take (that is covered in Chapter 19), but on the key concepts to pass along to clients so that they, the clients, can make informed decisions as we counsel them regarding treatment options, referral recommendations, or prognosis.

As has been addressed elsewhere in this book, it is important not to provide a diagnosis of IVDD/IVDH to the clients as an established fact prematurely. Though IVDH may be far and away the most likely etiology for many of the patients we see with signs of neck or back pain or paresis, we should advise clients that there are other possible causes. It can be embarrassing or worse to subsequently find that the patient's signs were due to non-disc-related disease and to not have informed the client of this possibility (see Chapters 9, 20, and 21).

As outlined in the chapter on "when should dogs be referred for surgery" (Chapter 19), as well as the chapter on "history, neurologic examination, and neurolocalization" (Chapter 10), we at the outset have to formulate a recommended plan of action for the client based on our assessment of the patient. Concomitant with this formulated plan is the need to convey to the client what our reasoning is (e.g., conservative treatment initially or emergency referral?), as well as our expected results or alternative plans should we not achieve those expected results.

Advances in Intervertebral Disc Disease in Dogs and Cats, First Edition. Edited by James M. Fingeroth and William B. Thomas.
© 2015 ACVS Foundation. Published 2015 by John Wiley & Sons, Inc.

Imaging

The issue of taking plain radiographs on patients with suspected IVDD/IVDH is addressed elsewhere (Chapter 19). When the clinician elects to take survey radiographs, he or she should be clear in communicating to the client that the main objective in taking such images is to help rule out or reduce concern for other possible causes for the patient's signs (such as fracture, obvious infiltrative disease in the bone, obvious changes that might suggest discospondylitis, etc.) rather than to "prove" that the patient has IVDD or IVDH. It can be misleading to conclude that normal radiographs rule out IVDD, or that lesions that support a diagnosis of IVDD (such as narrowed disc spaces, calcified discs, spondylosis, etc.) somehow confirm the diagnosis of IVDH as the cause for the current signs. It can also undermine the clinician's relationship of trust with the client to point out a particular lesion on a plain radiograph, explain to the client that "the x-ray shows that the dog has a ruptured disc at T12–T13," only to later find out that the lesion was elsewhere or of some other pathology.

Crate/cage rest

Cage rest or similar confinement is the bedrock of conservative care for dogs with suspected IVDH where surgery is deemed not immediately necessary. It is imperative that the clinician *explicitly* describes the conditions and duration of such confinement. Many clients may be under the misapprehension that "cage rest" means keeping the dog crated—except when it's not and may not appreciate just how restrictive this limitation should be. This is especially true if the patient has minimal signs or signs that seem to be rapidly improving after only a few days. The veterinarian should describe in detail exactly what activity outside the crate is permissible, how the pet should be handled when outside the crate or cage, and the minimum time of such confinement regardless of perceived improvement.

The crate should be large enough for the pet to stand up and lay down comfortably. Most important is a top that is low enough to prevent the patient from attempting to stand up on the pelvic limbs. The crate is placed in a quiet room where there is minimal activity. Having the crate in a busy room, such as the kitchen or family room, often leads to the pet becoming more anxious and barking in an attempt to get out of the crate to be with the family members the pet can see and hear. This behavior is also stressful for the client and may even persuade the client to stop confinement prematurely.

The patient is kept confined except to go outside to urinate and defecate. For that, the pet is carried outside and placed on the ground with a leash and harness to eliminate and then carried back to the crate. Even 30 min of unrestricted activity can negate several days of confinement.

Clients should also be educated as to what signs to look for that might suggest deterioration in patient status, and which should prompt an immediate call to the veterinarian. Any progression in neurologic deficits such as worsening ataxia, paresis, or pain is an indication for reevaluation. The veterinarian or veterinary staff should periodically contact the client to ensure the patient is not getting worse and find out if the client is having any trouble complying with recommendations.

In addition to explaining *how* to provide restricted activity, it is critical to explain *why*. Many clients are personally familiar with back pain; about two-third of adults suffer back pain at some point in their life and disc extrusion accounts for only 4 per cent of these cases. The majority (95%) of human patients with back pain recover with conservative therapy, and prolonged strict bed rest is not recommended for uncomplicated back pain in human patients [1]. Clients will often extrapolate their experience to their pet's condition and thereby underestimate the need for strict confinement in dogs with potential disc extrusion. Hence, it is helpful to explain the differences between people with back pain and dogs with disc disease. People with back pain rarely suffer acute paralysis, whereas severe, even potentially permanent paralysis is a real risk in dogs with disc extrusion. Dogs with neck or back pain due to IVDD typically have torn annular fibers in the affected disc space. As with any damaged ligament, the annulus can heal with time provided further stress on the annulus is minimized. Therefore, the goal of confinement is to reduce stress on the damaged disc to allow healing and hopefully prevent further disc extrusion that could lead to spinal cord injury and the need for surgery. Confining the pet is not easy for the client. If they understand the reasons for this treatment, clients are more likely to comply with the veterinarian's recommendations.

With adequate client education, most patients with mild signs of IVDD can be managed successfully at home. However, after discussing recommendations with the client, the veterinarian may come to feel the client is unlikely to comply fully with cage rest at home. In those cases it is usually best to recommend hospitalization for a few days to watch for any neurologic worsening, provide good analgesia, and ensure the patient is adequately confined.

Paretic or paralyzed patients

The ante is raised when dogs have neurologic deficits and not just discomfort to manage. Clients need to understand in lay terms what is transpiring at the level of the spinal cord (see Chapters 3, 14, 15, and 19), and why there is concern about acting properly (type and timing of treatment) to hopefully prevent irreversible spinal cord injury and permanent paralysis. The clinician must convey the urgency of the case based on his assessment of the "time–sign graph" (Chapter 19) and suggest referral for definitive imaging and possible surgery when appropriate. As such a recommendation is made, the attending veterinarian should guard against making overly specific conclusions, such as the nature and level of the lesion based on radiographs (see the text on imaging), the absolute certainty of surgery being necessary (until so determined by advanced imaging findings combined with assessment of the patient's neurologic status and prognosis), the type of advanced imaging to be used (unless already established), or the speed with which each of these steps needs to be accomplished. It is best and more suitable to simply explain to the client that you feel conservative care may not be the proper course from this point on, and that you feel the patient's needs would best be met through the process of referral, and what might be accomplished thereafter.

At the same time, there are some important aspects to discuss with the client prior to referral for advanced imaging and potential surgery.

The process

The client should be provided with information regarding the person or institution to which they are being referred. To facilitate this, it is preferable for the attending clinician to communicate directly with the doctor or referral institution before sending the client and patient, in order to discuss any special logistical concerns and to permit the receiving hospital time to prepare for what may be an emergency disruption of an already established schedule. Referral hospitals and university teaching hospitals are not "black boxes"; they are facilities staffed by our colleagues and coworkers, and they no more appreciate a "surprise" emergency admission than any of us enjoy a sudden alteration of our carefully made plans for the day.

The need for any medication should be discussed with the referral specialist and the client instructed accordingly. For example, many surgeons would prefer the patient not receive aspirin prior to surgery. However, it is not uncommon for a client to administer aspirin to their pet for pain. Hence, preemptive warning against administering over-the-counter medication can help avoid future complications. Unless fasting is medically contraindicated, the client is instructed not to feed the pet a large meal soon before presentation to the referral center in case general anesthesia will be performed soon after admission.

With respect to advanced imaging, the attending doctor might ask whether it will be via myelography, CT, or MRI (or "to be determined") so as to avoid improperly suggesting to the client one modality and the client later being told a different modality is recommended. Similarly, the attending veterinarian should explain that the patient is being referred for *evaluation* for potential surgery. There are a number of reasons the referral specialist might decide surgery is not indicated or at least not indicated on an emergent basis. For example, the neurologic status may change from the time of the attending veterinarian's examination or further diagnostic investigation may reveal a disease other than IVDH. Conflicting recommendations from different veterinarians are confusing for the client, so while it is important for the client to know what to expect at the referral hospital, it is also helpful not to paint the referral specialist into a corner by promising specific procedures that the specialist may feel are not indicated.

Bladder management

If a pet is paralyzed, it is common for them to also have associated loss of normal bladder control. In the more common case of upper motor neuron deficits to the pelvic limbs, this usually implies a tendency for urine retention and reflexive overflow incontinence. The attending veterinarian should anticipate this, explain the concern to the client, and empty the bladder (manual expression or catheterization) as needed until and again just prior to referral. It is also important but frequently overlooked by the attending veterinarian to address the issue of bladder management with the client before committing them to referral. Clients of course are focused on the limb paralysis and any associated discomfort. It is incumbent on the veterinarian to also inform the client that there may be a period of time—even after any surgery—where the pet might continue to be unable to ambulate and might also still require assistance with bladder emptying. This is a crucial piece of client communication since, depending on patient size and/or client time or physical limitations, some clients may not be able to care for and manage a dog or cat that requires manual expression or catheterization. This in turn may have an impact on the client's decision to pursue referral and further care, and is best determined before the client travels to another institution or incurs much greater expense. The client education about bladder management needs to be reinforced as well at the receiving end of the referral chain (i.e., by the surgeon and affiliated personnel), in order to be sure that this very key concept is understood before making any final commitment to advanced imaging or surgery.

Costs

As always with referrals for any reason it is important for the client to have some idea of their impending financial obligation before committing to the process. This includes not only the estimated cost but also the availability or unavailability of any payment plans. Unfortunately, in veterinary medicine the emergent nature of any condition does not obviate the need for the client to take financial responsibility, since third party payment

is the exception rather than the rule. Referral practices and universities do not usually have funds they can commit to assisting those that cannot pay for services, even when done under the auspices of a teaching hospital setting. So there is little point in making an "emergency referral," only to have the client face the agonizing prospect of euthanasia or return to the primary care hospital once they arrive at the referral institution, unable to afford the recommended care. Such information is only a phone call away, and at least allows the attending veterinarian to provide the client with a reasonable estimated range of costs before actually making the referral. Either over- or underestimating the costs can have an adverse effect on outcome. If the attending veterinarian guesses too low, the client may face "sticker shock" when seen at the referral institution, and may have to abandon plans to continue. Conversely, if the attending veterinarian suggests an inappropriately high estimated cost, this might discourage a client from pursuing treatment that they in reality could have afforded. This same phone call can be used to alert the referral institution that a patient may be coming their way, and should be followed up with another call to verify whether and when they should expect to see the patient, after the attending doctor has discussed the issues with the client and the client has indicated how he or she wants to proceed.

Prognosis

The attending veterinarian should of course provide the client with his or her best estimation of the patient's chances for full or nearly full recovery, and what an approximate time line might be. As with the cost estimate, it is preferable to avoid providing an either overly optimistic or pessimistic prognosis. If the attending veterinarian is unsure, he or she should say so to the client, and see whether the receiving doctor or institution can provide a more accurate assessment. While statistics can guide such discussion with the client, it is always important that clients understand and accept that there are some factors that cannot be known (e.g., the severity of spinal cord injury prior to treatment), or fully controlled (e.g., the degree of possible iatrogenic injury caused during decompressive surgery), which can affect outcome and delay or lessen the chances for neurologic recovery. Clinicians should bear in mind that "prognostic indicators" such as the presence or absence of nociception ("deep pain") distal to the lesion are not objective measures (see Chapter 11), and so only provide a rough idea as to prognosis.

Also included in the discussion with clients regarding prognosis is an explanation that most dogs and cats do not appear to suffer the same psychological negatives that we associate with humans who suddenly lose function in their limbs. While long term or indefinite management of a paraplegic dog or cat may be difficult for some, there are many instances where paralyzed dogs and cats have seemingly enjoyed a good quality of life so long as their physical needs (e.g., bladder management, prevention of sores, ambulating with carts, etc.) were met [2]. Therefore, in circumstances where the prognosis for recovery seems poor, or where clients are unable to afford a recommended intervention, there may be alternatives to euthanasia, and the client should at least be provided the opportunity to consider or try management of a paralyzed pet at home.

Conclusion

The goal for veterinarians when counseling clients with dogs suspected of having IVDD/IVDH should be to provide those key pieces of information that will allow each client to understand the salient aspects of their pet's condition, and to make informed decisions that take into account the pet's needs as well as the client's capabilities with respect to logistical, financial, emotional/psychological, and physical requirements for ongoing care. In this way, and regardless of client choices or outcome, we have served our role as health care professionals and met our obligations to both client and patient alike.

References

1. Kinkade S. Evaluation and treatment of acute low back pain. Am Fam Physician. 2007 Apr 15;75(8): 1181–8.
2. Bauer M, Glickman N, Glickman L, Toombs J, Golden S, Skowronek C. Follow-up study of owner attitudes toward home care of paraplegic dogs. J Am Vet Med Assoc. 1992 Jun 15;200(12):1809–16.

Section IV

Nonsurgical and Adjunctive Medical Management of IVDD

Not all patients affected by IVDD need surgery. And some that might best be served by surgery may only be managed nonoperatively owing to client decisions not to pursue recommended surgical intervention. Dogs that do receive surgical treatment require appropriate preoperative and postoperative care. There is also a great deal of controversy regarding some of the nonoperative and pharmacologic interventions available. In this section, we attempt to address some of these areas of controversy, and provide as much scientific evidence as possible to guide the veterinarian in making proper treatment choices.

23 Steroid Use in Intervertebral Disc Disease

Joseph M. Mankin and Franck Forterre

Introduction

Glucocorticoids have been used in cases of intervertebral disc disease managed both medically and surgically since the 1960s and have been shrouded in controversy for at least the past 15 years. While clinical improvement can be seen in certain cases, the use of steroids is not without risk and potential detriment to the patient. Most physicians and veterinarians today prescribe steroids in this setting, not because of an understanding of the evidence surrounding their use, but largely because the practice has been so common over a long period of time [1]. In this chapter, we will address the reasons steroids can be useful, the controversy surrounding them, and their effects in our patients.

Pathophysiology

One of the effects of acute spinal cord injury (SCI) is reduction in blood flow to the neural tissue. As reperfusion occurs, highly reactive free radicals are liberated. These free radicals cause damage to the plasma membrane of cells by the process of lipid peroxidation. This phenomenon is key in irreversible tissue loss following spinal cord trauma and ischemia [2].

The potentially beneficial mechanism of action of glucocorticoids in SCI is inhibition of this lipid peroxidation as well as hydrolysis, processes that lead to damage of both neuronal and microvascular membranes [3]. This inhibition is postulated to be due to the steroids' high lipid solubility and ability to intercalate into artificial membranes between the hydrophobic polyunsaturated fatty acids of the membrane phospholipids and limit the chain reaction of lipid peroxidation throughout the phospholipid bilayer [4–6]. This is the so-called "membrane stabilization" phenomenon that steroids are known for. In addition to the primary action of glucocorticoids at physiologic doses, some formulations, such as methylprednisolone sodium succinate (MPSS) and lazeroids (21-aminosteroids), can exert a number of other actions on the spinal cord when given at suprapharmacologic doses, including maintenance of tissue blood flow, maintenance of aerobic energy metabolism, improved reversal of intracellular calcium accumulation,

Advances in Intervertebral Disc Disease in Dogs and Cats, First Edition. Edited by James M. Fingeroth and William B. Thomas.
© 2015 ACVS Foundation. Published 2015 by John Wiley & Sons, Inc.

reduction of neurofilament degradation, and enhanced neuronal excitability and synaptic transmission [3, 5, 7].

Another effect of methylprednisolone is inhibition of phospholipase A_2 formation, inhibiting arachidonic acid release as well as prostaglandin $F_{2\alpha}$ and thromboxane A_2, which can produce anti-inflammatory effects. Dexamethasone has historically been used frequently for SCI, based on the fact that it is such a potent glucocorticoid and has a high anti-inflammatory potency. However, as an inhibitor of lipid peroxidation it is only slightly more potent than methylprednisolone, as well as having fewer antioxidant properties [5, 6]. Due to these findings, both animal and human studies have focused on methylprednisolone for SCI in the past two decades.

In cases of chronic spinal cord compression, both blood flow and oxygen levels can be better maintained without intervention due to the slow, progressive nature of the process. The most common pathology in these cases is predominantly demyelination and axonal swelling, with white matter edema occurring later. Glucocorticoids are effective against this vasogenic edema, accounting for the clinical response seen in chronic cases [8].

Justification of steroid use based on human literature

Initial studies

Starting in 1979, three National Acute Spinal Cord Injury Studies (NASCIS) were conducted to determine the efficacy of MPSS as a treatment modality for acute SCI. The first study compared a standard dose of MPSS to high-dose MPSS, with sensory and motor assessments being performed at admission, 6 weeks, 6 months, and 1 year after injury. The results showed no significant difference between the two groups [2, 7].

The second study compared groups receiving high-dose MPSS, a placebo, or an opioid antagonist (Naloxone). Once again, sensory and motor assessments were conducted at admission, 6 weeks, 6 months, and 1 year after injury. Results showed improved sensory function at 6 months, but no significant difference at 1 year. There was no difference in motor score between treatment groups at any time point. However, with *post hoc*

stratification of patients by time to treatment, patients receiving steroids within 8 h had a statistically significant improvement in motor score at 6 months and 1 year [9].

The third NASCIS was performed on those patients receiving therapy within 8 h, and the groups consisted of MPSS bolus with 24 h infusion, MPSS bolus with 48 h infusion, and MPSS bolus followed by Tirilazad, a lazeroid drug that has similar lipid peroxidation effects without the glucocorticoid activity. There was no significant difference in motor score between treatment groups at any time point. Using *post hoc* analysis, patients treated with 48 h infusion of MPSS starting between 3 and 8 h of injury had higher motor scores at 6 weeks and 6 months, but not at 1 year [10].

Follow-up studies and reassessment

Since the results of NASCIS trials have been published, there has been significant controversy over the results. There have been many criticisms of the studies including the study design, determination of timing of therapy, and the statistical analysis performed. The use of *post hoc* analysis of subgroups raises the possibility that the statistically significant results were random events. The fact that only right-sided motor scores were reported, while bilateral sensory scores were reported, has raised questions. The statistics performed were only done on one-third of the patients enrolled due to exclusion criteria, which reduced the power of the study. In addition, there was not a standard medical or surgical treatment regimen for patients in the study.

The higher motor and sensory scores for patients receiving methylprednisolone do not necessarily correlate with significant, life-altering improvement as the functional scores remained the same. In addition, those differences in recovery were only seen in those patients with complete SCI (i.e., loss of both motor function and sensation).

Several other studies have been performed, but none could reproduce the findings from the initial studies. However, there has been evidence that those treated with methylprednisolone have an increased risk of complications including pneumonia, sepsis, and death due to respiratory complications [11–14].

The controversy surrounding the results has brought into question the use of steroids as standard of care. In fact, many hospitals no longer use steroids in cases of spinal trauma.

Animal models/studies

Initial animal models in SCI included rat and feline models. From these studies, the benefits of steroids were examined as a precursor to human studies for MPSS. Initial results showed that high-dose MPSS was effective in improving functional neurologic recovery in these experimental models [15, 16]. Despite those studies, obtaining comparable results in clinical cases has proven to be quite elusive.

When comparing dexamethasone to a placebo in feline models, it was found that dexamethasone was no more effective [17]. In cases of presumed thoracolumbar intervertebral disc herniation (IVDH), results suggested that glucocorticoid administration was negatively associated with success. It was also associated with low owner-reported quality of life. The potential causes for these results could be due to direct effects of glucocorticoids on the spinal cord, systemic glucocorticoid side effects, or the fact that some dogs with presumed herniation may have had other causes for their myelopathy wherein steroids would be contraindicated [18]. In a study of patients with disc-associated wobbler syndrome (DAWS; see Chapter 7), where there is disc protrusion instead of extrusion, a treatment protocol of prednisone and cage rest was instituted. Those patients that were treated with glucocorticoids prior to diagnosis had significant improvement when compared to treatment with nonsteroidal anti-inflammatory drugs (NSAIDs) or a combination of both [19]. This improvement is probably attributable to diminishing vasogenic edema, which results in return of function without removal of the mass [8].

The administration of glucocorticoids has been associated with significant side effects, especially in cases of spinal cord disease. Patients with acute SCI are at an increased risk of gastrointestinal (GI) hemorrhage and ulceration [20, 21]. Side effects associated with steroid use include vomiting, diarrhea, and potentially fatal GI hemorrhage, ulceration, and perforation [22, 23]. When the high-dose MPSS protocol was studied in canine patients, those that received it had a significantly increased cost for that hospital stay, and had more GI complications than those receiving other steroids [24]. In a further study, dogs receiving dexamethasone were found to be 3.4 times as likely to develop adverse effects, 3.5 times as likely to develop diarrhea, and 11.4 times as likely to have urinary tract infections compared to dogs treated without dexamethasone [25].

With all of the controversy surrounding the human NASCIS, it is difficult to extrapolate their results to our patients. When examined closely, the benefit perceived in humans was very slight, with the result being minimal motor improvement. It is hard to discern what function that would correlate to in our patients, and if that effect would even be perceptible (in some humans there was increased digital motor function; such a benefit in dogs would be clinically insignificant). Another limitation in extrapolating the human trials to our patients has to do with the temporal effects of steroid administration. The human studies routinely showed either no benefit or worsened outcomes when patients received steroids more than 8h after SCI. Unfortunately for veterinarians, it is not always possible to identify the precise time of onset of disc-induced SCI in our patients, so we may find ourselves treating dogs with steroids well beyond any time frame where they might have had any potential benefit. Until we have prospective, blinded, large-scale studies in our patients with naturally occurring SCI, we cannot advocate using high-dose MPSS in our patients.

Recently, epidural infiltration with methylprednisolone acetate for medical treatment of degenerative lumbosacral stenosis in dogs has been described. Since local inflammation is a well-known component associated with compression in degenerative lumbosacral stenosis, it is a short logical step to deposit an anti-inflammatory drug at the inflamed location. The results from epidural infiltration were comparable to those of dorsal decompressive surgery and comparable to those of human studies of similar lesions, with rapid amelioration of clinical signs in most patients and a long-term recovery rate of approximately 50–75% [26]. Dogs in this study had pain and/or lameness but those with neurologic deficits such as loss of proprioception or incontinence were excluded.

Current uses and recommendations

Even with the controversy surrounding the use of steroids in cases of suspected IVDH, they can still be used judiciously in appropriate situations. Patients that might benefit from the anti-inflammatory properties are those that are amenable to being managed medically; the prime example being mainly cases of ambulatory paraparesis in a first-time offender with other major differentials ruled out, or patients with cervical pain where IVDH is the top differential. The key to safely using these medications is to use them at an anti-inflammatory dose for a short, tapering period. A typical recommended protocol is to use a short-acting medication such as prednisone at 0.5–1.0 mg/kg/day for 5 days, decreasing by 50% for 5 days and then going to an every-other-day regimen for five treatments. It is best to avoid long-acting formulations such as methylprednisolone acetate (Depo-Medrol) or dexamethasone, since the medication may have to be withdrawn if side effects are seen, if the patient's condition worsens, or if there is another underlying cause of the neurologic disease rather than IVDH. If drugs such as dexamethasone are utilized, it is also imperative to use much lower doses than prednisone and to taper off the drug more quickly, so as to avoid some of the aforementioned potentially catastrophic side effects. Moreover, because of its long half-life, there is no physiologic advantage to reducing dexamethasone to every-other-day treatment as there is with prednisone. In addition, in some experimental models of spinal cord damage, with administration of long-term steroids, there was not only a decrease in demyelination but also interference with remyelination, showing both positive and negative effects [27].

When steroids (or any medical management) are used in lieu of surgery for treating presumptive IVDH, it is key for these patients to have strict cage confinement during the medical management period, as the anti-inflammatory effects of the steroids can reduce the patient's discomfort, cause them to have an increase in activity, and potentially result in further disc herniation and resultant worsening of clinical signs.

Based on initial experimental animal models that showed improved neurologic function and neuroprotective effects in animals treated with steroids prior to or just after SCI [28], there is some consideration in their use prior to an invasive spinal cord surgery. Typically, this is considered in surgeries that will result in significant spinal cord manipulation or handling, such as repair of vertebral body fractures/subluxations or with intradural spinal cord tumor removal, but some also consider their use for disc removal surgery. There is no clinical evidence justifying steroid use in these scenarios, and the side effects and increased risk associated with steroid use are still present. However, there may be a theoretical benefit in some cases, so their preemptive use by some surgeons in cases of unavoidable anticipated spinal cord manipulation is understandable, even if not scientifically validated.

Conclusion

There is a significant amount of controversy over the use of glucocorticoids in humans and subsequently in our animal patients as well. We understand why they might be helpful in cases of acute SCI based on experimental models, but producing convincing results in clinical cases has not been consistently accomplished at this point. Our patients can benefit from their use (particularly in those with chronic spinal cord compression), but only in carefully selected acute cases, and with appropriate, short-term use.

References

1. Hurlbert RT. The role of steroids in acute spinal cord injury. An evidence based analysis. Spine 2001;26:39–46.
2. Sharp NJ, Wheeler SJ. Small Animal Spinal Disorders. 2005, Elsevier Limited, Philadelphia, PA.
3. Bracken MB, Shepard MJ, Holford TR, et al. Administration of Methylprednisolone for 24 or 48 hours or Tirilazad Mesylate for 48 hours in the treatment of acute spinal cord injury. JAMA 1997; 277(20):1597–1604.
4. Demoupoulis HB, Flamm ES, Pietronigro DD, et al. The free radical pathology and the microcirculation in the major central nervous system disorders. Acta Physiol Scand Suppl 1980;492:91–119.
5. Hall ED. The neuroprotective pharmacology of methylprednisolone. J Neurosurg 1992;76:13–22.
6. Hall ED, Springer JE. Neuroprotection and acute spinal cord injury: a reappraisal. NeuroRx 2004; 1:80–100.

7. Bracken MB, Shepard MJ, Collins WF, *et al.* A randomized, controlled trial of methylprednisolone or naloxone in the treatment of acute spinal cord injury. NEJM 1990; 322(20):1405–11.

8. Platt SR, Abramson CJ, Garosi LS. Administering corticosteroids in neurologic diseases. Compend Contin Ed Pract Vet 2005;27(3):210–227.

9. Bracken MB, Shepard MJ, Collins WF, *et al.* Methylprednisolone or naloxone treatment after acute spinal cord injury: 1-year follow up data. Results of second National Acute Spinal Cord Injury Study. J Neurosurg 1992;76:23–31.

10. Bracken MB, Shepard MJ, Holford TR, *et al.* Methylprednisolone or tirilazad mesylate administration after acute spinal cord injury: 1-year follow up. Results of the third National Acute Spinal Cord Injury randomized controlled trial. J Neurosurg 1998;89:699–706.

11. Pandya KA, Weant KA, Cook AM. High-dose methylprednisolone in acute spinal cord injuries: proceed with caution. Orthopedics 2010;33(5):327–31.

12. Hurlbert RJ. Methylprednisolone for acute spinal cord injury: an inappropriate standard of care. J Neurosurg 2000;93:1–7.

13. Sayer FT, Kronvall E, Nilsson OG. Methylprednisolone treatment in acute spinal cord injury: the myth challenged through a structured analysis of published literature. Spine J 2006;6:335–43.

14. Coleman WP, Benzel E, Cahill DW, *et al.* A critical appraisal of the reporting of the national acute spinal cord injury studies (II and III) of methylprednisolone in acute spinal cord injury. J Spinal Disord 2000;13(3):185–199.

15. Means ED, Anderson DK, Waters TR, *et al.* Effect of methylprednisolone in compression trauma to the feline spinal cord. J Neurosurg 1981;55:200–8.

16. Behrmann DL, Bresnahan JC, Beattie MS. Modelling of acute spinal cord injury in the rat Neuroprotection and enhanced recovery with methylprednisolone, U-74006F and YM-14673. Exp Neurol 1994;80:97–111.

17. Hoerlein BR, Redding RW, Hoff EJ, *et al.* Evaluation of dexamethasone, DMSO, mannitol and solcosyl in acute spinal cord trauma. JAAHA 1983;19:216–25.

18. Levine JM, Levine GJ, Johnson SI, *et al.* Evaluation of the success of medical management for presumptive thoracolumbar intervertebral disk herniation in dogs. Vet Surg 2007;36:482–91.

19. De Decker S, Bhatti SFM, Duchateau L, *et al.* Clinical evaluation of 51 dogs treated conservatively for disc-associated wobbler syndrome. JSAP 2009;50:136–42.

20. Moore RW, Withrow SJ. Gastrointestinal hemorrhage and pancreatitis associated with intervertebral disc disease in the dog. J Am Vet Med Assoc 1982;180:1443–7.

21. Davies M. Pancreatitis, gastrointestinal ulceration and hemorrhage and necrotizing cystitis following the surgical treatment of de-generative disc disease in a Dachshund. Vet Rec 1985;116:398–9.

22. Toombs JM, Caywood DD, Lipowits AJ, *et al.* Colonic perforation following neurosurgical procedures and corticosteroid therapy in four dogs. JAVMA 1980; 177:68–72.

23. Neiger R, Gaschen F, Jaggy A. Gastric mucosal lesions in dogs with acute intervertebral disc disease: characterization and effects of omeprazole or misoprostol. JVIM 2000;14:33–6.

24. Boag AK, Otto CM, Drobatz KJ. Complications of methylprednisolone sodium succinate therapy in dachshunds with surgically treated intervertebral disc disease. JVECC 2001;11(2):105–10.

25. Levine JM, Levine GJ, Boozer L, *et al.* Adverse effects and outcomes associated with dexamethasone administration in dogs with acute thoracolumbar intervertebral disk herniation: 161 cases (2000–2006). JAVMA 2008;232:411–7.

26. Janssens, L, Beosier Y, Daems R. Lumbosacral degenerative stenosis in the dog. The results of epidural infiltration with methylprednisolone acetate: a retrospective study. Vet Comp Orthop Traumatol 2009;22:486–91.

27. Triarhou LC, Herndon, RM. The effect of dexamethasone on L-α-Lysophosphatidyl choline (Lysolecithin)—induced demyelination of the rat spinal cord. Arch Neurol 1986;43:121–5.

28. Hall ED, Braughler JM. Glucocorticoid mechanisms in acute spinal cord injury: a review and therapeutic rationale. Surg Neurol 1982;18(5):320–7.

24 Nonsteroidal Anti-inflammatory Drugs, Muscle Relaxants, Opioids, and Other Treatments for Primary and Adjunctive Medical Management of Intervertebral Disc Herniation

James M. Fingeroth, Franck Forterre, Núria Vizcaíno Revés, and William B. Thomas

Nonsteroidal anti-inflammatory drugs

Historically, corticosteroids have been the main pharmacologic agent utilized in the treatment of intervertebral disc disease (IVDD), including patients with pain only as well as those with neurologic deficits (Chapter 23). The widespread dependence on steroids in the past was based on both the believed benefits of steroids and the paucity of safe and effective alternatives. Recently, as the efficacy and safety of steroids has been studied more closely and plethora of canine-specific and anti-cyclooxygenase (COX)-specific drugs have become available, there has been an increasing shift toward the use of nonsteroidal anti-inflammatory drugs (NSAIDs) as first-line medical therapy for suspected IVDD patients, particularly those in which discomfort is the main sign. This remains however a controversial area in part because some patients treated initially with NSAIDs later develop neurologic deficits prompting a desire to switch the patient to a corticosteroid. It is well known that a combination of steroids and NSAIDs increases the risk of an adverse effect, and a "washout" period of several days is desirable before starting another NSAID or a steroid. A second reason for the ongoing controversy stems from widespread anecdotal experience by veterinarians that steroids seem to be generally effective and safe for the treatment of disc disease. Therefore, some practitioners perhaps look askance at publications that question the safety and efficacy of steroids. This form of clinical bias is not rare in any aspect of medicine. And judicious use of corticosteroids can certainly be beneficial in treating pain. Nonetheless, for dogs with neck pain or back pain and minimal or no neurologic deficits, NSAIDs can provide significant analgesia.

Mechanisms of action

COX is present in most body tissues and can become upregulated with a variety of stimuli. Two forms have been recognized traditionally, COX-1 and COX-2, and both are expressed in the spinal

Advances in Intervertebral Disc Disease in Dogs and Cats, First Edition. Edited by James M. Fingeroth and William B. Thomas.
© 2015 ACVS Foundation. Published 2015 by John Wiley & Sons, Inc.

cord [1–5]. Although both enzymes have similar functions, their patterns of expression are very different. COX-1 is expressed in many cell types and functions as a "housekeeping" enzyme with important roles in vascular hemostasis and gastroprotection. In contrast, COX-2 expression is primarily induced by factors such as endotoxins and cytokines, is expressed at sites of inflammation and produces prostaglandins that mediate inflammatory and pain responses. NSAIDs inhibit the biosynthesis of prostanoids though the inhibition of the COX. They can target both COX-1 and COX-2 or be COX-2 selective. COX-2 selective NSAIDs have been developed to reduce the adverse effects, especially when administered over a long period of time. Experimentally, prostanoid concentrations in gastric and duodenal tissues are not significantly affected by COX-2 selective drugs [6]. However, there are no studies demonstrating that they also reduce the renal or hepatic adverse effects [2].

Experimental animal and clinical human studies

In contrast to a number of studies evaluating steroids in patients with neurologic deficits due to spinal cord injury, studies of NSAIDs in patients with intervertebral disc herniation focus primarily on inhibition of the hyperalgesia caused by the sensitization of the peripheral afferent nerve and not on the spinal cord injury itself [7]. The role of the different epidural inflammatory components is still a subject of study both in animal models and humans. Studies of human patients reveal a predominant prevalence of macrophages and a minor role for mast cells in both acute and chronic disc herniation [8]. Furthermore acute lateral disc herniations are linked with the presence of T and B lymphocytes. Based on these observations, the type of inflammation might be dependent on the kind of herniation. One study evaluating the inflammatory properties of contained versus noncontained lumbar disc herniation in human patients demonstrated a higher concentration of leukotriene B4 and thromboxane B2 in cases of noncontained herniated disc material [9]. Similar observations have been made in animal studies. In a porcine model, disc injury without disc prolapse resulted in a modest inflammatory response

dominated by T lymphocytes, followed by a macrophage response that peaks 1 month after disc injury [10]. In rats, COX-2 contributes to an increased excitability of the spinal cord with peripheral inflammation [5].

In dogs, the cytologic and histopathologic appearance of extruded degenerate disc material is variable and can include some degree of inflammation and presence of dysplastic spindyloid cells [11]. Approximately 82% of the dogs with cervical or thoracolumbar disc extrusion have an inflammatory reaction in the epidural space at the site of extrusion [12]. This ranges from acute invasion of neutrophils to formation of chronic granulation tissue. The mononuclear inflammatory infiltrates consisted mostly of monocytes and macrophages and only few T and B cells. The degree of inflammation correlates with the degree of disc extrusion and associated epidural hemorrhage and the extent of calcification of the extruded disc material. Also, there is an inverse correlation between intensity of the epidural inflammation and outcome [12].

In light of these observations, experimental studies evaluating the effect of NSAIDs on nerve root dysfunction in model animals have been performed. In pigs, a nucleus pulposus-induced nerve root injury was created. Nerve root dysfunction was reduced with the administration of diclofenac but not ketoprofen. The authors suggested that the reason for this disparity in the response might be due to the different selectivity for the two COX types [13]. Similarly in dogs, incision of the nucleus pulposus decreased blood flow to the nerve root and dorsal ganglion and reduced nerve function, an effect that was blocked by simultaneous administration of indomethacin [14]. In another study, local application of nucleus pulposus to the nerve roots and/or mechanical compression resulted in functional and histological changes in nerve roots and the dorsal root ganglia. The combination of mechanical compression and chemical irritation from the nucleus pulposus caused more nerve root injury than each factor alone [15].

Canine clinical studies

There are only a few clinical studies of NSAIDs as part of a conservative treatment for IVDD in dogs. In a retrospective study of conservative treatment of dogs with presumptive thoracolumbar IVDH, dogs receiving NSAIDs were more likely to have higher quality of life than those who had not received these medications [16]. In another retrospective study, dogs with back pain and mild neurological deficits due to presumed thoracolumbar intervertebral disc herniation were managed medically with steroids or NSAIDs. Patients treated with NSAIDs had a lower rate or recurrence (33%) compared to those treated with steroids (66%) [17]. In a retrospective study of dogs with presumed cervical disc herniation treated conservatively, 49 per cent of patients recovered and administration of NSAIDs was significantly associated with a successful outcome [18].

Recommendations

NSAIDs are valuable as analgesics, either alone or as part of a multimodal analgesic plan. A multimodal analgesic approach is preferred for an adequate management of neuropathic pain [19]. To date, published studies of NSAID administration in dogs with disc disease are retrospective in nature, and there are no randomized controlled clinical trials evaluating efficacy and safety. However, based on clinical experience in human and veterinary patients as well as laboratory animal studies, NSAIDs can be considered as one component of conservative therapy in appropriate patients. The authors would recommend their use as part of a conservative treatment only in cases with acute signs of neck or back pain, with no to mild neurological deficits. These patients should be closely monitored for any worsening of the neurological status, and specific instructions about physical restraint should be given to the owner.

Commonly used NSAIDs in dogs include *aspirin, carprofen, etodolac, meloxicam, ketoprofen, deracoxib, firocoxib, meclofenamic acid, tepoxalin,* and *tolfenamic acid.* Selectivity of COX-2 versus COX-1 is often expressed as the COX-1/COX-2 inhibitory ratio. Because different studies use different techniques, there is considerable variability with respect to the COX-1/COX-2 inhibitory ratio for the various products. And in veterinary studies, there is no convincing evidence that drugs with higher COX-1/COX-2 ratios produce fewer gastrointestinal or renal adverse effects than drugs with low ratios [20]. NSAID administration should

be only considered in normotensive, well-hydrated patients with a normal hepatic, renal, gastrointestinal, and hemostatic function. In addition, NSAIDs should not be combined with corticosteroids and two or more NSAIDs should not be administered concurrently.

Acetaminophen (paracetamol)

Acetaminophen is not traditionally considered an NSAID because it does not have significant anti-inflammatory activity at typical doses and is only a weak inhibitor of COX-1 and COX-2. A third COX isoenzyme, COX-3, has been identified in the canine brain, although this may be a variant of COX-1, rather than a distinct isomer [21]. The analgesic and antipyretic actions of acetaminophen are related to COX-3 inhibition [21]. Acetaminophen is occasionally used as an analgesic in dogs as a stand-alone medication or in combination products containing codeine, hydrocodone, or tramadol. Acetaminophen is contraindicated in cats at any dosage because toxic metabolites are formed in this species, causing methemoglobinemia, hematuria, and icterus that can be fatal.

Muscle relaxants

Because nerve root impingement from a herniated disc may induce abnormal firing patterns resulting in spasm of muscles served by those nerve roots, or the experience of pain may cause a patient to voluntarily tense groups of muscles, some of the discomfort associated with IVDH may be attributable to such muscle pain. This phenomenon has been well documented in humans, especially those with lumbar pain [22]. It stands to reason therefore that alleviation of muscle spasm might contribute to overall improvement in patient comfort, even if there yet remains some discomfort associated with direct nerve root compression or inflammation.

There are numerous strategies for trying to relieve muscle spasm and discomfort. Manipulative therapies, including physiatry, chiropractic, and massage would all fit into this category. Studies in human patients suggest that some patients indeed derive benefit from such interventions, but it is difficult to rule out placebo effect or the possibility of self-limiting disease that only appears to improve as a consequence of treatment. And we do not know whether such symptoms in dogs are the same as they are in humans with neck pain or back pain, or respond in any similar manner. In addition to manipulative therapies there is increasing use of energetic treatment of muscle pain with such devices as deep ultrasound and therapeutic lasers. Here again, the data in humans are equivocal at best, and very scant in veterinary medicine, beyond testimonials and belief. There are also numerous over-the-counter topical products marketed to humans for relieving "sore" or "aching" muscles, but these neither have much supporting evidence for their efficacy in humans nor any reported widespread use in veterinary patients.

Skeletal muscle relaxants are divided into two categories: (1) antispastic (for conditions associated with increased muscle tone, such as chronic upper motor neuron paresis) and (2) antispasmodic agents (for musculoskeletal conditions such as neck or back pain). Antispasmodic agents (e.g., methocarbamol, diazepam) are preferred for neck and back pain, because there is sparse evidence to support the use of antispastic agents (e.g., baclofen, dantrolene) for musculoskeletal conditions [23]. *Methocarbamol* is probably the most widely used antispasmodic drug in veterinary medicine. Despite its widespread use over many years, there is a dearth of controlled studies that prove it has any usefulness in dogs with neck or back pain from any cause, including IVDH [24]. The main side effect is sedation [23, 25]. In some instances this may be perceived to be an added benefit for dogs as it may permit the dog to rest better, and the altered sensorium may lessen the symptoms associated with painful stimuli. *Diazepam* is a benzodiazepine with anxiolytic, sedative, and skeletal muscle relaxant effects. Benzodiazepines are effective for short-term treatment in human patients with neck and back pain [23]. As with methocarbamol, we are unaware of published studies assessing efficacy in the setting of symptomatic IVDD.

In summary, there is neither a body of evidence to support nor refute the use of muscle relaxants in general, nor data that suggest that any one product is superior to another. Muscle relaxants are rarely if ever prescribed alone for the treatment of presumptive IVDH, and this makes it even more difficult to determine if their inclusion in a treatment protocol contributes to amelioration of signs. Therefore, it remains largely a matter of conjecture and personal preference by the veterinarian whether to employ such treatment.

Opioids

Opioids, defined as all drugs that are chemical derivatives of compounds derived from opium, are some of the most effective analgesics used in veterinary medicine. They interact with various types and subtypes of opioid receptors present in the central and peripheral nervous system. This directly inhibits the ascending transmission of nociceptive information arising from the dorsal horn cells and activates pain-control circuits that descend from the brain to the spinal cord. In addition, these drugs interact with opioid receptors in sensory nerves. Thus, opioids mediate both central and peripherally mediated analgesia [26].

Opioid agonists exert analgesia by maximal activation of mu (μ) receptors. They are superior analgesics and the drugs of choice for moderate to severe pain. Opioid agonists include morphine, oxymorphone, hydromorphone, meperidine, methadone, fentanyl, and codeine. *Morphine* provides effective analgesia for 2–4h. It produces moderate sedation, and vomiting and panting are common side effects. When administered intravenously (IV), morphine can induce histamine release related to the rate and quantity of drug injected. Therefore, small quantities are injected slowly when using IV administration [27]. *Oxymorphone* is approximately 10 times as potent as morphine, with a similar duration of analgesia. Vomiting is rare and oxymorphone does not cause histamine release. *Hydromorphone* is approximately 5–7 times as potent as morphine and induces a greater degree of sedation than oxymorphone and has a slightly shorter duration of action. It does not stimulate release of histamine when given IV. *Meperidine* (Demerol) is less potent than morphine and produces less sedation but has similar side effects. Panting is rare after administration of meperidine, but this drug is even more likely to cause histamine release compared to morphine and should not be used IV. It has a short duration of action (0.5–2.0h). *Methadone* is 1.0–1.5 times as potent as morphine and provides analgesia for about 4h. Methadone does not cause histamine release and can be given

IV. *Fentanyl* is a potent analgesic with a relatively short duration of action and rapid onset of action (2–3 min). Thus, fentanyl is well suited for continuous rate IV infusion to control severe pain [27]. A transdermal fentanyl preparation (adhesive patch) is also available, which provides sustained therapeutic plasma fentanyl concentrations over a period of at least 4 days and is effective for postoperative pain in dogs [28].

Codeine tablets are available as a sole ingredient or in combination with other drugs, including acetaminophen. In dogs, the active metabolite codeine-6-glucuronide probably accounts for most of the analgesic effects. Codeine is only 0.05 as potent as morphine so it is used for mild pain [29]. Codeine formulations with acetaminophen cannot be safely administered to cats because of acetaminophen toxicity. *Hydrocodone* is only available as combination products, such as hydrocodone with acetaminophen or homatropine. Hydrocodone is twice as potent as morphine with a 6–8 h duration [27]. A potential advantage is its ability to be administered orally, compared to the parenteral route typically required for morphine.

Butorphanol is an agonist–antagonist that exerts analgesia by acting as an agonist on the kappa (κ) receptors while acting as an antagonist on *μ* receptors. It exerts a ceiling effect whereby increasing doses do not cause additional adverse effects but it also has limited analgesic efficacy [26]. It is effective for mild to moderate pain with a duration of activity of 2–6 h [27].

Buprenorphine is an opioid partial agonist that binds *μ* receptors but produces only limited clinical effect and is only effective for treating mild to moderate pain. The peak effect does not occur until about 45–60 min after IV administration with analgesia lasting about 6 h.

Tramadol is a synthetic opioid and weak *μ* receptor agonist. It also inhibits neuronal reuptake of norepinephrine and serotonin. These mechanisms all contribute to analgesic activity. It is effective for control of moderate to severe pain. Tramadol is tolerated well in dogs, although sedation, nausea, and anorexia are occasionally noticed [29]. It should not be used with other drugs that affect serotonin reuptake or metabolism because of the risk of serotonin toxicity. These include monoamine oxidase inhibitors (selegiline), tricyclic antidepressants (TCAs), and selective serotonin reuptake inhibitors (fluoxetine, paroxetine). In dogs, serotonin syndrome causes tremor, rigidity, myoclonus, seizures, hyperthermia, salivation, and even death [29].

In summary, opioids are effective for ameliorating many types of pain. Here again we lack controlled studies that prove such efficacy specifically for IVDH-induced pain. As with all discussions regarding opioids, issues that must be considered include specific receptor-type affinities, whether drugs are pure agonists or mixed agonists–antagonists, route of delivery (oral, injectable, transdermal, etc.), and the cost/time associated with inventorying, dispensing, and record keeping for such drugs.

Gabapentin and pregabalin

Gabapentin and *pregabalin* are synthetic branched-chain amino acids that inhibit calcium influx-mediated release of excitatory neurotransmitters, including substance P [30]. Gabapentin and pregabalin are used as antiseizure drugs in people and animals, but both drugs also reduce neuropathic pain, with pregabalin having a steeper dose–response relationship and greater treatment effect [31]. In human patients, gabapentin and pregabalin were initially used to treat chronic pain but recently have been used for more acute pain, such as postoperative pain [32]. In human patients with acute back pain and radiculopathy, gabapentin is associated with small improvements in pain scores compared with placebo [33]. Gabapentin use has increased significantly in veterinary medicine over the past several years. Although there are no clinical trials evaluating its safety and efficacy as an analgesic agent in dogs it has anecdotally been used to treat many types of pain, including neck and back pain in animals with IVDH.

Amantadine

Amantadine is an antiviral drug that was originally approved to treat influenza A in people. Later, it was realized the drug also blocks N-methyl-D-aspartate (NMDA) glutamate receptor. NMDA receptors are important in central nervous system sensitization and hyperalgesia. Amantadine is not expected to provide analgesic effects as a sole therapy, but may enhance the analgesic effects of NSAIDs, opioids, or gabapentin/pregabalin [29]. Although there are no controlled studies evaluating efficacy of amantadine in veterinary patients with IVDD, amantadine improved pain control in dogs with osteoarthritis refractory to NSAIDs compared to placebo [34].

TCAs

TCAs, such as *amitriptyline*, are sometimes used to treat chronic back pain in human patients although there are no clinical trials evaluating TCAs for acute back pain. TCAs produce analgesia through multiple mechanisms, including serotonin and norepinephrine reuptake inhibition, NMDA antagonism, and voltage-gated, sodium channel blockade, enhancing activity of adenosine and GABAB receptors, and they have anti-inflammatory effects [29]. There are no clinical trials evaluating these agents in IVDH in dogs although there are anecdotal reports of using amitriptyline in dogs with presumed neuropathic pain [35].

Summary

In addition to the list of drugs briefly discussed earlier, there are numerous other agents, including analgesics, anti-inflammatories, and psychotropic drugs (such as antidepressants, mood elevators, etc.) that have been touted by various veterinary practitioners as being "useful" when included in a multimodal approach to trying to relieve discomfort associated with presumed IVDH. Lacking conclusive data for any of these, it is reasonable for clinicians to consider various combinations, based on a rational consideration of each drug's pharmacodynamics and potential interactions (both synergistic and antagonistic), in their treatment protocol. But as has been stated elsewhere in this text, the clinician attempting to palliate signs associated with presumptive IVDH assumes the responsibility for making an ongoing assessment of efficacy, and for not simply revising the medication protocol if there is abject failure for the patient to respond in a timely and appropriate manner. The recommendation to pursue definitive diagnostic imaging (to verify IVDH as the cause for the signs and to precisely localize the lesion) and surgery where appropriate, should never be far from the veterinarian's mind when advising clients and treating pets with presumptive IVDH.

Conclusions

Regardless of analgesic protocols selected, one of the most important aspects of management for the nonsurgically treated dog with suspected IVDH is to enforce *strict rest*. This recommendation is somewhat at odds with current protocols for treating low back pain in humans, where controlled mobility is encouraged. However, we need to recall that most humans with low back pain have muscle soreness and often no disc herniation, and moreover, even those people who have disc herniations at L3–L4, L4–L5, or L5–S1 (the most common levels) are at no risk for spinal cord injury and paralysis because of the location of the lesion relative to the termination of the spinal cord (see Chapter 3). This contrasts sharply with our chondrodystrophoid canine population, where the preponderance of disc herniations occurs in the area of the thoracolumbar junction and where, as a result, spinal cord injury and paralysis loom as real threats. While disc herniation in these patients is a spontaneous event that may be unassociated with any particular movement or activity, once a disc has begun to herniate there is clearly an increased risk for movement to cause further protrusion or extrusion, with potentially severe consequences. Therefore, restricting movement in the hope that there will be a combination of resorption of any extruded disc and scarring/stabilization of the bulging or torn annulus fibrosus is the strategy employed when attempting to resolve signs associated with IVDH in patients for whom surgery is not planned immediately. The use of analgesics may achieve the goal of making the patient more comfortable, but the masking or amelioration of pain might have the deleterious consequence of instigating the animal to resume more normal activity with the attendant risk of exacerbating disc herniation. It is therefore prudent to always insist on a period of strict crate confinement, with activity limited to short leash walks to void urine and feces (and carrying patients to the designated spot when feasible) *regardless of any perceived "resolution" of the signs of discomfort.* We generally recommend a period of at least 2–3 weeks of such confinement irrespective of perceived clinical improvement during that time period.

References

1. Lascelles BD, King S, Roe S, Marcellin-Little DJ, Jones S. Expression and activity of COX-1 and 2 and 5-LOX in joint tissues from dogs with naturally occurring coxofemoral joint osteoarthritis. J Orthop Res. 2009;27(9):1204–8.
2. KuKanich B, Bidgood T, Knesl O. Clinical pharmacology of nonsteroidal anti-inflammatory drugs in dogs. Vet Anaes Anal. 2012;39(1):69–90.
3. Willingale HL, Gardiner NJ, McLymont N, Giblett S, Grubb BD. Prostanoids synthesized by cyclo-oxygenase isoforms in rat spinal cord and their contribution to the development of neuronal hyperexcitability. Br J Pharmacol. 1997;122(8):1593–604.
4. Beiche F, Brune K, Geisslinger G, Goppelt-Struebe M. Expression of cyclooxygenase isoforms in the rat spinal cord and their regulation during adjuvant-induced arthritis. Inflamm Res. 1998 Dec; 47(12):482–7.
5. Seybold VS, Jia YP, Abrahams LG. Cyclo-oxygenase-2 contributes to central sensitization in rats with peripheral inflammation. Pain. 2003 Sep;105(1–2): 47–55.
6. Wooten JG, Blikslager AT, Marks SL, Law JM, Graeber EC, Lascelles BD. Effect of nonsteroidal anti-inflammatory drugs with varied cyclooxygenase-2 selectivity on cyclooxygenase protein and prostanoid concentrations in pyloric and duodenal mucosa of dogs. Am J Vet Res. 2009 Oct;70(10):1243–9.
7. Ferreira AJ, Correia JH, Jaggy A. Thoracolumbar disc disease in 71 paraplegic dogs: influence of rate of onset and duration of clinical signs on treatment results. J Small Anim Pract. 2002 Apr;43(4):158–63.
8. Habtemariam A, Virri J, Grönblad M, Seitsalo S, Karaharju E. The role of mast cells in disc herniation inflammation. Spine. 1999;24(15):1516.
9. Nygaard ØP, Mellgren SI, Østerud B. The inflammatory properties of contained and noncontained lumbar disc herniation. Spine. 1997;22(21): 2484–8.
10. Kanerva A, Kommonen B, Grönblad M, Tolonen J, Habtemariam A, Virri J, et al. Inflammatory cells in experimental intervertebral disc injury. Spine. 1997;22(23):2711–5.
11. Royal AB, Chigerwe M, Coates JR, Wiedmeyer CE, Berent LM. Cytologic and histopathologic evaluation of extruded canine degenerate disks. Vet Surg. 2009;38(7):798–802.

12. Fadda A, Oevermann A, Vandevelde M, Doherr M, Forterre F, Henke D. Clinical and pathological analysis of epidural inflammation in intervertebral disk extrusion in dogs. J Vet Int Med. 2013;27:924–34.
13. Cornefjord M, Olmarker K, Otani K, Rydevik B. Nucleus pulposus-induced nerve root injury: effects of diclofenac and ketoprofen. Eur Spine J. 2002; 11(1):57–61.
14. Arai I, Mao G-P, Otani K, Konno S, Kikuchi S, Olmarker K. Indomethacin blocks the nucleus pulposus-induced effects on nerve root function. Eur Spine J. 2004;13(8):691–4.
15. Takahashi N, Yabuki S, Aoki Y, Kikuchi S. Pathomechanisms of nerve root injury caused by disc herniation: an experimental study of mechanical compression and chemical irritation. Spine. 2003; 28(5):435–41.
16. Levine JM, Levine GJ, Johnson SI, Kerwin SC, Hettlich BF, Fosgate GT. Evaluation of the success of medical management for presumptive thoracolumbar intervertebral disk herniation in dogs. Vet Surg. 2007 Jul;36(5):482–91.
17. Mann F, Wagner-Mann CC, Dunphy ED, Ruben DS, Rochat MC, Bartels KE. Recurrence rate of presumed thoracolumbar intervertebral disc disease in ambulatory dogs with spinal hyperpathia treated with anti-inflammatory drugs: 78 cases (1997–2000). J Vet Emerg Crit Care. 2007;17(1):53–60.
18. Levine JM, Levine GJ, Johnson SI, Kerwin SC, Hettlich BF, Fosgate GT. Evaluation of the success of medical management for presumptive cervical intervertebral disk herniation in dogs. Vet Surg. 2007 Jul;36(5):492–9.
19. Mathews KA. Neuropathic pain in dogs and cats: if only they could tell us if they hurt. Vet Clin North Am Small Anim Pract. 2008 Nov;38(6):1365–414, vii–viii.
20. Papich MG. An update on nonsteroidal anti-inflammatory drugs (NSAIDs) in small animals. Vet Clin North Am Small Anim Pract. 2008; 38(6):1243–66.
21. Chandrasekharan N, Dai H, Roos KLT, Evanson NK, Tomsik J, Elton TS, et al. COX-3, a cyclooxygenase-1 variant inhibited by acetaminophen and other analgesic/antipyretic drugs: cloning, structure, and expression. Proc Natl Acad Sci U S A. 2002;99(21): 13926–31.
22. Cailliet R. Low Back Syndrome. Philadelphia: FA Davis; 1981.
23. See S, Ginzburg R. Choosing a skeletal muscle relaxant. Am Fam Physician. 2008 Aug 1;78(3): 365–70.
24. Rowe ET, Christian CW. Clinical experiences with use of methocarbamol to control muscular spasms in treatment of spinal lesions in dogs. Vet Med Small Anim Clin. 1970 Nov;65(11):1082–4 passim.
25. Plumb DC. Plumb's Veterinary Drug Handbook. 7th ed. Ames: Wiley-Blackwell; 2011.

26. Lamont LA, Mathews KA. Opioids, nonsteroidal anti-inflammatories and analgesic adjuvants. In: Tranquilli WJ, Thurman JC, Grimm KA, editors. Lumb & Jones' Veterinary Anesthesia and Analgesia. 4th ed. Ames: Blackwell; 2007. pp. 241–71.

27. Pascoe PJ. Opioid analgesics. Vet Clin North Am Small Anim Pract. 2000 Jul;30(4):757–72.

28. Linton DD, Wilson MG, Newbound GC, Freise KJ, Clark TP. The effectiveness of a long-acting transdermal fentanyl solution compared to buprenorphine for the control of postoperative pain in dogs in a randomized, multicentered clinical study. J Vet Pharmacol Ther. 2012 Aug;35 Suppl 2:53–64.

29. KuKanich B. Outpatient oral analgesics in dogs and cats beyond nonsteroidal antiinflammatory drugs: an evidence-based approach. Vet Clin North Am Small Anim Pract. 2013;43(5):1109–25.

30. Lamont LA. Adjunctive analgesic therapy in veterinary medicine. Vet Clin North Am Small Anim Pract. 2008;38(6):1187–203.

31. Bockbrader HN, Wesche D, Miller R, Chapel S, Janiczek N, Burger P. A comparison of the pharmacokinetics and pharmacodynamics of pregabalin and gabapentin. Clin Pharmacokinet. 2010; 49(10):661–9.

32. Dauri M, Faria S, Gatti A, Celidonio L, Carpenedo R, Sabato AF. Gabapentin and pregabalin for the acute post-operative pain management. A systematic-narrative review of the recent clinical evidences. Curr Drug Targets. 2009;10(8):716–33.

33. Chou R, Huffman LH. Medications for acute and chronic low back pain: a review of the evidence for an American Pain Society/American College of Physicians clinical practice guideline. Ann Intern Med. 2007;147(7):505–14.

34. Lascelles BD, Gaynor JS, Smith ES, Roe SC, Marcellin-Little DJ, Davidson G, et al. Amantadine in a multimodal analgesic regimen for alleviation of refractory osteoarthritis pain in dogs. J Vet Intern Med. 2008 Jan–Feb;22(1):53–9.

35. Cashmore RG, Harcourt-Brown TR, Freeman PM, Jeffery ND, Granger N. Clinical diagnosis and treatment of suspected neuropathic pain in three dogs. Aust Vet J. 2009 Jan–Feb;87(1):45–50.

Neuroprotective Treatments for Acute Spinal Cord Injury Associated with Intervertebral Disc Herniation

25

Jonathan M. Levine

Introduction

Medical treatments for spinal cord injury (SCI) are typically classified as neuroprotective, regenerative, or plasticity inducing [1]. Neuroprotective strategies attempt to mitigate acute secondary SCI. Regenerative strategies facilitate the remyelination and regrowth of axons through injured areas as well as the development of new cellular constituents. Plasticity-inducing treatments focus on altering function or connectivity of existing parenchyma in order to improve outcomes. In some instances, therapeutics may have mechanisms of action that encompass more than one of these three categories.

To date, a limited number of neuroprotective therapies have been systematically evaluated in dogs with acute SCI resulting from intervertebral disc herniation (IVDH). This chapter will review modern, accepted means of developing and testing novel therapeutics, define commonly used outcome matrices, and review published clinical trial data. This chapter will not address glucocorticoids, which are among the mostly commonly used and controversial neuroprotective agents, as these are discussed in detail in another chapter (see Chapter 23).

Animal models: The first step

Typically, potential treatments for SCI are first investigated in animal injury models. The advantages of using preclinical SCI models are that these systems are inexpensive, are easily reproducible, induce relatively homogeneous parenchymal changes, permit histologic assessment of injury at established time points, and have well-characterized functional outcomes [2]. The majority of rodent injury models induce contusive SCI by use of an impactor that rapidly deforms the plane of the spinal cord in a reproducible manner [3]. Clip and crush models are also used by some investigators.

Promising neuroprotective agents are identified based on pathomechanisms or targets that have been characterized in rodent models. These drugs are then delivered in model systems to determine safety and efficacy. The assessment of efficacy is typically performed using a placebo group, with or without investigator blinding; outcomes such as histologic lesion volume, gait scores, or electrophysiological responses are assessed. There are weaknesses in this approach. For example, rodent models do not mimic lesion heterogeneity, all

Advances in Intervertebral Disc Disease in Dogs and Cats, First Edition. Edited by James M. Fingeroth and William B. Thomas.
© 2015 ACVS Foundation. Published 2015 by John Wiley & Sons, Inc.

primary injury mechanisms, and variation in timing seen in naturally occurring disease [4, 5]. Additionally, many preclinical rodent studies are not externally validated. Recent evidence from the National Institutes of Health "Facilities of Research—Spinal Cord Injury" project suggests that when independent replication of rodent studies is performed previously detected outcome associations often are not present or significantly smaller in magnitude. This unfortunate reality has been borne out with neuroprotectives such as erythropoietin, Nogo-66 antagonists, and minocycline [6–8].

Clinical trials

Drugs that show promise in animal models— preferably in multiple studies from independent laboratories—are then taken to clinical trials. When a drug is introduced into clinical trials in animals

or humans with naturally occurring SCI, this is done in phases. Phase I studies usually involve a small number of subjects (10–20) with the primary goals being establishing dose and safety data. Phase II studies (20–200 subjects) continue to evaluate safety at a preset dose and also gather preliminary data regarding efficacy over a limited number of outcome measures. Phase II studies may be controlled or uncontrolled, may utilize blinding, and always are performed at a single institution. Phase III investigations are performed following encouraging phase II data; they are randomized, double-blinded, placebo-controlled studies that use a multi-institutional population. Meta-analysis is a technique that allows data from several similarly constructed trials to be combined to address issues such as efficacy and toxicity. In human medicine, this type of synthesis is often performed to help set standards of care. Figure 25.1 summarizes the "pipeline" algorithm for studying prospective therapeutic agents.

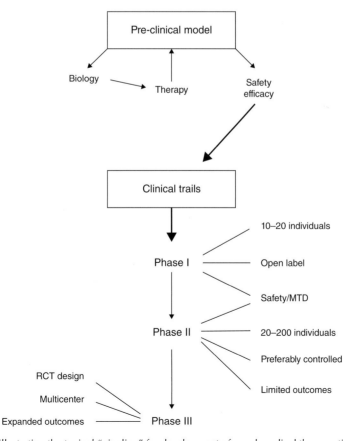

Figure 25.1   Schematic illustrating the typical "pipeline" for development of novel medical therapeutics.

Neuroprotectives studied in models

The breadth and number of neuroprotective drugs currently under investigation in animal models is staggering [9]. Some of the more thoroughly evaluated therapeutics include minocycline, polyethylene glycol (PEG), hypothermia, magnesium, erythropoietin, nonsteroidal anti-inflammatory drugs, anti-CD11d antibodies, estrogen, progesterone, matrix metalloproteinase antagonists, and various antioxidants. In most instances, results in models have been conflicting, divergent in their magnitude, not replicated independently, or available in only one species/system.

Outcomes in dogs with IVDH

Using valid outcome measures is central to generating accurate data concerning the effect of any intervention for SCI. In general, these assessments should have strong intra- and interobserver agreement, correlate with some anatomic measure of injury severity (e.g., histopathology or imaging), and predict or be associated with recovery milestones. In dogs with IVDH, behavioral assessments have been the predominant means of assessing outcomes following SCI. Typically, these have included the subjective assessment of response to nociceptive stimuli and the use of ordinal gait scores. At the time of this writing, the only ordinal gait scores that have been formally validated in dogs include the 14-point motor score, Modified Frankel Score (MFS), and Texas Spinal Cord Injury Score (TSCIS) [10, 11]. Computed gait analysis may offer several advantages over traditional gait scores, including the generation of truly continuous data and enhanced ability to detect subtle changes within dogs that have similar degrees of disability [12]. Electrophysiology, urodynamics, and advanced imaging have been used to a very limited extent as outcome endpoints. Proxy quality-of-life measures are a potential additional avenue by which to measure outcome.

Available clinical trial data in dogs with IVDH

To date, the author is aware of only two published, prospective clinical trials that have assessed neuroprotective treatments in dogs with IVDH. There are several reports in this population, however, on plasticity/regenerative therapies. Despite the paucity of trial data, work is ongoing at several institutions to assess novel neuroprotectives.

PEG

PEG has received attention in recent years as a neuroprotective treatment for dogs with IVDH-associated SCI. The effects of PEG are believed to be mediated by the agent's ability to penetrate the central nervous system and act as a surfactant. The surfactant properties of PEG may permit fusion of transected axons and sealing of disrupted myelin [13]. PEG was first studied in guinea pig models of SCI, where it was shown to enhance conduction of evoked potentials through lesions and facilitate parenchymal sparing [14–16]. More recent investigations performed by independent investigators have shown modest to no positive effects in behavioral or histologic outcomes in rodent models when PEG alone was compared to saline placebo [17]. In most experimental models, PEG was delivered minutes to a few hours after injury, which might maximize effects.

In 2004, Laverty et al. conducted an open-label study examining outcomes following PEG delivery in dogs with thoracolumbar IVDH-associated SCI [18]. The study included 19 paraplegic dogs lacking deep nociception that were delivered PEG IV within 72h of SCI. Behavioral outcomes including ambulation, response to nociceptive stimuli, and ordinal neurological score were recorded and compared to a historical control group of matched injury severity. The study identified statistically significant differences between treatment and control animals across these parameters at follow-up times ranging from 3 days to 6–8 weeks after SCI. For example, at 6–8-week follow-up, the mean ordinal gait score (range, 1–5) in the PEG group was 2.3 (2=stepping at the limit of detection, at best a few steps before falling), whereas the control group was 1.3 (1=complete inability to step).

While data concerning PEG delivery in dogs with IVDH-associated SCI are encouraging, they need to be viewed cautiously. As Laverty et al. utilized an historical control group, the potential exists for selection bias and record abstraction bias. The neurologic gait scores in the investigation were not formally validated, and intergroup differences could have been affected by rater variability. Additionally, as investigators were not blinded the results in study dogs may have been enhanced by placebo effect. Currently, a phase III trial in dogs with thoracolumbar IVDH lacking deep nociception comparing outcomes following PEG, saline, or methylprednisolone sodium succinate delivery is ongoing; it is likely that data from this work will answer important questions concerning PEG, at least in a group with behaviorally complete SCI.

N-Acetylcysteine

In 2008, Baltzer et al. investigated the effects of N-acetylcysteine (NAC) in dogs with thoracolumbar IVDH with and without pelvic limb deep nociception [19]. The intervention was attempted as NAC is capable of penetrating the central nervous system, has antioxidant properties, has a high safety margin, and was previously shown in a rodent model of SCI to improve motor recovery. In addition, the investigators had previously demonstrated that markers of oxidative stress were increased in the urine of dogs with IVDH. The investigation was a phase I/II trial with blinding and randomization that used an ordinal scale to grade behavioral outcome. It included 52 enrollees with 34 having data available for evaluation at the 42-day post-SCI time point. There were no differences in outcome between study groups. This negative result may be due to the very abbreviated neurological score (only three grades) which was utilized, which may have limited the ability to detect subtle differences in gait; the small number of dogs studied; the variable timing of injury relative to drug delivery (0–7 days); or a true lack of effect.

Conclusions

Clearly, very limited data exist concerning the effect of neuroprotective agents in dogs with IVDH-associated SCI. In humans with traumatic SCI, neuroprotective treatments have been largely elusive. Dobkin has estimated that more than 60 phase II and III clinical trials have been performed in people with SCI, with only 1–2 showing promise. Whether translational biologists and veterinarians will face the same challenges treating dogs with IVDH is unknown. As trials are contemplated,

careful attention must be paid to developing strategies in preclinical models, using appropriate and valid outcome measures, and designing trials with adequate power, limited opportunity for bias, and appropriate inclusion/exclusion criteria.

Editors' Note: It is critical that veterinarians, as scientists, appreciate the requirements for validating therapies for any disease, as outlined here by Dr. Levine. An all-too-common problem faced by clinicians is the premature and widespread dissemination of preliminary study data by the media, often hyped with breathless and dramatic headlines ("New 'miracle' breakthrough treatment!"), that inspires both our clients and ourselves to believe that we now have a new tool for combating a clinical problem such as IVDH-induced SCI, especially when such problems are so frustrating for all. It is our duty however to maintain our skepticism and to fully understand the "pipeline" and requirements for dubbing any new treatment as "proven" before we seek to incorporate it into our clinical practice.

References

1. Levine JM, Levine GJ, Porter BF, Topp K, Noble-Haeusslein LJ. Naturally occurring disk herniation in dogs: an opportunity for pre-clinical spinal cord injury research. J Neurotrauma. 2011 Apr;28(4):675–88.
2. Kwon BK, Okon EB, Tsai E, Beattie MS, Bresnahan J, Magnuson DS, et al. A grading system to objectively evaluate the strength of preclinical data of acute neuroprotective therapies for clinical translation in spinal cord injury. J Neurotrauma. 2011 Aug;28(8):1525–43.
3. Young W. Spinal cord contusion models. Prog Brain Res. 2002;137:231–55.
4. Courtine G, Bunge MB, Fawcett JW, Grossman RG, Kaas JH, Lemon R, et al. Can experiments in nonhuman primates expedite the translation of treatments for spinal cord injury in humans? Nat Med. 2007 May;13(5):561–6.
5. Tator CH. Review of treatment trials in human spinal cord injury: issues, difficulties, and recommendations. Neurosurgery. 2006 Nov;59(5):957–82; discussion 82–7.
6. Pinzon A, Marcillo A, Pabon D, Bramlett HM, Bunge MB, Dietrich WD. A re-assessment of erythropoietin as a neuroprotective agent following rat spinal cord compression or contusion injury. Exp Neurol. 2008 Sep;213(1):129–36.
7. Pinzon A, Marcillo A, Quintana A, Stamler S, Bunge MB, Bramlett HM, et al. A re-assessment of minocycline as a neuroprotective agent in a rat spinal cord contusion model. Brain Res. 2008 Dec 3;1243:146–51.

8. Steward O, Sharp K, Yee KM, Hofstadter M. A re-assessment of the effects of a Nogo-66 receptor antagonist on regenerative growth of axons and locomotor recovery after spinal cord injury in mice. Exp Neurol. 2008 Feb;209(2):446–68.

9. Kwon BK, Okon E, Hillyer J, Mann C, Baptiste D, Weaver LC, et al. A systematic review of non-invasive pharmacologic neuroprotective treatments for acute spinal cord injury. J Neurotrauma. 2011 Aug;28(8):1545–88.

10. Levine GJ, Levine JM, Budke CM, Kerwin SC, Au J, Vinayak A, et al. Description and repeatability of a newly developed spinal cord injury scale for dogs. Prev Vet Med. 2009;89:121–7.

11. Olby NJ, De Risio L, Munana KR, Wosar MA, Skeen TM, Sharp NJH, et al. Development of a functional scoring system in dogs with acute spinal cord injuries. Am J Vet Res. 2001;62:1624–8.

12. Hamilton L, Franklin RJM, Jeffery ND. Development of a universal measure of quadrupedal forelimb-hindlimb coordination using digital motion capture and computerised gait analysis. BMC Neurosci. 2007;8:77–87.

13. Borgens RB. Cellular engineering: molecular repair of membranes to rescue cells of the damaged nervous system. Neurosurgery. 2001 Aug;49(2):370–8; discussion 8–9.

14. Borgens RB, Shi R. Immediate recovery from spinal cord injury through molecular repair of nerve membranes with polyethylene glycol. FASEB J. 2000 Jan;14(1):27–35.

15. Borgens RB, Shi R, Bohnert D. Behavioral recovery from spinal cord injury following delayed application of polyethylene glycol. J Exp Biology. 2002 Jan;205(Pt 1):1–12.

16. Duerstock BS, Borgens RB. Three-dimensional morphometry of spinal cord injury following polyethylene glycol treatment. J Exp Biol. 2002 Jan;205(Pt 1): 13–24.

17. Kwon BK, Roy J, Lee JH, Okon E, Zhang H, Marx JC, et al. Magnesium chloride in a polyethylene glycol formulation as a neuroprotective therapy for acute spinal cord injury: preclinical refinement and optimization. J Neurotrauma. 2009 Aug;26(8):1379–93.

18. Laverty PH, Leskovar A, Breur GJ, Coates JR, Bergman RL, Widmer WR, et al. A preliminary study of intravenous surfactants in paraplegic dogs: polymer therapy in canine clinical SCI. J Neurotrauma. 2004;21:1767–77.

19. Baltzer WI, McMichael MA, Hosgood GL, Kerwin SC, Levine JM, Steiner JM, et al. Randomized, blinded, placebo-controlled clinical trial of N-acetylcysteine in dogs with spinal cord trauma from acute intervertebral disc disease. Spine 2008 Jun 1;33(13):1397–402.

26 The Use of Discography and Nucleolysis in Dogs

James F. (Jeff) Biggart

Discography

Discography is the imaging of the intervertebral disc by radio-opaque contrast material introduced percutaneously into the nucleus pulposus. It is primarily a diagnostic technique testing the integrity of the annulus and nucleus. Traditionally, physicians and veterinarians use this technique to diagnose herniated discs in the last several lumbar spaces of the vertebral canal. Access to the vertebral canal has traditionally been dorsally, between the facets of the cranial and caudal lamina over a disc space. To avoid penetration of the spinal cord and dura mater, a more lateral or dorsolateral approach has been used [1, 2].

Advantages

This technique is minimally invasive with the use of fluoroscopy. Used in conjunction with nucleolysis, both diagnosis and treatment of herniated discs can be accomplished with one needle placement.

It aids in the diagnosis of disc herniation in cases of suspected false negative myelograms without requiring surgical exploration of these suspected disc levels. Herniations within large areas devoid of myelographic contrast due to spinal cord swelling may be identified.

Disadvantages

In veterinary patients, discography requires general anesthesia, negating one value found in humans, namely, where disc injection can reproduce clinical symptoms in a conscious patient and aid in lesion localization. Classically, fluoroscopy is necessary for needle placement; however, needle placement can be accomplished successfully with newer high-definition digital radiographic systems. In addition, with the advent of magnetic resonance imaging, it is possible to distinguish normal-appearing discs from those that have undergone degeneration (with and without herniation) using a completely noninvasive methodology (see Chapter 16).

Advances in Intervertebral Disc Disease in Dogs and Cats, First Edition. Edited by James M. Fingeroth and William B. Thomas.
© 2015 ACVS Foundation. Published 2015 by John Wiley & Sons, Inc.

Discographic patterns

Normal discs demonstrate a contrast pattern of a small, oval, pearl-like image of the nucleus pulposus (Figure 26.1). Depending on the volume of the contrast material injected, complete or incomplete filling of the nucleus pulposus may be the result. Introduction of contrast material into a normal disc with an intact annulus is difficult, as a volume of the nucleus must be replaced by contrast material. Since this is a closed confined space, considerable pressure may be needed to introduce additional material [3].

Abnormal discs can demonstrate several patterns after contrast introduction.

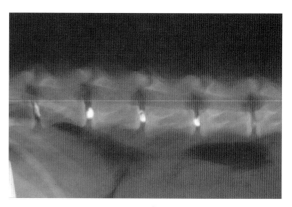

Figure 26.1   Normal discograms.

Collapsed discs

Long-standing disc disease may produce complete collapse of the intervertebral space leaving minimal space between the end plates for contrast deposition. Generally, these discs have minimal annular confinement of the nucleus and contrast may leak into adjacent tissues, resulting in no useful images (Figure 26.2).

Protruded discs

Contrast leaks into the annulus with bulging outside the traditional confines of the annulus (Figure 26.3).

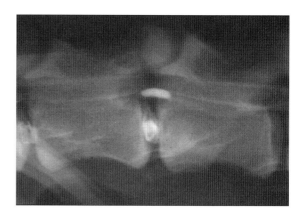

Figure 26.2   Protruded discogram.

Extruded discs

Contrast leaks through the annulus but is still contiguous with the disc space (Figures 26.4 and 26.5).

Sequestered discs

Contrast leaks into the vertebral canal with no continuity with the disc space (Figure 26.6).

Intravascular discograms

These patterns are seldom seen without continuously recorded dynamic fluoroscopy. Further study is needed, but these patterns may be related to and help explain the etiology of fibrocartilaginous emboli with spinal cord infarction (see Chapter 9), ascending/ descending myelomalacia (see Chapter 12), and possibly other spinal cord pathologies.

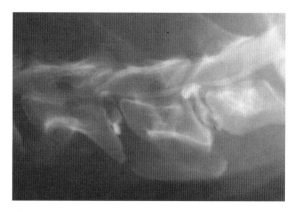

Figure 26.3   Protruded discogram.

A. End plate penetration
Contrast media extrudes into the adjacent vertebral body medullary spaces. This produces an instantaneous and very transient blush of contrast into the vertebral body.

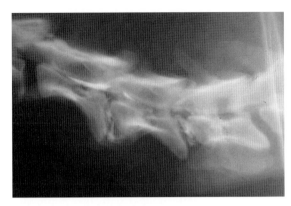

Figure 26.4   Extruded discogram.

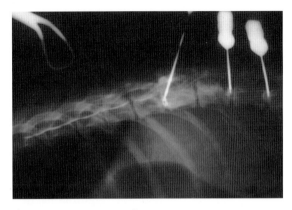

Figure 26.7   Intravenous discogram.

C. Intra-arterial discograms

Contrast medium flows into the arterial system of the vertebral canal and vertebral body, characterized by a tortuous pattern without obvious connection to the vertebral canal.

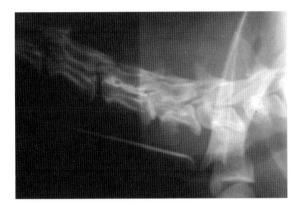

Figure 26.5   Extruded discogram.

Nucleolysis

Nucleolysis (chemonucleolysis, discolysis, disc injection, intradiscal therapy) is the enzymatic dissolution of the nucleus pulposus of the intervertebral disc. The technique involves percutaneously placing needles into the nucleus with the deposition of proteolytic enzymes such as chymopapain or collagenase. The goal is to have these enzymes follow the path of the herniated disc, mix with and dissipate the disc in the vertebral canal, and thus relieve pressure on the spinal cord and nerve roots.

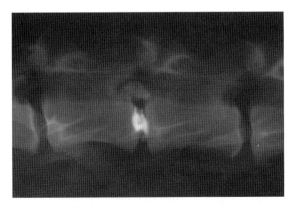

Figure 26.6   Sequestered discogram.

B. Intravenous discograms

Contrast flows into the vertebral venous sinuses in the ventral vertebral canal. This is a very transient pattern with flow toward the heart (Figure 26.7).

Historical perspectives

Early in the development of nucleolysis, controversy arose when two human cases of transverse myelitis were produced by radiologists who inadvertently placed chymopapain into the subarachnoid space following posterior transdural discograms. The risk for this error was reduced by development of a more lateral approach avoiding the spinal cord altogether. However, the medicolegal damage was done, and controversy ensued as to whether radiologists, orthopedists, neurologists or other specialists should perform this procedure. The U.S. Federal

Drug Administration became involved as it had oversight for the use of these enzymes and their clinical application. Clinical outcome reports revealed a success rate of between 70 and 80% for nucleolysis using these enzymes, which, by comparison to traditional surgical outcomes, was less than an ideal result. Eventually legal issues reduced the use of chymopapain and collagenase in the United States to such a point that production of the enzymes was unprofitable and clinical availability ceased. The popularity of this type of minimally invasive procedure continued in Canada and Europe, however. The finding that failed nucleolysis did not preclude later surgery, and that nearly 70% of patients avoided surgery, encouraged the continued use of these enzymes as a treatment for disc herniation in humans [4].

Use of nucleolysis in dogs

Indications

Any of the indications for surgical removal of herniated discs also may apply to nucleolysis (i.e., pain, paresis, or paralysis). Chemical dissolution of herniated discs can be as effective in removing disc material from the vertebral canal as surgical excision. Generally, patients who have been conservatively treated unsuccessfully for at least 2 weeks for pain or those with more acute paresis/paralysis are potential candidates for this procedure. Early treatment is preferable to delayed treatment as a soft, freshly herniated disc is more porous and spongy, which enables better penetration by the enzyme than in older, more consolidated lesions. Mixing of the enzyme within the interstices of the herniated disc promotes better dissolution than simply coating the disc surface as might happen with a more chronic herniation. Patients successfully treated conservatively but with recurrence of pain or paresis after cessation of treatment can also be effectively treated in a more permanent way by nucleolysis (or surgery). Patients with neurological impairment are more successfully treated with early nucleolysis or surgery than if treatment is delayed. Proteolytic enzymes can remove herniated disc material as effectively as surgery, but as with surgery, delayed treatment before spinal cord decompression may

result in a poorer outcome or slower neurologic recovery. There are some indications where nucleolysis might be preferable to surgical decompression. Sick or debilitated animals can be treated with this percutaneous, minimally invasive procedure as anesthesia does not have to be as deep as required for surgery, and the procedure usually does not take longer than 15 or 20 min for most patients, once anesthesia has commenced. Animals with potential bleeding disorders, such as Doberman pinschers with von Willebrand's disease, or patients with hyperadrenocorticism may be more safely treated with this minimally invasive procedure. Both cervical disc herniations and thoracolumbar herniations can be treated with nucleolysis, and in the author's opinion, with equal effectiveness as with surgery. Since all of the canine discs can be injected successfully, some of the surgical difficulties in accessing certain parts of the vertebral canal may be avoided.

Contraindications

Patients known to have sensitivity to proteolytic enzymes are susceptible to anaphylactic shock. While this is a common concern in human disc disease treatment, as exposure to proteolytic enzymes is prevalent, no reports of anaphylaxis have been reported in dogs or cats to the author's knowledge. Enzymatic leakage into the subarachnoid space or spinal cord is a serious potential complication. Dural integrity is important and may be compromised by prior durotomies, and tears secondary to disc herniation. Punctures of the dura during myelography represent a potential hazard if enzymes are deposited adjacent to these areas [5].

Advantages

Multiple discs can be treated with nucleolysis during a single anesthesia, both as a primary treatment for an extruded disc and prophylactic treatment of adjacent discs to try to prevent subsequent herniations (i.e., "chemical fenestration"; discussed later in the chapter). In dogs with apparent spine pain, but where radiographic site location is ambiguous, multiple discs can be treated without the morbidity associated with imprecise surgical exploration.

Patients with myelograms that reveal multiple segments of swollen spinal cord can have multiple discs injected without resorting to multiple level or wrong-sided laminectomy. Where disc herniation is still suspected despite a negative myelogram (and advanced imaging is not available), it may be possible to identify the lesion with discography and then treat with subsequent enzyme injection.

Another potential advantage of chemonucleolysis is that localization of the herniation to a particular side is unnecessary, as the enzyme will typically follow the path of the rupture wherever the displaced nucleus ends up. On the other hand, there are differences between the more typical contained herniation common in humans and the more explosive extrusions seen particularly in chondrodystrophoid dogs. The latter may no longer have a preserved connection or path between the disc space and the extruded material (sequestration). Hence, it is possible that therapeutic use of nucleolysis in chondrodystrophoid dogs with sequestered disc material might be less effective than in dogs and humans with more well-preserved connection between the disc space and the herniated nucleus, and that the chief value for nucleolysis in chondrodystrophoid dogs may be in prevention of further disc herniation at treated sites. The enzyme may reach the herniated components even if they are sequestered away from the site of herniation. However, the more localized the herniated material is to the site of annular tear, the more likely the enzyme will fully concentrate there and achieve the goal of dissolution and decompression. However, the entire dose of enzyme does not necessarily have to be adjacent to the herniated material to be effective, so more research is needed to determine the fate of extruded disc material within the vertebral canal after injection of proteolytic enzymes. To the author's knowledge there have not been randomized, prospective studies comparing nucleolysis with surgical decompression, so the personal impression that nucleolysis can be as effective as surgery (or vice versa) remains anecdotal.

Lateral disc herniations not associated with the vertebral canal can be effectively treated with nucleolysis. These lateral herniations may not be evident with standard radiography or myelography (see Chapter 30 on cervical disc disease).

Disadvantages

Despite the near-instantaneous biochemical reaction of the enzyme with the nucleus pulposus, resolution of the neurologic signs may be prolonged in comparison with surgery. It is uncertain whether the enzyme takes longer to remove the nucleus material, but postoperative pain and weakness may be worse in 25–30% of patients treated with nucleolysis. This occurs in fewer than 10% of surgically treated patients. This worsening is temporary and usually resolves within 7–10 days, but is still worrisome to both the veterinarian and the client. When surgical patients are worsened after surgery, it is assumed that the surgery itself resulted in added trauma to the spinal cord or nerve roots. The reason for worsening of signs after nucleolysis is not determined. One possibility is that there is contact with nerve roots (extruded disc material typically impinges on or envelops the nerve roots), and degradative enzymes may induce radicular pathology, even though these enzymes are thought to be nontoxic to nerve roots, or enzymes may gain access to the intradural space where the nerve roots penetrate the dura.

Verification of the amount of disc removal by enzymatic dissolution is difficult. In surgery, visual confirmation of disc removal is straightforward. With nucleolysis, posttreatment diagnostic imaging is needed to verify disc resorption and spinal cord decompression. Since we are unsure as to how rapidly these processes occur, the timing for such confirmatory imaging is uncertain. In the clinical setting, reimaging patients generally occurs only with failure. And since these patients usually recover to the same degree that surgical patients do in the author's experience, this verification has not been pursued routinely.

Herniations with fibroid, cartilaginous, bony, and scar formation components are not amenable to proteolytic enzyme treatment. Chronic herniations have an abundance of these components and surgical decompression may be necessary.

Technique

Under fluoroscopic or digital radiographic control, the enzymes are introduced into the nucleus with double spinal needles (18 gauge needle placed into the outer annulus with a 22 gauge needle placed inside this larger needle penetrating the annulus into the nucleus). The enzyme follows the path of the herniation, mixing with the nucleus material in the vertebral canal as well as the normally located nucleus pulposus. Radiographic contrast material mixed with or added as a separate injection follows the enzyme, marks the trail of the injection, and verifies mixing with the herniated disc. Once the enzyme leaves the tip of the needle in the nucleus, there is no control over its movement. It is anticipated that it will follow the path of least resistance, presumably the path of the herniated disc nucleus. How much of the enzyme mixes with the disc material in the vertebral canal is unknown and probably variable. However, very little of the enzyme has to contact the offending nucleus to effect volume reduction. Since many successful treatments of herniations in dogs have presumably involved sequestered disc material, it appears that very little of the enzyme needs to be in contact with the nucleus to be effective [6–8].

Enzymes

Chymopapain

Chymopapain is the most common enzyme used in human and veterinary medicine. It is derived from the papaya plant by extracting crude papain from papaya latex. Papain is a mixture containing proteolytic enzymes, one of which is chymopapain. However, this enzyme has been unavailable for clinical use for the past decade because of the aforementioned medicolegal issues. It works quite well in the degenerated chondrodystrophic canine disc, which has a higher proportion of mineralized content than human discs or discs from nonchondrodystrophoid dogs. Postinjection pain and muscle spasm are minimal compared to collagenase. With removal of the hygroscopic ground matrix (see Chapters 1 and 2), the nucleus releases water, resulting in decreasing the intradiscal pressure. Water binding property of the ground substance is provided by the protein disaccharide polymer, which is depolymerized by chymopapain.

Disc space collapse is noted within a few days [7,8]. Annular changes occur minimally and end plate changes are few. The nucleus will rehydrate and the disc space will rewiden in about 20–25% of cases. About half of chymopapain injected mineralized discs will demineralize based on radiographs. Complete demineralization is not necessary for successful results. Currently the dose is between 2 and 300 units per disc, depending on the size of the disc space and the amount of disc material in the vertebral canal. While multiple discs can be injected, the more enzyme present in the vertebral canal, the more chance for postinjection pain, weakness, and muscle spasm. Injecting five to six discs at one time has been my usual maximum. Interestingly, clinical improvement often occurs far in advance of complete radiographic demineralization. Usually within 6–8 weeks, demineralization has occurred radiographically.

Collagenase

Collagenase is the only enzyme that is currently available for intradiscal proteolytic use. It has stronger demineralization properties than chymopapain and routinely collapses disc spaces within several days. Most discs remain collapsed and few discs rewiden as they tend to do more often with chymopapain. Postinjection pain, weakness, and muscle spasm occur with about a 15–20% higher incidence than with chymopapain. Pain can usually be controlled with anti-inflammatory drugs, muscle relaxants, sedation, and other analgesic modalities. Usually within 3 or 4 days, these patients are better and most are pain-free and neurological deficits decrease or resolve by 14–16 days postinjection. Vertebral end plate changes are minimal, but sclerosis and spondylosis are common. Clinical signs associated with these postinjection changes have not been appreciated. Disc demineralization occurs 92% of the time without rewidening. Presumed sequestration of extruded discs has not negatively influenced this outcome in the experience of the author. Utilizing lower doses of collagenase appears to minimize the postinjection side effects of pain, muscle spasm, and weakness [9].

Chondroitinase ABC

Clinical trials using this enzyme have been insufficient to demonstrate efficacy or toxicity. Its mode of action is based on splitting disaccharide bonds, and it has an affinity for chondroitin sulfate.

Toxicity to vessels and nerves is minimal. It may take 5 days to see radiographic evidence of disc space collapse with this agent [10].

Toxicity

None of the enzymes commonly used are especially toxic to tissue, except with dural penetration. An intact dura acts as a barrier to enzyme-produced toxic spinal cord injury. The annulus, end plates, and nerve roots all purportedly tolerate these enzymes well. Tissues in the epidural space are also accommodating. Penetration of the dura into the subarachnoid space by enzyme can be catastrophic however. Diapedesis occurs with capillary wall integrity loss. Transverse myelopathy is the usual result and appears to be permanent, at least in humans. Canine disc herniation seldom causes dural penetration and thus proteolytic enzymes are usually safe [11]. Anaphylaxis with chymopapain is a concern in the human field. There have been no reported allergic reactions in dogs. Canine patients are seldom exposed to papain products (meat tenderizers, contact lens cleaners, etc.). Anaphylaxis has not been associated with collagenase, a common enzyme found throughout mammalian tissue.

Clinical response following injection

It takes 1–5 days for the disc space to collapse radiographically. The annulus and dorsal longitudinal ligament bulge up into the vertebral canal as a result of this disc space collapse. After 4–6 weeks, the initially unstable collapsed disc becomes more stable due to scar formation. After 4–6 months, the ventral vertebral canal is virtually flat as the initial redundancy of these tissues subsides due to contraction and decreased motion. Virtually all collapsed disc spaces, due to facet mechanics and other aligning anatomy, collapse in such a manner that normal vertebral canal alignment is maintained. The initial annular and ligamentous redundancy produced with disc space collapse decreases the vertebral canal diameter and may produce clinical signs. Worsening of the neurological signs sometimes seen with both nucleolysis and surgical decompression can be vexing and requires good communication between the veterinarian and the client to help the patient and client through the period of time before clinical improvement is observed.

Approximately 30–40% of collagenase-injected patients will have increased pain or weakness compared to their preinjection status. Usually, the nadir occurs within the first 2 days after injection. Most dogs have slight improvement by the week after injection, and by 10–12 days after injection significant improvement usually occurs. By 14 days after injection, I find 90–95% of these patients are clinically improved enough for the owners to be encouraged sufficiently to allow them the 6 weeks necessary to determine a final outcome. The method by which disc irritation or compression of neurological tissues is treated, whether by mechanical surgery or the biochemistry of nucleolysis, does not seem to influence the outcome. Removal of the pathological tissue and compressive effect is the important task (see Chapter 28) [5].

Chemical prophylactic fenestration

Surgical fenestration is performed by creating a window in the (lateral) annulus (usually with a scalpel blade) and then removing nucleus with an instrument. Initially this was used as a primary treatment for dogs with disc herniations, predicated on the theory that by reducing the intradiscal pressure, a reduction in the amount of annulus pressing on the spinal cord would ensue. Failure of this technique is attributed to most of the herniated disc material in dogs being sequestered, or at least beyond the reach of instruments placed within the disc space, and is not affected by manipulations within the intervertebral disc space [12].

Results of chemical fenestration in dogs

I evaluated more than 3000 cases of thoracolumbar disc herniation over the past 30 years. Approximately 1100 cases were presented with clinical signs occurring after the client reported prior surgical fenestration. The previously fenestrated discs were specifically identified and confirmed based on surgical reports from other hospitals and my own records. Eight hundred and twenty-one (75%) of these previously fenestrated discs had normal radiographic width. One hundred and forty (13%) were narrowed. Forty-three (4%) had evidence of herniation. One hundred and seventy (15%) had narrowed disc spaces without confirmation of previous fenestration or herniation. Eighteen patients (1.6%) had both laminectomy and fenestration of the herniated disc level. Since these patients were not followed continuously after fenestration, it is not possible to determine the effectiveness of fenestration on preventing subsequent disc herniation. But it is suggested by these personal data that surgical fenestration does not always prevent subsequent herniation or recurrent clinical signs in all patients.

Eight hundred and ninety-one patients were presented with clinical signs of disc herniation and were treated with chymopapain. These patients were followed for a minimum of 5 years, and the radiographic appearance of these discs assessed periodically, with recurrence of disc herniation recorded. Eight hundred and fifteen (91%) of these discs narrowed initially and remained narrowed throughout the study period without new signs of herniation. Three discs had recurrent herniations after the patients recovered successfully from the original injection treatment. Sixty discs (7%) rewidened without evidence of herniation.

One thousand and ten patients were treated with collagenase and similarly followed for 5 years. These patients presented with signs of disc herniation. Nine hundred and seventy (96%) had posttreatment disc space collapse and did not rewiden. Thirty-one (3%) rewidened without signs of herniation. Nine collagenase-treated discs (<1%) subsequently herniated, and these were successfully treated with reinjection or surgery.

Critical statistical analysis is lacking and these were not blinded, controlled studies. Nonetheless, it appears that surgical fenestration may be less effective for prophylaxis of disc herniation when compared to chemical fenestration and that collagenase is associated with less rewidening and subsequent herniation than chymopapain [13].

Nucleolysis and spondylomyelopathy in Doberman pinschers

Because "wobblers" disease can be associated in part with disc degeneration (disc-associated wobbler disease—"DAWS"; see Chapter 7), it is conceivable that nucleolysis could play a role in the treatment of that condition. Although one surgical technique is vertebral distraction (i.e., widening the disc space and stretching redundant ligamentous structures that impinge on the spinal cord), the author has investigated use of nucleolysis over the past 25 years, speculating that dissolution of the nucleus might result in a stable fibrous-type "fusion" of the adjacent vertebrae and thus reduce vertebral motion segment instability. Among the advantages to using nucleolysis in this setting are the minimal morbidity compared with more typical distraction–fusion methods, the minimal risk for hemorrhage in patients with bleeding disorders (e.g., von Willebrand's disease), and the ability to use minimal anesthesia in patients that may have concurrent cardiac disease. Prior nucleolysis also does not preclude later surgery if needed, and clients may be more willing to pursue a percutaneous treatment than surgery. I have been encouraged by my results over the years, but also note that, as with standard surgical methods, outcome is largely predicated on preoperative status, with better outcomes in dogs with less severe neurologic signs at the time of treatment. My results are not published, and so remain speculative, but at least warrant further investigation.

References

1. Sisson AF, LeCouteur RA, Ingram JT, Park RD, Child G. Diagnosis of cauda equina abnormalities by using electromyography, discography, and epidurography in dogs. J Vet Intern Med. 1992 Sep–Oct;6(5):253–63.
2. Barthez PY, Morgan JP, Lipsitz D. Discography and epidurography for evaluation of the lumbosacral junction in dogs with cauda equina syndrome. Vet Radiol Ultrasound. 1994;35:152–7.
3. Wrigley RH, Reuter RE. Canine cervical discography. Vet Radiol 1984;25:274–9.
4. Morrison PC, Felts MS, Javid MJ, Nordby EJ. Overview of chemonucleolysis. In: Savitz MH, Chiu JC, Yeung AT, editors. The Practice of Minimally Invasive Spinal Technique. Richmand, VA: AAMISMS Education; 2000. pp. 19–28.
5. Biggart JF, Gill GR. Discolysis: an introduction. Calif Vet. 1984;38:10–11,25.

6. Kahanovitz N, Arnoczky SP, Sissons HA, Steiner GC, Schwarez P. The effect of discography on the canine intervertebral disc. Spine (Phila Pa 1976). 1986 Jan–Feb;11(1):26–7.

7. Bailey CS. Chymopapain chemonucleolysis. In: Kirk RW, Bonagura JD, editors. Kirk's Current Veterinary Therapy XI (Small Animal Practice). Philadelphia: WB Saunders; 1992. pp. 1018–20.

8. Biggart JF. Discography for diagnosis of neurological disease. In: Bojrab MJ, editor. Current Techniques in Small Animal Surgery, Fourth Edition. Baltimore, MD: Williams and Wilkins; 1998. pp. 809–13.

9. Biggart, JF. Collagenase: toxicity and efficacy. Proc Abbott Soc 1985;16:56–65.

10. Fry TR. Evaluation of chondroitinase abc for chemonucleolysis of canine lumbar intervertebral discs. Vet Surg 1990;19:65.

11. Biggart JF. Collagenase vs. chymopapain. Proceedings of the International Intradiscal Therapy Society. Aberdeen, Scotland. International Intradiscal Therapy Society; 1994:34.

12. Fingeroth JM. Fenestration. Pros and cons. Probl Vet Med. 1989;1:445–66.

13. Biggart JF. Results of discolysis in the treatment of 125 patients with herniated discs. Vet Surg 1988; 17:29.

27 Medical Management and Nursing Care for the Paralyzed Patient

James M. Fingeroth and William B. Thomas

Even with an accurate diagnosis and specific therapy such as surgery, if subsequent nursing care is inadequate, the patient with intervertebral disc herniation (IVDH)-induced paralysis will not recover optimally and may suffer unnecessary discomfort or pain or even fatal complications. This chapter reviews basic principles of nursing care in the recumbent patient, and applies equally to those being managed medically and those recovering from surgery.

Bladder management

A critical aspect of caring for a paralyzed patient is early assessment of the animal's ability, or lack thereof, to void urine voluntarily. Urine retention is too often overlooked during initial evaluation. This can lead to unnecessary discomfort for the animal and predispose to secondary problems such as urinary tract infection (UTI) and detrusor atony. The failure to identify and initiate early intervention for this problem probably stems from several factors. These include being overly focused on limb dysfunction and forgetting to consider the likelihood of concomitant urinary dysfunction, and misinterpreting overflow incontinence as voluntary micturition.

An early part of client communication/education should also touch on the need for bladder management, as this may be something the clients have to learn and assume control over once a pet is discharged from the hospital. As a rule of thumb, most dogs and cats recover voluntary control over micturition concomitant with recovery of voluntary/purposeful appendicular motor function (even if yet nonambulatory).

Control of micturition

Micturition is the process of storing and periodically voiding urine. This involves a complex series of neural pathways that controls the urinary bladder and urethra. The primary control center for micturition is located in the pons. Other brain regions, including the forebrain and cerebellum, are important for voluntary storage of urine and initiation of voiding. Axons projecting from the micturition center travel caudally in the spinal

Advances in Intervertebral Disc Disease in Dogs and Cats, First Edition. Edited by James M. Fingeroth and William B. Thomas.
© 2015 ACVS Foundation. Published 2015 by John Wiley & Sons, Inc.

cord to the lumbar and sacral segments that innervate the bladder and urethra.

Sympathetic neurons in the lumbar spinal cord segments (L1–L4 in the dog, L2–L5 in the cat) provide axons to the hypogastric nerves that innervate the detrusor muscle in the bladder (β-adrenergic receptors) and the smooth muscle of the urethra (α-adrenergic receptors). These act to inhibit detrusor muscle contraction and increase urethral tone during the storage phase of micturition.

Parasympathetic neurons in the sacral spinal cord segments innervate the detrusor muscle via the pelvic nerves and act to contract the detrusor muscle during voiding. General somatic efferent neurons in the sacral segments innervate the skeletal muscle of the urethra via the pudendal nerves. This provides voluntary contraction of the urethra that is important in storage of urine.

During storage, sympathetic tone predominates to relax the detrusor muscle to accommodate filling with urine against a closed outlet provided by a contracted urethra. As the bladder becomes full, stretch receptors in the bladder are activated and project sensory information along the spinal cord to the brain so that the animal is aware of bladder distension. Conscious voiding occurs by voluntary release of inhibition of the micturition center in the pons. Parasympathetic tone predominates during voiding. Impulses travel along the spinal cord to the lumbar and sacral segments to relax the urethra in coordination with contraction of the detrusor muscle [1, 2].

Upper motor neuron bladder

In most cases of intervertebral disc herniation, the spinal cord lesion is cranial to the sacral spinal cord segments. If the lesion is severe enough, it damages the ascending sensory pathways and descending motor pathways responsible for micturition and prevents voluntary voiding. Detrusor and urethral tones are increased because of loss of inhibition from the brain. The bladder becomes full and feels firm and turgid, and there is substantial resistance to manual evacuation of the bladder. There may be inconsistent leakage of urine from an overly full bladder (overflow incontinence). This syndrome is referred to as an upper motor neuron (UMN) bladder.

Over a period of days to weeks, some patients will develop a variable degree of reflex voiding. Bladder distension activates neurons in the sacral segments that serve to contract the detrusor muscle and relax the urethra. However, this voiding is involuntary and occurs only to the point where detrusor stretching is sufficiently relieved. At that point, the situation returns to *status quo ante*, where the bladder still retains urine. In some cases, this reflex is stimulated by abdominal pressure such as picking up the patient. It is critical to not mistake this reflex and incomplete voiding as evidence of voluntary micturition.

Lower motor neuron balder

Much less common in patients with disc herniation is a lesion affecting the sacral spinal cord segments or nerve roots. This results in loss of voluntary micturition accompanied by decreased tone in the detrusor muscle and urethra. The bladder feels flaccid and is easily expressed. Overflow incontinence is common when the bladder is distended and the patient often leaks urine spontaneously or in response to abdominal pressure. This syndrome is called a lower motor neuron (LMN) bladder [1, 2].

In some cases, smooth muscle sphincter tone (innervated by the hypogastric nerve) may be preserved and become static such that outflow resistance is preserved [1]. In these patients, it may be difficult to manually express the bladder. Therefore, the assessment of urethral tone alone is not always an accurate way to localize spinal cord lesions. These patients often have decreased anal tone and absent perineal reflexes and may have loss of sensation in the perineum and tail. These findings are more reliable in localizing the lesion to the sacral segments and nerve roots, and underscore the need to assess anal tone and perineal reflexes when evaluating paralyzed patients.

Management of urine retention

Animals with severe paresis or paralysis should be suspected of having micturition compromise as well. Urine retention increases the risk of UTI, and overdistension of the bladder can damage the detrusor muscle resulting in persistent atony [1, 3]. Patients may leak urine due to decreased urethral tone (LMN bladder) or overflow incontinence (UMN) or incompletely void urine due to reflex voiding. Therefore, finding urine in the patient's cage or bedding is not a reliable indicator that the animal can urinate voluntarily. If possible, the patient is taken outside and given adequate time to urinate voluntarily. Even if the patient voids, the bladder is palpated to assess residual volume. Normal residual volume after voiding is 0.2–0.4 ml/kg (usually <10 ml total) [1]. It may be difficult to palpate the bladder in obese patients or painful patients with increased abdominal muscle tone. In those cases, ultrasound is useful to assess bladder size. In general, the bladder should be assessed every 6 h, but this is adjusted as necessary in individual patients. For example, patients receiving intravenous fluid therapy or corticosteroids often have increased urine volume and require more frequent assessment.

In patients that do not urinate voluntarily or have excess residual volume, the first step is to attempt manual bladder expression. This is performed outside, over absorbent bedding, or over a drain. Expression can be done with the patient in lateral recumbency or supported in a standing position, whichever is more comfortable. Place a hand on each side of the abdomen, just caudal to the last rib. Gently palpate the abdomen by advancing your hands medially and caudally until you can feel the bladder. Then apply slow, steady pressure with the flat portions of the hands and fingers to completely empty the bladder. If the patient starts to tense the abdominal muscles, release pressure until the patient relaxes and then start again. Never try to "overpower" the patient.

If the bladder cannot be comfortably expressed, the next step is catheterization. Sedation is often helpful for patient comfort. For male patients, a sterile, soft urethral or feeding tube is premeasured from the tip of the penis to 2–4 cm cranial to the pubis to ensure appropriate length to reach the urinary bladder. The patient is physically restrained in lateral recumbency with the aid of an assistant. The penis is exposed and the urethral opening cleansed with antiseptic solution. Wearing sterile gloves, the lubricated sterile catheter is passed into the urethral opening and into the urinary bladder. The bladder is emptied with a syringe until urine can no longer be obtained [4].

Female patients are positioned in lateral or sternal recumbency, and the perivulvar region is clipped, cleaned, and prepared with antiseptic.

A stylet is often useful. A light and a sterile vaginascope or an otoscope with a sterile speculum is helpful in visualizing the urethral papilla. The catheter is inserted through the papilla and into the bladder to a premeasured length in a sterile fashion.

In females or other patients where catheterization is expected to be difficult or uncomfortable for the patient, it is often beneficial to place an indwelling silicone Foley urinary catheter. In patients undergoing diagnostic imaging and/or surgery, this can be accomplished under general anesthesia at the time of imaging or surgery. Once urine flows from the catheter, the balloon at the tip of the catheter is inflated with sterile saline and the catheter connected to a sterile, closed urine collection system. Urine is aseptically drained from the collection system two to four times daily and urine volume recorded. The exposed portion of the catheter is cleaned daily with antiseptic solution. Once the patient has recovered strong motor function in the pelvic limbs, or one anticipates being able to accomplish manual bladder emptying, the urinary catheter may be removed and the patient observed for voluntary urination.

Although urethral catheterization carries a risk of introducing bacteria, one study did not find a statistically significant difference in the rate of UTI in patients managed with intermittent catheterization or indwelling catheterization, compared to manual expression [4]. A longer duration of catheterization is associated with a progressive increase in the risk for UTI, so catheterization is stopped as soon as the patient is able to urinate voluntarily [2, 4]. Empiric antibiotic therapy for prophylaxis during the period of indwelling catheterization is generally contraindicated because this increases the risk of UTI and antibiotic resistance [5].

Pharmacologic treatment of urine retention

Pharmacologic treatment is most effective when started early in the course of treatment and used for short periods of time. Drug therapy is helpful in altering detrusor and urethral tone, but no drug will restore voluntary urination in a patient with spinal cord disease. Drug therapy is only one component of management and not a substitute for other therapies such as manual bladder expression or catheterization. Commonly used drugs are described in Table 27.1.

Table 27.1   Drugs used to manage urine retention

Drug	Action	Dose	Possible adverse effects
Diazepam	Centrally acting skeletal muscle relaxation	Dog: 2–10 mg q8 h, PO Cat: 1–2.5 mg/cat q8 h, PO	Sedation Paradoxic excitement Hepatic necrosis (cats)
Dantrolene	Direct-acting skeletal muscle relaxation	Dog: 1–5 mg/kg q8 h, PO Cat: 2 mg/kg q8 h, PO	Sedation GI upset
Phenoxybenzamine	Smooth muscle relaxation	Dog: 5–20 mg q12–24 h, PO Cat: 2.5–5 mg q12–42 h, PO	Hypotension Tachycardia GI upset
Prazosin	Smooth muscle relaxation	Dog: 1 mg per 15 kg q8–12 h, PO Cat: 0.25 q12–24 h, PO	Hypotension Mild sedation

Pharmacologic manipulation of outlet resistance may be directed at smooth or skeletal muscle components of the urethra. Drugs to decrease urethral tone are most commonly used in patients with UMN bladders to facilitate manual bladder expression. Phenoxybenzamine is a nonselective α-adrenergic antagonist that decreases urethral resistance. It is administered orally at dosage of 5–20 mg every 12 or 24 h in dogs or 2.5–5 mg every 12 or 24 h in cats. Side effects can include gastrointestinal upset and hypotension. It often takes several days of therapy for clinical effects to become apparent. Phenoxybenzamine is considered obsolete for the treatment of functional urethral obstruction in human patients, following the advent of selective α-1 antagonists, and concerns regarding the potential carcinogenicity of phenoxybenzamine. This has limited the availability of the drug in certain regions and resulted in an increase in price [6].

Prazosin is a readily available and inexpensive selective α-1 antagonist. It is administered orally at 1 mg per 15 kg every 8 or 12 h in dogs and at 0.25 mg per cat every 12 or 24 h [1]. Side effects are similar to those of phenoxybenzamine, especially hypotension. To decrease the risk of hypotension, half the calculated dose is often administered for the first few days of treatment as the patient is monitored for signs of hypotension, such as lethargy or syncope.

Skeletal muscle relaxants provide additional relaxation of the urethra in patients with UMN bladders, especially in male dogs and in cats, which have greater proportions of skeletal muscle in the urethra. In dogs, diazepam is administered orally at 2–10 mg per dog every 8 h. The dose for cats is 1–2.5 mg orally every 8 h [1]. In patients that are managed with manual bladder expression, the dose is administered 30– 60 min prior to attempting bladder expression. The most common side effect is mild sedation. Some cats have developed hepatic failure after receiving oral diazepam for several days. Clinical signs include anorexia, lethargy, ataxia, and jaundice [7]. Cats that receive diazepam should have baseline liver function tests, and the drug should be discontinued if clinical signs of toxicity develop.

Dantrolene is a direct-acting skeletal muscle relaxant that has been used to reduce urethral pressure. It is administered orally at 1–5 mg/kg every 8 h (dogs) or 2 mg/kg every 8 h in cats [1]. Potential adverse effects include sedation, hypotension, and gastrointestinal upset [1].

UTI

UTI is a common complication of thoracolumbar disc-induced spinal cord disease, occurring in 27–42% of patients [3–5, 8]. Risk factors for the development of UTI include loss of ambulation, inability to voluntarily urinate, duration of inability to urinate, and body temperature less than 35 °C during anesthesia [4, 5, 8]. Perioperative administration of cefazolin decreased the risk of UTI in one study [8]. *Escherichia coli* and *Enterococcus* sp. are the most common isolates. Others include *Klebsiella pneumoniae, Staphylococcus intermedius, Streptococcus* sp., *Enterobacter* sp., *Acinetobacter* sp., and *Proteus mirabilis*. Many UTIs are occult, with no clinical signs and no hematuria or pyuria detected on urinalysis [4, 8]. Given the high incidence of UTI and the frequency of occult infections, one of the authors (WT) routinely collects urine for culture at the time of surgery and again once the patient regains voluntary urination and any catheterization has ceased. Any confirmed UTI is treated with a 10-day course of antibiotic chosen on the basis of susceptibility testing. Several days after antibiotic therapy is discontinued, another urine sample is submitted for culture to ensure the infection is eradicated.

Defecation

Although both urinary continence and fecal continence are affected with the disturbance of sphincter function of both UMN and LMN, there is less concern generally with the fecal continence in dogs and cats. Animals with lesions cranial to S2 may well have some degree of constipation, but we rarely recognize overt signs of discomfort in patients with fecal retention, and the reflexive emptying of stool appears to occur with much less effort than with urine emptying. Quite often, one will observe defecation simultaneously with manual bladder expression, presumably because the stimulation provided during manual expression initiates a reflexive impulse in the pudendal nerves that subserve both bladder/urethral and anal sphincter relaxations. The propulsive peristaltic nature of ingesta and fecal transit through the gastrointestinal tract also probably influences the movement of stool through the anal sphincter despite hypertonicity/hyperreflexia. As with LMN urine incontinence described earlier, the key nursing care element is prevention of fecal soiling and subsequent dermatitis, as the patient may be unaware of (and unable to move away from, due to paralysis) any bowel movement.

With both LMN fecal and urinary incontinence, the patient is likely to become soiled with excretions. Nursing care thus demands minimizing the dermatologic effects from such soiling. Fecal soiling can be combated by frequent examination and cleansing, shaving the perineum, and wrapping the tail. Appropriate salves can also be employed to soothe irritated skin.

Hydration and nutrition

Patients with acute paralysis associated with IVDH may have anxiety and discomfort. These may adversely affect intake of food and water. A short period of hyporexia or anorexia is probably not harmful to most patients, but dehydration is anathema for patients with spinal cord injury, as this may cause a reduction in spinal cord blood flow in a situation where spinal cord circulation in the injured segments may already be tenuous. It is therefore always a consideration as part of the early and ongoing nursing care and management of patients with IVDH and neurologic deficits to provide intravenous fluid support.

Adequate nutrition is important to slow catabolism and provide precursors for optimal immune function, tissue repair, and drug metabolism. The resting energy requirement (RER) is estimated by the following formulas:

$$Dogs: RER \, kcal \, / \, day = 33 \times body \, weight \, in \, kg$$

$$Cats: RER \, kcal \, / \, day = 44 \times body \, weight \, in \, kg$$

Recording the food intake of patients is important in determining if assisted feeding is necessary. Nutritional support is considered for any patient with inadequate food intake for more than 3 days. Patients that cannot or will not eat but have a normally functioning gastrointestinal tract should receive enteral feeding support. Nasoesophageal tubes are generally used for short-term support (3–7 days). A 5 French (cats, small dogs) or 8 French (larger dogs) silicone or polyurethane feeding tube is placed through the nasal cavity into the distal esophagus. Gastrotomy tubes are recommended for long-term use if needed.

Liquid foods, such as CliniCare (Abbott Animal Health; Abbott Park, IL, United States), are used for small-diameter nasogastric tubes. Blended pet foods are suitable for larger diameter feeding tubes. Feed an amount equal to the patient's RER in the first 24 h if tolerated. Diets should be warmed to room temperature but no higher than body temperature before feeding. Infuse food over a period of at least 1 min to allow gradual gastric expansion. Salivating, gulping, retching, and vomiting may occur when too much food has been infused or when the infusion rate is too fast. Feeding is stopped at the first sign of retching or salivating. If the patient is volume sensitive, initially feed a third of RER and then increase the amount fed by a third every 24 h until reaching an adequate dose. Patients that cannot tolerate bolus feeding without vomiting benefit from slow continuous-drip administration by pump or gravity flow of food [9].

Recumbency and decubital sores

The inability to rise and walk predisposes patients to discomfort from lying in one position for extended periods, and may also predispose to decubital sores. An important part of nursing care is therefore provision of suitable substrates for the patient to lie on, and frequent shifting or position or recumbent side. Mobilization of paralyzed patients and physical therapeutic interventions are covered in Chapter 38.

Decubital sores are most common over bony prominences, such as the ischium and greater trochanter. Moist skin increases the risk of decubital sores so the skin should be kept clean and dry. Recumbent patients are kept on appropriate bedding such as sheepskin, foam or air mattresses, or trampolines. Sheepskin minimizes friction, absorbs moisture, and can be laundered. Air mattresses evenly distribute pressure but can be punctured by the patient's nails, are difficult to clean, and do not absorb moisture. Therefore, air mattresses are covered with sheepskin or other suitable material. Trampolines are excellent for large recumbent patients. They consist of a frame of plastic tubing that supports fiberglass netting. The trampoline distributes the patient's weight evenly and the netting allows drainage of urine away from the patient's skin [10].

Doughnut-shaped bandages can be placed over bony prominences to prevent or treat decubital sores. Medical therapy for decubital ulcers includes topical antibiotic preparations and enzymatic debriding agents. Preparation-H can be used as it helps stimulate wound healing [10]. Systemic antibiotics, frequent wound lavage, wet-to-dry bandaging, or surgery is indicated for more severe wounds [10].

Respiratory care

Recumbent patients are at risk of developing several respiratory complications, including atelectasis and pneumonia. Patients with severe lesions of the cervical spinal cord segments may develop respiratory paresis. Such complications can quickly become life threatening, so respiratory function is monitored closely. The rate and quality of respiration are assessed, the chest is auscultated frequently, and the results are recorded to detect any trends. Respiratory paresis is initially evident as decreased intercostal movement. More severe paresis is manifested as paradoxical chest movement where the chest wall moves inward on inspiration, instead of outward.

Pulse oximetry and blood gas analysis are indicated anytime respiratory compromise is suspected or anticipated. With respiratory paresis, $PaCO_2$ often increases (hypoventilation) before there are changes in PaO_2 or pulse oximetry (hypoxemia). Chest radiographs are obtained when pneumonia is suspected.

Recumbent patients are turned every 4 h to minimize atelectasis. Keeping the patient propped sternally or supported with a sling is also helpful. Nasal oxygen therapy is administered in patients with decreased respiratory function. Pneumonia is treated with systemic antibiotics, nebulization, and coupage. Mechanical ventilation is necessary in patients with substantial respiratory paresis or severe pneumonia. This is labor intensive and is best administered in a facility with continuous nursing care and clinicians experienced in critical care.

Summary

Veterinarians must be attuned to the various potential problems in paralyzed patients, and avoid becoming too focused on only the ambulation deficits that typically form the client's chief complaint, and which are the most obvious, but not necessarily the most significant functional loss the pet faces. This awareness is particularly important in those instances where the patient is not going to be referred to a specialty center for advanced imaging or surgical treatment, when there is going to be any delay of more than 1–2 h before referral, or when the hospital offers less than 24 h care. By having in mind the urinary, fecal, and respiratory problems that might accompany a paralyzed patient and addressing these early on (both with the patient and with the client), the attending veterinarian will be doing much to improve patient comfort, health, recovery, and client understanding of what management entails.

References

1. Lane IF. Diagnosis and management of urinary retention. *Vet Clin North Am Small Anim Pract.* 2000;30(1):25–55.
2. de Lahunta A, Glass E. *Veterinary Neuroanatomy and Clinical Neurology.* 3rd ed. St. Louis, MO: Saunders Elsevier; 2009.
3. Olby NJ, MacKillop E, Cerda-Gonzalez S, *et al.* Prevalence of urinary tract infection in dogs after surgery for thoracolumbar intervertebral disc extrusion. *J Vet Intern Med.* Sep–Oct 2010;24(5):1106–1111.
4. Bubenik L, Hosgood G. Urinary tract infection in dogs with thoracolumbar intervertebral disc herniation and urinary bladder dysfunction managed by manual expression, indwelling catheterization or intermittent catheterization. *Vet Surg.* Dec 2008;37(8):791–800.
5. Bubenik LJ, Hosgood GL, Waldron DR, Snow LA. Frequency of urinary tract infection in catheterized dogs and comparison of bacterial culture and susceptibility testing results for catheterized and noncatheterized dogs with urinary tract infections. *J Am Vet Med Assoc.* Sep 15 2007;231(6):893–899.
6. Fischer JR, Lane IF, Cribb AE. Urethral pressure profile and hemodynamic effects of phenoxybenzamine and prazosin in non-sedated male beagle dogs. *Can J Vet Res.* Jan 2003;67(1):30–38.
7. Center SA, Elston TH, Rowland PH, *et al.* Fulminant hepatic failure associated with oral administration of diazepam in 11 cats. *J Am Vet Med Assoc.* Aug 1 1996;209(3):618–625.
8. Stiffler KS, Stevenson MA, Sanchez S, Barsanti JA, Hofmeister E, Budsberg SC. Prevalence and characterization of urinary tract infections in dogs with surgically treated type 1 thoracolumbar intervertebral disc extrusion. *Vet Surg.* Jun 2006;35(4):330–336.
9. Remillard RL. Nutritional support in critical care patients. *Vet Clin North Am Small Anim Pract.* Sep 2002;32(5):1145–1164, viii.
10. Tefund MB, Dewey CW. Nursing care and physical therapy for patients with neurologic disease. In: Dewey CW, ed. *A Practical Guide to Canine and Feline Neurology.* 2nd ed. Ames: Wiley-Blackwell; 2008:559–584.

Section V

Surgical Management of Intervertebral Disc Herniation

There is an enormous body of literature regarding the role of surgery for dogs and cats with intervertebral disc herniation, and an equally enormous body of literature that describes a myriad of approaches and intraoperative procedures thought to be most suitable or helpful, both diagnostically/prognostically and therapeutically. Since this is not a surgical atlas we do not focus heavily on the mechanics and techniques of spinal disc surgery per se. Instead, we address surgery from a more philosophical standpoint: What are our goals? What are the pitfalls? How do we decide which surgical approach is most suitable? And given the concern about recurrent IVD-related signs in a given patient, we discuss the rationale, results, and pros and cons of prophylactic procedures aimed at reducing the number of re-operations. Although surgery may be the key *initial* step in returning a patient affected by disc herniation to normal function, all will be for naught if there is a failure to properly manage and rehabilitate the patient during the recovery phase. In this section, we also present some of the key concepts that should be borne in mind and applied clinically when the patient leaves the operating room. Needless to say, these same principles and interventions apply equally to those patients that are managed nonoperatively.

28 What Constitutes Spinal Cord Decompression?

James M. Fingeroth

When patients are referred for surgical treatment of suspected intervertebral disc (IVD) disease, there are some assumptions made that may not always be applicable in every case, or which can mislead both the referring veterinarian and the surgeon.

It has already been established elsewhere in this text that clinical signs may be suggestive of an intervertebral disc etiology; however, in the absence of definitive imaging studies that correlate with the neurologic examination, it remains only a speculation that IVD disease (IVDD) is the underlying problem. Moreover, it has been demonstrated throughout the text that one must be careful to distinguish IVD *disease* (wherein we may find evidence based on signalment, the neurologic exam, or plain radiographic findings) from actual disc *herniation* (Figure 28.1). It is only for the latter cases that surgery is felt to have a therapeutic role. Furthermore, it has been demonstrated elsewhere in the text that not all disc herniations result in lingering compression of the spinal cord or nerve roots. This is critically important, since the main thrust of surgery for disc disease is predicated on the concept of decompression (Figure 28.2). The

issue of concussive versus compressive spinal cord injury is addressed in Chapter 15, and it is on that basis that we utilize surgery to treat the latter in hopes of more rapidly reversing the effects of spinal cord injury and preventing further parenchymal changes that could lead to permanent paralysis.

Therefore, the first issue to be confronted at the time of surgical referral is to establish whether there is persistent spinal cord and/or nerve root *compression* that can be treated. This determination is made using some of the advanced imaging techniques described in Chapter 16. If the surgeon observes that there is a compressive lesion that correlates with the presenting signs, it is appropriate at that point to move forward and take the patient to the operating room.

An all too common misconception, perhaps reinforced by terminology in the literature that describes such things as a "dorsal decompressive laminectomy," is that the laminectomy (or ventral slot, or hemilaminectomy, etc.) is itself a decompressive procedure. There is some limited merit to this viewpoint when one considers that most disc herniations leave masses of disc material ventral

Advances in Intervertebral Disc Disease in Dogs and Cats, First Edition. Edited by James M. Fingeroth and William B. Thomas.
© 2015 ACVS Foundation. Published 2015 by John Wiley & Sons, Inc.

(A)

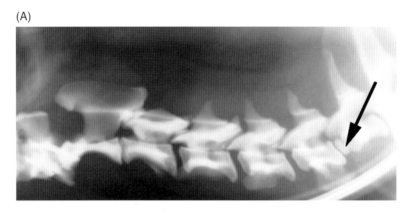

(B)

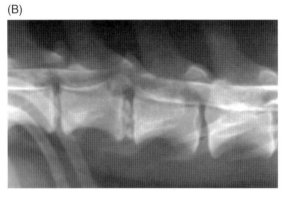

Figure 28.1 (A) Lateral radiograph of the cervical spine of a dog with signs of a cervical myelopathy. Note the mineralized intervertebral disc at C6–C7 (arrow). This is clearly an example of intervertebral disc *disease* (IVDD). However, note also the collapsed disc space at C2–C3. This too represents radiographic evidence of IVDD. Subsequent imaging confirmed that spinal cord compression was occurring from disc *herniation* at the C2–C3 level. One has to be careful to avoid seeing evidence of IVDD on plain radiographs and concluding that clinical signs are due to that lesion. In particular, the presence of mineralization confined to within the disc space only indicates IVDD and not necessarily IVDH. (B) In this instance from a lumbar spine, there is mineralized disc material both in the disc space and within the vertebral canal, and the myelogram confirms that this is herniated disc material causing spinal cord compression.

or ventrolateral to the dural tube, thus causing displacement of the dural tube and contained spinal cord dorsally toward the laminar bone. It is conceivable that some measure of pressure relief is achieved in some cases when this overlying bone is removed. However, it is important to remember that the dural tube and spinal cord are not free-floating within the vertebral canal. These structures are anchored in their position by the nerve roots that emerge and exit the foramina on either side. Hence, when a mass of material is located in the vertebral canal adjacent to the dural tube, there is a limited ability of the dural tube/ spinal cord to shift away from the mass, whether overlying bone is present or not. Moreover, the dural tube and spinal cord are not rigid struc-

tures. So when there is an impinging mass, it tends to create a focal zone of deformation within the dura/spinal cord in addition to any generalized shift of the entire circumference of the dural tube. This is readily evident when hemilaminectomies are done and the position of the dural tube and underlying mass can be visualized *in situ*. Though the bone has been removed, and some disc material has possibly been evacuated from just subjacent to that bone removal, it is not until the vast majority of disc material has been carefully removed from around the dural tube and nerve roots that one begins to see the dural tube return to its more normal position, and without an obvious area of displacement from its usual linear orientation.

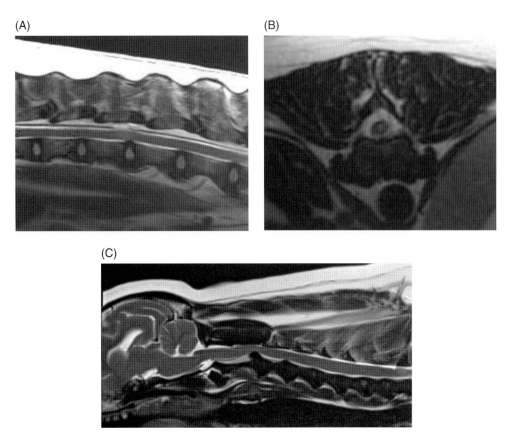

(A)

(B)

(C)

Figure 28.2 (A) Sagittal and (B) transverse MR images of the spine of a dog that presented with acute paraplegia. There is extradural material in the vertebral canal consistent with hemorrhage from where the T13–L1 intervertebral disc extruded, but note that there is no residual nucleus pulposus material seen in the canal and that the spinal cord itself is not compressed. This is consistent with ANNPE (acute noncompressive nucleus pulposus extrusion) and would not likely be benefited by surgery since the spinal cord injury in this case is predominantly due to contusion. (C) Sagittal MR image of the cervical spine of a dog presented for severe and unremitting neck pain. Note the marked focal spinal cord compression at C2–C3 from an extruded intervertebral disc. This dog would more clearly benefit from spinal cord and nerve root decompressive surgery, irrespective of signs being limited to discomfort (i.e., no neurological deficits). This dog likely has very minimal contusive spinal cord injury, but has severe spinal cord compression.

The key point here is that decompression is predicated on *mass* removal and not just *bone* removal. Any of the techniques commonly used for disc surgery (dorsal laminectomy, hemilaminectomy, pediculectomy, facetectomy, foraminotomy, partial corpectomy, ventral slot, etc.) should only be thought of as ways to access the offending mass of disc and not of any intrinsic value from merely removing bone. The choice of procedure is therefore based on the location of the compressive mass, and the surgeon's judgment as to the best way to access that mass with the least morbidity for the patient. Part of that judgment is recognition that spinal cord manipulation is potentially

harmful (particularly in a spinal cord that may already be compromised by decreased perfusion and other alterations as outlined elsewhere in this text), and therefore trying to choose a surgical approach that allows access to extruded disc with the least need for any contact with or manipulation of the dural tube.

Another related misconception centers on the presence of spinal cord swelling when there has been disc-induced concussion with or without compression. There seems to be an inherent image in the mind of many veterinarians that this swelling, occurring as it does within the closed confines of the bony vertebral canal, can be at least partially relieved by creating an opening in the surrounding bone, akin to removing an overly tight pair of shoes and feeling relief. Unfortunately, there is no evidence that this analogy is appropriate. In this way, the spinal cord behaves differently from the brain, where swelling and increased intracranial pressure may be relieved via varying degrees of bone and dura mater removal (the latter being more intimately associated with the calvarial bone than is the dura mater in the spine). The spinal cord is contained within the lepto- and pachymeninges. These, especially the latter (the dura mater), are relatively noncompliant membranes that only stretch to a very limited degree when the spinal cord within swells centripetally. So, while one may posit that durotomy or even piotomy might result in some degree of mechanical decompression of the spinal cord (and the role/value of these procedures is addressed in Chapter 33), it is evident that even the most extensive laminectomy and facetectomy will serve no useful role in relieving this internal pressure within the dural tube and spinal cord itself, and veterinarians should be cautious in ever assuming otherwise.

29 General Principles of Spinal Surgery for Intervertebral Disc Herniation

James M. Fingeroth and Brigitte A. Brisson

Goals

As outlined in Chapters 15 and 28, the fundamental purpose of therapeutic surgery is alleviation of compression and mechanical distortion of the spinal cord and nerve roots. Spinal cord compression results in varying degrees of neurologic deficits at and distal to the site of the lesion, while nerve root compression (especially dorsal root and ganglion compression) is felt to underlie much of the discomfort associated with intervertebral disc herniation (IVDH). To achieve these goals, the surgeon should have adequate clinical and imaging data that demonstrate the vertebral level of the lesion and whether there is lateralization to one side or the other. Armed with these data, the surgeon can select what he or she feels is the best bone removal approach that will provide sufficient access for removal of the extruded disc, with minimal iatrogenic trauma to the spinal cord.

A good rule of thumb when doing spinal disc surgery is to *try to avoid any direct contact with or manipulation of the dural tube and contained spinal cord*. While not always achievable in clinical practice, this guiding philosophy should always be forefront in the mind of the spinal surgeon, and every effort should be made to minimize such contact/manipulation if it cannot be avoided outright. The normal spinal cord is sensitive to contact/manipulation and can become injured (with corresponding neurologic deficits) as a consequence [1, 2]. This sensitivity/ vulnerability is only accentuated in an already compromised spinal cord that has sustained the effects of concussion and compression from a herniated disc.

Procedures

The reader is referred to other surgical texts and atlases for more detailed descriptions of the various techniques used to access the vertebral canal for removal of herniated disc material.

It is of course imperative that the proper spinal location be approached. In ventral approaches to the cervical spine, common landmarks for counting intervertebral disc spaces include palpation of the

Advances in Intervertebral Disc Disease in Dogs and Cats, First Edition. Edited by James M. Fingeroth and William B. Thomas.
© 2015 ACVS Foundation. Published 2015 by John Wiley & Sons, Inc.

(A)

(B)

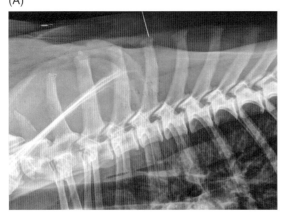
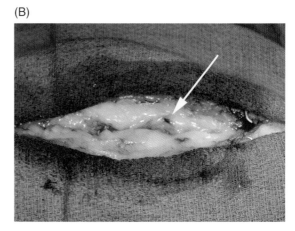

Figure 29.1 (A) Lateral radiograph depicting a hypodermic placed percutaneously into a dorsal spinous process (in this example, at T4). The needle is placed approximately at the location where the approach to the vertebral canal is planned, based on palpation, and then the needle hub aseptically cut off. The radiograph then serves to identify the precise location of the needle, which can then be used during the surgical dissection to assure that the proper site for laminectomy is being approached. As long as the needle is placed within the dimensions of the surgical incision, it need not be placed exactly at the intended level. Care should be taken to secure the needle's tip securely into the bone and to avoid dislodging it during the balance of patient preparation and transport to the operating room or during draping and dissection. (B) As an alternative or adjunct to leaving the hypodermic needle *in situ* after confirming its location radiographically, a small aliquot of sterile methylene blue, USP, can be injected into the dorsal spinous process, and the needle removed if desired. During dissection, the dye can be observed as shown here and used to determine the correct location for the laminectomy. The advantage of leaving the needle in place is that it provides both tactile and visual cues during draping, incision, and dissection. The disadvantage is that the needle can become dislodged, and though usually found in close proximity to the radiographed spinous process, some uncertainty is introduced. The use of dye mitigates this problem. *Source*: Photos courtesy of Dr. William Thomas.

midline ridge on the ventral arch of the atlas and the larger transverse processes of the C6 vertebrae. For dorsal approaches to the cervical vertebrae, the distinct spinous process of the axis (C2) and the much taller spinous process of T1 (compared with C7 or spinous processes more cranially) are reliable landmarks. In the thoracolumbar spine, palpation of the ribs and transverse processes can be used, but this can require larger incisions and may be difficult in obese patients. An alternative is to radiographically identify vertebrae using a hypodermic needle. The needle (20–25 gauge, depending on patient size) is usually placed aseptically into a dorsal spinous process close to the anticipated surgical site after the initial clip and prep for surgery and then radiographed with the patient in lateral recumbency to identify the precise vertebra in which the needle is located. Either the needle can be drilled securely into the spinous process, the needle hub can be aseptically cut off with the balance of the needle left below the skin (to be found by palpation in the operating room and then guiding the incision), or else a small aliquot of dye (e.g., methylene blue) can be injected into the dorsal aspect of the spinous process and identified visually after incising the skin (Figure 29.1). The needle or dye need not be at the precise proper level of the disc herniation; once one knows the location of the needle or dye, the vertebrae can be counted cranial or caudal as needed to identify the proper location for dissection. When MRI has been used for diagnostic imaging, these radiographs also serve to verify the vertebral and costal formula for the particular patient, as some dogs may have more or fewer lumbar vertebrae or ribs than standard. Although this can be assessed using various MRI sequences (the dorsal view is often best for this), some surgeons prefer radiographic images for this purpose.

Instrumentation

Because of the small size of many of our patients and the need for precise and delicate manipulations within the vertebral canal, it is generally helpful to have both excellent *lighting* and some degree of *magnification*. The former can be achieved with the use of appropriate overhead lighting fixtures, possibly augmented by the use of fiber-optic light sources on a head-mounted device that can be focused directly in the surgeon's field of view. Magnification is usually achieved with loupes; the power of magnification is at the discretion of the surgeon when purchasing loupes. 2.5X is usually sufficient without creating too small a field of view.

Hemostasis is best achieved through the use of *bipolar electrocautery*, with the bayonet size chosen based on patient size. Bipolar cautery reduces electrical current transmission near or through the neural tissues and also can remain effective under a small amount of fluid such as blood. Tamponade is also important for hemostasis and maintaining a clear operative field. *Paper-based "gauze" squares* (3×3 or 4×4) are effective, especially if opened up and moistened and the corners are used. Cotton gauze may be too likely to shed small fibers and may also be more abrasive if applied to the soft tissues. There are also *"cottonoid" neurosurgical patties* of various dimensions and sizes produced that can be used for blotting and tamponade. For more troublesome bleeding where the source cannot be readily grasped or cauterized, hemostasis can be aided by the use of *clot-provoking adjuncts* underneath any sponge or cottonoid patty. Such adjuncts include small pieces of muscle or fat harvested from the surgical field or synthetic substrates such as cellulose sponge material (e.g., Gelfoam, Surgifoam). Critical to hemostasis and visualization is active wound suction. Adson or Frazier tips of various diameters should be available (along with stylets for clearing any obstructions), with a gradual progression from larger to smaller diameters as one works closer to the neural structures. By placing the moistened tip of a sponge or cottonoid patty (possibly with underlying adjunct) and then holding the suction tip directly against the sponge, one can achieve both tamponade (the tip applies pressure) and faster clotting, as the offending source is drawn to the sponge. When attempting to control venous sinus hemorrhage, gentle tamponade with Gelfoam/Surgifoam or a cottonoid tip applied to the laminectomy site and combined with flooding the surgical field with saline can also promote hemostasis by creating a slightly higher pressure environment compared with the low pressure venous system.

Sterile, warmed *saline lavage solution* should be available in a bowl or cup and a *bulb syringe* used to flush away debris, cool the bone during high-speed burring, and maintain moist tissues.

Besides standard operating instruments, a selection of *self-retaining retractors* is helpful for exposing the vertebral column. *Periosteal elevators* are used to elevate the epaxial muscles from the bone (thoracolumbar spine) or the longus colli muscles ventrally (cervical spine). Bone removal for hemilaminectomy or dorsal laminectomy can be done entirely with manually operated *rongeurs*, and it can be useful to have familiarity with this in case power tools are unexpectedly unavailable. However, it is more common to perform these procedures (and ventral slots) with *high-speed power drills* (usually compressed air driven but in some cases battery driven) and a series of *burs* in various shapes and sizes, combined with rongeurs and *curettes*. The goal is to define and accurately create the desired bony window (usually by progressing from larger to smaller instruments) without exposing the neural structures or vessels within the intervertebral foramen or vertebral canal to either excess thermal energy or direct contact with instruments. Where possible, the surgeon should operate all these instruments with two hands, with the hands suitably stabilized to prevent any uncontrolled movement. For dorsal approaches, the ideal is to create the window down to but not through the endosteum that lines the inner cortex of the lamina and pedicle and then to incise and remove this final layer with the aid of a #11 scalpel, curettes, and small rongeurs. The thinned inner cortical bone and endosteum can be elevated with a bent 22 gauge hypodermic needle used as a hook to facilitate incising with the scalpel. Some surgeons prefer to drill while the field is simultaneously irrigated (to dissipate heat), while others prefer to alternate drilling and lavaging in sequential steps so that visualization during drilling is not impeded by working under water. Bone dust created during high-speed drilling should be lavaged and aspirated.

Manipulation of the disc material within the vertebral canal is usually accomplished with a variety of small instruments, with the goal again being able to grasp or sweep disc material toward the surgeon without impacting the dural tube. Each surgeon tends to identify particular instruments he or she feels works best in achieving these aims.

Decompression

As outlined in Chapter 28, true decompression is only achieved when the neural structures are no longer distorted by extruded disc material. So the goal with every surgery is evacuation of all extruded disc material until such point as the dural tube and nerve roots are completely restored to their normal dimensions and position. In some cases, this might require working directly adjacent to these structures with a degree of aggression (as in the case of chronic, hard disc material that adheres to the dura), while in others being willing to accept leaving some extruded disc material behind if adequate decompression has been achieved, and further removal might unnecessarily subject the spinal cord to further iatrogenic trauma. Since signs of discomfort are largely attributable to radiculopathy, it is important for the surgeon to ensure that the nerve roots are decompressed along with the dural tube itself. In the case of ventral slots in the cervical region, this might require gentle probing of the foramina, while in the thoracolumbar spine this might entail foraminotomy. In either location, it should be remembered that the nerve roots are accompanied by radicular vessels and also that the vertebral venous sinuses deviate abaxially over each intervertebral disc. Hence, exploration and decompression of nerve roots is accompanied by some increased risk for iatrogenic vascular injury and brisk hemorrhage. Magnification and precise placement of instruments lessens the risk for untoward hemorrhage or nerve root injury.

Fenestration

Details regarding the efficacy of prophylactic fenestration are covered in Chapters 18 and 35. Regardless of any decision by the surgeon to pursue elective fenestration at sites cranial and caudal to the level of decompression, it is highly recommended by the authors that the intervertebral disc *at* the level of decompression be fenestrated. For ventral slots, this is automatically accomplished during the drilling procedure. For thoracolumbar discs, this is usually done as the final step after decompression is complete and prior to closure. For thoracolumbar surgery, the disc space can be approached dorsolaterally or laterally, and fenestration done manually or with power [3–6]. The goal is to remove all remaining nucleus pulposus that has the potential to herniate dorsally through the ruptured annulus following decompressive surgery, which could cause further spinal cord injury/compression. It is also helpful to remove any bulging or torn annulus fibrosus that might be causing distortion of the dural tube. As one performs thoracolumbar fenestration, one needs to be cognizant of the location of the nerve roots with their radicular vessels, the vertebral venous sinus, and the great vessels (aorta and caudal vena cava) ventral to the vertebral column.

Closure

Chapter 34 discusses the various schemes used for covering laminectomy and ventral slot defects. For laminectomies, the epaxial muscles are usually not sutured themselves, but the overlying thoracolumbar fascia is securely sutured (muscle fascia may be closed separately prior to thoracolumbar fascia). This is followed by the fat layer, subcutaneous layer, and skin. An adhesive/occlusive bandage may be applied at the surgeon's discretion for the initial 12–48 h. For ventral slots, the longus colli muscles and fascia are apposed, followed by the strap muscles, subcutaneous tissue and platysma muscle, and skin.

References

1. Forterre F, Gorgas D, Dickomeit M, Jaggy A, Lang J, Spreng D. Incidence of spinal compressive lesions in chondrodystrophic dogs with abnormal recovery after hemilaminectomy for treatment of thoracolumbar disc disease: a prospective magnetic resonance imaging study. Vet Surg. 2010 Feb;39(2):165–72.
2. Waters DJ. Spinal surgery. In: Lipowitz AJ, Caywood DD, Newton CD, Schwartz A, editors. Complications in Small Animal Surgery. Baltimore: Williams & Wilkins; 1996. p. 541–62.
3. Flo GL, Brinker WO. Lateral fenestration of thoracolumbar discs. J Am Anim Hosp Assoc. 1975;11:619–26.
4. Forterre F, Dickomeit M, Senn D, Gorgas D, Spreng D. Microfenestration using the CUSA excel ultrasonic aspiration system in chondrodystrophic dogs with thoracolumbar disk extrusion: a descriptive cadaveric and clinical study. Vet Surg. 2011;40(1):34–9.

5. Holmberg D, Palmer N, VanPelt D, Willan A. A comparison of manual and power-assisted thoracolumbar disc fenestration in dogs. Vet Surg. 1990;19(5):323–7.

6. Morelius M, Bergadano A, Spreng D, Schawalder P, Doherr M, Forterre F. Influence of surgical approach on the efficacy of the intervertebral disk fenestration: a cadaveric study. J Small Anim Pract. 2007;48(2):87–92.

30 Cervical Disc Disease: Ventral Slot versus Hemilaminectomy versus Dorsal Laminectomy

Amy E. Fauber

Introduction

Once a patient with a cervical intervertebral disc herniation has been deemed a surgical candidate, the surgeon is faced with several options on how to operate. A general rule of thumb is to establish a goal of mass (disc) removal, as this is ultimately the decompressive element of surgery. A challenging decision comes when the herniated disc material is lateralized and residual material may remain in the intervertebral foramen without a carefully planned and executed approach. In these instances, it is not always clear which approach will best allow for spinal cord and nerve root decompression. Also challenging is the current lack of biomechanical studies comparing the instability created by these different approaches or the clinical significance of any such instability.

Ventral approach and ventral slot

The ventral slot is one of the most widely used approaches for spinal cord decompression in veterinary patients with cervical intervertebral disc herniation. Using this procedure, it is very easy to access displaced disc material located within the ventral aspect of the vertebral canal (see Figure 30.1). This procedure was first described in dogs as an alternative to the dorsal approach for laminectomy or hemilaminectomy [1]. Either a ventral midline dissection or a paramedian dissection to the ventral cervical spine can be used. For the midline approach, a ventral midline incision is made and the approach is continued on the midline between the paired sternothyroideus and sternohyoideus muscles. The trachea, carotid sheath, and esophagus are retracted to the left to expose the paired longus colli muscles immediately ventral to the vertebrae [2]. For the paramedian approach, a ventral midline skin incision is made, but the dissection is continued paramedian, between the right sternocephalicus muscle and right sternothyroideus muscle [3]. The sternohyoideus and sternothyroideus muscles, trachea, esophagus, and carotid sheath are all retracted to the left. The paramedian approach may make it less likely to disrupt tracheal blood supply, the right carotid sheath, and the recurrent laryngeal nerve [3]. With either of these ventral approaches, the correct site for the

Advances in Intervertebral Disc Disease in Dogs and Cats, First Edition. Edited by James M. Fingeroth and William B. Thomas.
© 2015 ACVS Foundation. Published 2015 by John Wiley & Sons, Inc.

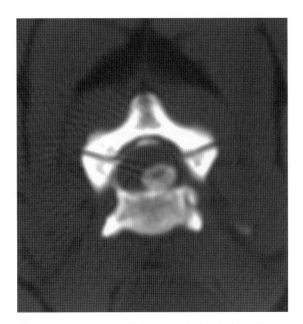

Figure 30.1   Transverse CT image at the level of C4–C5 demonstrating a ventral disc extrusion.

ventral slot is identified by palpating the large transverse processes of C6 and the ventral midline process of C1 and then, using these landmarks, palpating the caudal ventral processes of the cervical vertebrae that mark each interspace between C2–C3 and C7–T1. It is important to review preoperative imaging to identify any anatomical variations in vertebral formula or transitional vertebrae. The longus colli muscle is divided along the midline to expose the ventral aspects of the vertebral bodies and intervertebral disc. A high-speed burr is used to create an opening ("slot") in the vertebral bodies, centered over the disc space and extending to the dorsal longitudinal ligament. Due to the angulation of the intervertebral disc and end plates, the slot should be centered initially over the caudal aspect of the cranial vertebra rather than over the ventral annulus, with the caudal extent of the slot at the cranial end plate of the caudal vertebra. As the burring is continued dorsally, the slot will end up being centered on the dorsal aspect of the intervertebral disc. This will help avoid disruption of the paired vertebral venous plexus, which deviates laterally over each disc space, and thus reduce the risk for hemorrhage, which can be quite severe and interfere with completion of the disc removal and decompression. After penetrating the dorsal cortex of the vertebral

body, the dorsal longitudinal ligament is separated or excised, and the herniated disc material is removed from the vertebral canal using instruments such as a right-angle nerve root retractor passed gently along the ventral aspect of the vertebral canal.

Complications of the ventral slot include hemorrhage from the vertebral venous plexus, instability of the vertebral bodies, erosion of the dorsal tracheal membrane from sutures in the longus colli, and poor decompression due to the limited visibility through the slot created [1, 4–7]. The reason the ventral approach is confined to a slot, and not a larger window that would permit more visualization and room for manipulation of instruments, is because of the potential for vertebral collapse and fracture from an overly aggressive degree of bone removal from the vertebral bodies. This is less a problem in human anterior approaches owing to the short but wide morphology of cervical vertebrae in that species, compared with the long but narrow cervical vertebrae in dogs. The small size of the resultant windows created in dogs, along with the small overall size of many veterinary patients, means that there is very little working room for either visualization or manipulation of instruments in our patients. So while the ventral approach provides the most direct route to ventrally herniated disc material, and without the degree of dissection required for dorsal approaches, it comes with the trade-off of very limited working space. The use of magnification and good lighting can mitigate some of these inherent limitations, but this remains one of the limiting aspects to this approach in dogs.

Dorsal approach and dorsal laminectomy

A dorsal approach to the cervical spine has been described and used for decompression of ventral disc displacements if there is a combined ventral disc displacement and dorsal compression (see Figure 30.2). For this approach, a dorsal midline incision is made from the spinous process of C2 extending caudally to the spinous process of T1 [8]. The median raphes of the cleidocervicalis and trapezius muscles are sharply incised, and the paired biventer cervicis muscles are divided to expose the nuchal ligament. The nuchal ligament is retracted laterally to allow continuation of the approach

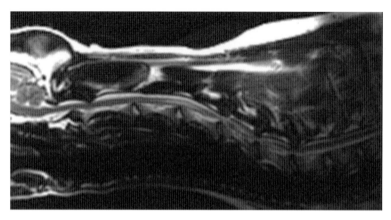

Figure 30.2   Midsagittal T2-weighted MRI image of the cervical spine demonstrating ventral spinal cord compression from disc protrusion at C4–C5 and C5–C6 and also dorsal spinal cord compression from misshapen dorsal laminae from C4–C7.

ventrally. The rectus capitis, spinalis et semispinalis cervicis and multifidus muscles are then divided and elevated from the spinous processes and laminae of the targeted cervical vertebrae. The lamina and potentially portions of the spinous processes are then removed after identification of the interarcuate ligament. The laminae can be safely removed to the level of the medial extent of the articular processes. The ligamentum flavum is removed to expose the epidural fat and spinal cord. Ventral disc extrusions will not be visualized because the spinal cord obscures them and they are inaccessible without manipulation/retraction of the spinal cord. However, good outcomes have been reported in small dogs despite not removing the extruded disc material, possibly as a result of restoration of normal blood flow to the spinal cord [9]. Nonetheless, use of dorsal laminectomy for ventral midline lesions violates the principle of decompression that only truly results from mass removal, and must be undertaken with this potential limitation in mind. The dural tube is anchored within the vertebral canal by the nerve roots, and while some decompression may be achieved by alleviating contact between the displaced dorsum of the dural tube and the lamina, there may still be a considerable amount of spinal cord deformation and compression ventrally that is not at all relieved by simple laminectomy. Disc retrieval and decompression via a dorsal approach are more likely when the disc extrudes ventrolaterally and can be accessed by passing instruments in the spaces laterally between the dural tube and the

pedicles. Very gentle and minimal retraction of the dural tube to one side can facilitate this maneuver.

Complications of this approach include hemorrhage from the sharp separation of the dorsal musculature, limited exposure to the ventral aspect of the vertebral canal and the intervertebral foramen, excessive manipulation of the spinal cord causing worsened neurologic deficits, seroma formation, and postoperative pain associated with the extensive soft tissue dissection [9, 10].

Dorsal approach and hemilaminectomy

To access more lateralized disc extrusions, a dorsal approach with a hemilaminectomy has been described and has reportedly been used with good to excellent outcomes in small-breed dogs [11]. The same approach as described for the dorsal laminectomy is performed; however, the dissection is continued slightly more laterally to allow exposure to the articular processes. To gain this exposure, the multifidus cervicis and complexus muscles are sharply transected from the articular processes to allow removal of the facet and lamina.

Complications of this approach include difficult visualization of the ventral aspect of the vertebral canal, hemorrhage from the sharp separation of the dorsal musculature and/or disruption of the vessels in the transverse foramina, nerve root damage, worsening of neurologic deficits, seroma formation, and postoperative pain associated with the extensive soft tissue dissection [4, 11–13].

Lateral approach and hemilaminectomy

To allow for better visualization of the ventral aspect of the vertebral canal as well as the foramen, a lateral approach has been described [14]. This approach was later modified to decrease postoperative discomfort associated with the incision into or transection of the cervical epaxial or extrinsic thoracic limb musculature [15]. In this modified approach, the brachiocephalicus and trapezius muscles are separated to expose the splenius and serratus ventralis muscles for caudal cervical lesions. For cranial cervical lesions the underlying muscles are exposed by bluntly dividing the brachiocephalicus muscle in a direction parallel to its fibers. The serratus ventralis muscle is bluntly dissected to allow exposure to the longissimus muscles. The transverse processes are palpated to determine the correct intervertebral foramen. The articular facet is exposed by creating a plane between the longissimus capitis and complexus muscles and then sharply transecting the longissimus capitis from the transverse processes. Once the muscles are retracted a hemilaminectomy can be performed.

Complications of this procedure include hemorrhage, seroma formation, and difficulty localizing the correct surgical site. Also, access is limited caudally to the level of C6–C7 without more extensive tissue dissection or forequarter amputation [15, 16].

Modified dorsal approach and hemilaminectomy

A modified dorsal approach to the cervical spine has been recently described [17]. A dorsal midline incision is made from C2 to T1. The median dorsal raphe of the splenius, trapezius, and rhomboideus is then sharply incised. Then rather than continue the approach on midline, the fascial plane lateral to the biventer cervicis muscle is bluntly dissected. This allows for palpation of the articular process and the spinous processes to determine the correct location for hemilaminectomy. The multifidus cervicis and complexus muscles are then elevated from the laminae and transected from the articular processes. The hemilaminectomy can then be performed. This approach has been used from C3–C4 to C7–T1. This modification has been suggested to decrease the amount of soft tissue dissection of the dorsal musculature, allow for better exposure of the ventral aspect of the vertebral canal when compared to the standard dorsal approach, and allow for more access to the most caudal cervical spine level (C7–T1) as compared to the other lateral approaches.

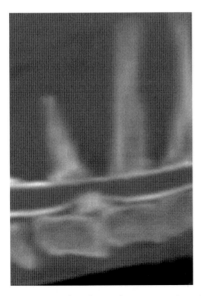 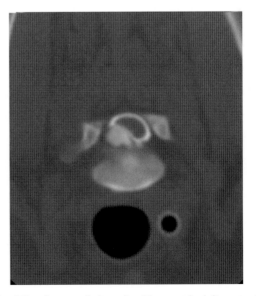

Figure 30.3   Transverse and midsagittal reconstruction of a CT/myelogram of a lateralized intervertebral disc extrusion at C7–T1.

Complications of the modified dorsal approach include hemorrhage and incorrect lesion localization. In the author's experience, it is important, when performing this approach to gain familiarity with the muscles and fascial planes and also differentiate between the palpation of the articular processes and the transverse processes.

Selection of surgical procedure

When evaluating imaging of a patient with intervertebral disc herniation, consideration for an approach that minimizes the need for manipulation of the spinal cord is strongly recommended. For disc extrusions into the ventral aspect of the vertebral canal (see Figure 30.1), a ventral slot procedure provides for the most direct access to the extruded disc material, with the limitations and caveats described earlier. For patients with ventral compression combined with dorsal compression (see Figure 30.2), a dorsal laminectomy should be considered. However, if lateral extrusion is present (see Figures 30.3 and 30.4), then a ventral slot or standard dorsal laminectomy will not allow for access to the intervertebral foramen

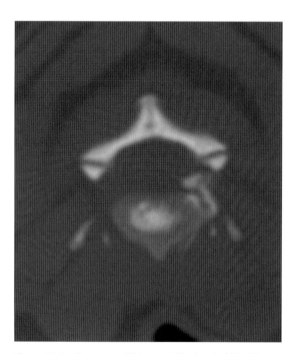

Figure 30.4 Transverse CT image at the level of C3–C4 demonstrating a lateralized foraminal disc extrusion.

or ventrolateral region of the vertebral canal. In these patients, a hemilaminectomy would be ideal, and the surgeon should consider performing a dorsal approach, modified dorsal approach, or modified lateral approach to complete the hemilaminectomy. In the author's experience, the modified dorsal approach is easy to perform for caudally located lesions, between C3–C4 and C7–T1, and the dorsal or lateral approach may be easier for more cranial lesions. Ultimately, the surgeon's familiarity with the anatomy and experience performing the surgery may be the best way of determining the most appropriate approach.

References

1. Swaim SF. Ventral decompression of the cervical spinal cord in the dog. J Am Vet Med Assoc. 1973 Feb 15;162(4):276–7.
2. Olsson SE. On disk protrusion in the dog (endochondrosis intervertebralis). Acta Orthop Scand. 1951;Suppl VIII:51–70.
3. Cechner P. Ventral cervical disc fenestration in the dog: a modified technique. J Am Anim Hosp Assoc. 1980;16:647–50.
4. Gilpin GN. Evaluation of three techniques of ventral decompression of the cervical spinal cord in the dog. J Am Vet Med Assoc. 1976 Feb 15;168(4):325–8.
5. Seim HB, III, Prata RG. Ventral decompression for the treatment of cervical disk disease in the dog: a review of 54 cases. J Am Anim Hosp Assoc. 1982;18:233–40.
6. Lemarie RJ, Kerwin SC, Partington BP, Hosgood G. Vertebral subluxation following ventral cervical decompression in the dog. J Am Anim Hosp Assoc. 2000 Jul–Aug;36(4):348–58.
7. Clements D, McGill S, Beths T, Sullivan M. Tracheal perforation secondary to suture irritation in a dog following a ventral slot procedure. J Small Anim Pract. 2003;44(7):313–5.
8. Funkquist B. Decompressive laminectomy for cervical disk protrusion in the dog. Acta Vet Scand. 1962;3:88–101.
9. Gill PJ, Lippincott CL, Anderson SM. Dorsal laminectomy in the treatment of cervical intervertebral disk disease in small dogs: a retrospective study of 30 cases. J Am Anim Hosp Assoc. 1996 Jan–Feb; 32(1):77–80.
10. Hoerlein B. The status of the various intervertebral disc surgeries for the dog in 1978. J Am Anim Hosp Assoc. 1978;14:563–70.
11. Tanaka H, Nakayama M, Takase K. Usefulness of hemilaminectomy for cervical intervertebral disk disease in small dogs. J Vet Med Sci. 2005;67(7):679.

12. Petit GD, Whitaker RP. Hemimlaminectomy for cervical disc protrusion in a dog. J Am Vet Med Assoc. 1963;143:379–383.

13. Felts JF, Prata RG. Cervical disk disease in the dog: intraforaminal and lateral extrusions. J Am Anim Hosp Assoc. 1983;19:755–60.

14. Lipsitz D, Bailey CS. Lateral Approach for cervical spinal cord decompression. Prog Vet Neurol. 1992;13:39–44.

15. Rossmeisl JH, Jr., Lanz OI, Inzana KD, Bergman RL. A modified lateral approach to the canine cervical spine: procedural description and clinical application in 16 dogs with lateralized compressive myelopathy or radiculopathy. Vet Surg. 2005 Sep–Oct;34(5):436–44.

16. Schmied O, Golini L, Steffen F. Effectiveness of cervical hemilaminectomy in canine hansen Type I and Type II disc disease: a retrospective study. J Am Anim Hosp Assoc. 2011;47(5):342–50.

17. Fauber AE, Bergman RL, editors. Modified dorsal approach to the lateral cervical spine. American College of Veterinary Surgeons Symposium; 2008; San Diego, CA.

Thoracolumbar Disc Disease: Dorsal Approaches versus Lateral versus Ventral Approaches. What to Do If I'm on the Wrong Side or Site (Level)?

31

Franck Forterre, Núria Vizcaíno Revés, and Luisa De Risio

Removal of the compressive disc material is the main objective of surgical treatment of thoracolumbar disc herniation [1]. Accurate clinical and imaging investigation, good preoperative planning, and surgical expertise minimize the chances of approaching the incorrect side or site and being unable to completely remove the herniated disc material.

Wrong site/level

There are several reasons the incorrect surgical site (i.e., intervertebral disc space cranial or caudal to the affected one) may be erroneously approached:

- Patients with vertebral and/or rib anomalies, such as transitional vertebrae, vestigial transverse process articulating with a rib, or abnormal number of ribs
- Lack of surgical expertise or mere surgeon's error
- Obese dogs whose standard anatomical landmarks (last rib, first transverse process, L6) might be difficult to palpate with certitude

- Limited information of affected site from preoperative diagnostic imaging, most commonly because of loss of myelographic contrast column over two or more adjacent intervertebral disc spaces

Approaching the incorrect site may be prevented by accurate imaging, by exposing and visualizing the anatomical landmarks intraoperatively (e.g., last rib, first transverse process, lumbosacral junction), by preoperative marking (e.g., needle, or methylene blue) of the target vertebra, or by using intraoperative fluoroscopy or radiography (e.g., for intervertebral disc herniations located two or more vertebral segments from the anatomical landmarks mentioned earlier). To mark the correct site, a hypodermic or spinal needle is placed percutaneously next to the appropriate spinous process with radiographic, fluoroscopic, or computed tomography (CT) confirmation. A small volume (0.1 ml) of sterile methylene blue is injected in the subcuteanous tissue overlying the spinous process and the needle withdrawn. Alternatively, the needle is securely placed into

Advances in Intervertebral Disc Disease in Dogs and Cats, First Edition. Edited by James M. Fingeroth and William B. Thomas.
© 2015 ACVS Foundation. Published 2015 by John Wiley & Sons, Inc.

the dorsal spinous process and then cut (preferably using a sterilized instrument) so that it no longer protrudes through the skin. This allows the skin to be aseptically prepared, and the surgeon identifies the needle after the skin is incised (see Figure 29.1).

If the incorrect site has been approached, extending the bone removal to the cranial (or caudal) intervertebral disc space generally permits removal of the herniated disc and adequate decompression of the spinal cord. A hemilaminectomy can be extended cranially or caudally without major concerns about spinal stability in the thoracolumbar region. Continuous hemilaminectomy of up to three adjacent vertebrae in the lumbar spine does not significantly decrease spine stiffness during flexion and extension [2]. Multiple continuous hemilaminectomies (up to six consecutive intervertebral disc spaces) in the thoracolumbar spine did not result in secondary postsurgical complications such as subluxations or chronic back pain [3]. Dorsal laminectomy could also be extended over two vertebral bodies without complications [4, 5]. At the cranial or midthoracic level, care should be taken to preserve the stabilizing supraspinous ligament [6]. However, when enlargment of a dorsal laminectomy over more than two vertebrae is performed, potential spinal instability should be taken into consideration since it has been biomechanically demonstrated that standard dorsal laminectomy already results in a marked increase in range of motion in flexion/extension [7].

Wrong side

The diagnostic and surgical errors that can sometimes lead to approaching the wrong side include:

- Incorrect labeling of the images
- Difficulty in performing or interpreting myelography
- Surgeon error

Incorrect labeling of myelographic images can occur by incorrect manual placement or accidental displacement of the right (or left) marker on the radiographic cassette. Similarly with CT or magnetic resonance imaging (MRI), when the left and right labelings are not modified in accordance with the position of the patient relative to the

standard assumption of the computer (e.g., head vs. tail in first or ventral vs. dorsal recumbency), the wrong side might be implicated. Difficulty in performing or interpreting myelography (e.g., poor contrast medium diffusion in the subarachnoid space, mixing of epidurogram and myelogram) is a well-recognized diagnostic problem. For example, when only ventrodorsal and lateral myelographic images are obtained, a 30–40% failure rate in determining the side of lateralization of the extruded disk might be expected. However, combining ventrodorsal and oblique myelographic views results in a 97–99% accurate localization of the side of intervertebral disc herniation [8–10]. Clinical signs may help in the interpretation of the myelography but are unreliable in indicating the side of the lesion [10, 11].

CT and MRI are far superior to myelography in determining the precise location of herniated disc material. Complete agreement between the MR imaging and surgical findings with regard to site and side of intervertebral disc herniation has been reported in the canine thoracolumbar spine [12]. However, despite the increase in diagnostic accuracy provided by CT and MRI, the surgeon can still accidentally approach the wrong side. This mistake is avoided if the surgeon and staff utilize a checklist before the start of surgery.

Recognition of being on the wrong side when performing hemilaminectomy is usually apparent when the inner cortical bone is removed. Instead of seeing evidence of contusion in the periosteum and then extruded disc material and/or hemorrhage in the vertebral canal, the surgeon encounters the dural tube displaced toward, rather than away from the hemilaminectomy defect. When the surgeon realizes she or he is on the incorrect side intraoperatively, the diagnostic imaging is reviewed thoroughly, including anatomical landmarks (e.g., kidney, spleen), to verify correctness of labeling. Ideally, this should be done preoperatively for each patient. If the surgical approach and bone removal have been performed on the wrong side because of diagnostic imaging error, the surgeon should approach the disc material and remove it without compromising spinal stability. The corrective surgical technique will depend on the initial surgical procedure that was used. The most common surgical techniques can be classified into three types: hemilaminectomy, partial corpectomy, and dorsal laminectomy.

Combination of these techniques might also be possible in some instances and may also help to solve the problem created by the wrong-sided approach.

Hemilaminectomy

Hemilaminectomy provides good access to and visualization of the lateral and ventrolateral aspect of the spinal cord and the nerve roots. Accordingly, hemilaminectomy better facilitates the removal of extruded disc and improves recovery compared to dorsal laminectomy [13]. In one study, dogs undergoing hemilaminectomy had a better neurological status immediately after surgery compared to those undergoing dorsal laminectomy [1]. Hemilaminectomy is an effective technique to decompress the thoracolumbar spinal cord and does not significantly affect spinal stability when performed unilaterally, which may be of advantage when the wrong level has been approached [7]. Generally, the removal of a contralaterally located herniated disc via hemilaminectomy is strongly discouraged because of the potential for excessive manipulation of the spinal cord and postsurgical neurological deterioration. In case of wrong-sided hemilaminectomy, contralateral foraminotomy, mini-hemilaminectomy, or pediculectomy should be considered. The decision is dependent on the location of the herniated disc material, and the stability of the affected segment (the thoracic spine being biomechanically more stable because of the stabilizing function of the ribs, intercapital ligaments, and the small intervertebral disc volume). If hemilaminectomy and fenestration have been performed on the wrong side and a contralateral hemilaminectomy is necessary to remove the extruded disc material, spinal stabilization should be strongly considered, such as using a vertebral body plate or pins/screws and bone cement [14]. Generally, in cases of a wrong-sided approach, less invasive techniques such as foraminotomy and mini-hemilaminectomy should be attempted first since they preserve the diarthrodial joint and cause less destabilization [15, 16]. Pediculectomy is less invasive and destabilizing than mini-hemilaminectomy, preserves both the articular process and the diarthrodial joint, and avoids the foramen and its blood vessels [17]. This procedure, however, results in limited exposure of

the vertebral canal, and might result in incomplete spinal cord decompression. In one study, 50% of the cases needed a conversion from a partial pediculectomy into a mini-hemilaminectomy in order to remove the extruded material [18]. Further, post-surgical instability has been described after performing bilateral mini-hemilaminectomy and pediculectomy because of a wrong-sided approach, possibly because of excessive thinning of the base of the facet joint, leading to fracture [19]. Therefore, careful postoperative evaluation and follow-up is mandatory to detect early clinical signs (pain, neurological worsening) in patients in which a bilateral approach was necessary. In case of clinical deterioration or lack of improvement, repeated imaging should be performed.

Another option for managing a wrong-sided hemilaminectomy is to extend the laminectomy to include the spinous process and dorsal lamina, but taking care to preserve the contralateral articular facet (Fingeroth, personal observation). This provides visualization and access similar to that achieved with the modified dorsal laminectomy described by Trotter [20]. Gentle bilateral manipulation of instruments from the wrong side (where the ventral aspect of the vertebral canal is visualized) and the correct side (where the ventrolateral aspect of the vertebral canal is accessible) can allow movement of herniated disc material into a position where it can be evacuated, and full decompression of the spinal cord and nerve roots achieved. However, there have been no studies of this technique to indicate either its success rate or complication rate.

Partial corpectomy

Partial lateral corpectomy provides access to the floor of the vertebral canal and has been recommended for chronic intervertebral disc protrusions [21, 22]. Since chronic disc protrusions are more frequently located in a midline position than acute extrusions, the wrong-sided approach has not yet been described as a complication of this procedure. However, its main disadvantage is that the surgeon has no or a limited visualization of the spinal cord [21, 22]. The main complication associated with partial lateral corpectomy is insufficient spinal cord decompression. If the exposure to the vertebral canal obtained with a ventral corpectomy needs to be extended and a hemilaminectomy is performed to provide better spinal cord decompression, spinal stabilization should be considered owing to potential weakening of that vertebral segment. A recent *in vitro* study showed significant spinal instability if partial lateral corpectomy was performed in combination with hemilaminectomy [17]. However, if the wrong site (level) has been chosen, a further corpectomy could be performed cranial or caudal to the first site without undue risk of complications, based on one clinical study that described up to three consecutive partial lateral corpectomies in a dog without any complication [22].

Dorsal laminectomy

Dorsal laminectomy provides good visualization of the dorsal but not the ventrolateral aspect of the vertebral canal and therefore is not the best approach for the majority of patients with intervertebral disc extrusion, even when "modified" techniques are used that provide better visualization of the ventrolateral aspects of the vertebral canal [20]. Since ventral and ventrolateral disc extrusions are most common, dorsal laminectomy may also result in incomplete disc removal and decompression and/or excessive manipulation of the spinal cord if complete removal of disc material is attempted [13]. Even with dorsal laminectomy, any remaining extruded disc material will exert some distortion and compression on the ventral aspect of the spinal cord and the nerve roots, which might slow recovery and result in persistent pain and neurological deficits.

Conclusions

With increased diagnostic accuracy provided by advanced imaging techniques (CT, MRI), wrong-sided approaches are expected to decrease in the future as these imaging modalities become more available. The problem that may remain will be wrong-level approaches, which can be easily prevented or solved as described previously. Where myelography is used, adding obliqued views as in the aforementioned should help reduce the incidence of wrong-sided approaches. In instances where the surgeon is still unable to confidently

diagnose the correct side, a limited approach (such as pediculectomy) should be considered so that the correct side can be determined before hemilaminectomy is performed. In case of delayed recovery or deterioration after decompressive surgery, residual or newly developed compression should always be suspected, and prompt diagnostic imaging reexamination is indicated.

References

1. Muir P, Johnson KA, Manley PA, Dueland RT. Comparison of hemilaminectomy and dorsal laminectomy for thoracolumbar intervertebral disc extrusion in dachshunds. J Small Anim Pract. 1995 Aug;36(8):360–7.
2. Corse MR, Renberg WC, Friis EA. In vitro evaluation of biomechanical effects of multiple hemilaminectomies on the canine lumbar vertebral column. Am J Vet Res. 2003 Sep;64(9):1139–45.
3. Tartarelli CL, Baroni M, Borghi M. Thoracolumbar disc extrusion associated with extensive epidural haemorrhage: a retrospective study of 23 dogs. J Small Anim Pract. 2005 Oct;46(10):485–90.
4. Funkquist B. Thoraco-lumbar disk protrusion with severe spinal cord compression in the dog III. Treatment by decompressive laminectomy. Acta Vet Scand. 1962;3:344–66.
5. Prata RG. Neurosurgical treatment of thoracolumbar disks: the rationale and value of laminectomy with concomitant disk removal. J Am Anim Hosp Assoc. 1981;17:17–26.
6. Aikawa T, Kanazono S, Yoshigae Y, Sharp NJ, Munana KR. Vertebral stabilization using positively threaded profile pins and polymethylmethacrylate, with or without laminectomy, for spinal canal stenosis and vertebral instability caused by congenital thoracic vertebral anomalies. Vet Surg. 2007 Jul;36(5):432–41.
7. Smith GK, Walter MC. Spinal decompressive procedures and dorsal compartment injuries: comparative biomechanical study in canine cadavers. Am J Vet Res. 1988 Feb;49(2):266–73.
8. Tanaka H, Nakayama M, Takase K. Usefulness of myelography with multiple views in diagnosis of circumferential location of disc material in dogs with thoracolumbar intervertebral disc herniation. J Vet Med Sci. 2004 Jul;66(7):827–33.
9. Gibbons SE, Macias C, De Stefani A, Pinchbeck GL, McKee WM. The value of oblique versus ventrodorsal myelographic views for lesion lateralisation in canine thoracolumbar disc disease. J Small Anim Pract. 2006 Nov;47(11):658–62.
10. Schulz KS, Walker M, Moon M, Waldron D, Slater M, McDonald DE. Correlation of clinical, radiographic,

and surgical localization of intervertebral disc extrusion in small-breed dogs: a prospective study of 50 cases. Vet Surg. 1998 Mar–Apr;27(2):105–11.

11. Smith JD, Newell SM, Budsberg SC, Bennett RA. Incidence of contralateral versus ipsilateral neurological signs associated with lateralised Hansen type I disc extrusion. J Small Anim Pract. 1997 Nov;38(11):495–7.

12. Naude SH, Lambrechts NE, Wagner WM, Thompson PN. Association of preoperative magnetic resonance imaging findings with surgical features in Dachshunds with thoracolumbar intervertebral disk extrusion. J Am Vet Med Assoc. 2008 Mar 1;232(5):702–8.

13. McKee WM. A comparison of hemilaminectomy (with concomitant disk fenestration) and dorsal laminectomy for the treatment of thoracolumbar disk protrusion in dogs. Vet Rec. 1992;130:296–300.

14. Downes CJ, Gemmill TJ, Gibbons SE, McKee WM. Hemilaminectomy and vertebral stabilisation for the treatment of thoracolumbar disc protrusion in 28 dogs. J Small Anim Pract. 2009 Oct;50(10):525–35.

15. Jeffery ND. Treatment of acute and chronic thoracolumbar disc disease by "mini hemilaminectomy." J Small Anim Pract. 1986;29:611–9.

16. Bitetto WV, Thacher C. A modified lateral decompression technique for treatment of canine intervertebral disk disease. J Am Anim Hosp Assoc. 1986;23:409–13.

17. Hill TP, Lubbe AM, Guthrie AJ. Lumbar spine stability following hemilaminectomy, pediculectomy, and fenestration. Vet Comp Orthop Traumatol. 2000;13:165–71.

18. McCartney W. Comparison of recovery times and complication rates between a modified slanted slot and the standard ventral slot for the treatment of cervical disc disease in 20 dogs. J Small Anim Pract. 2007 Sep;48(9):498–501.

19. Arthurs G. Spinal instability resulting from bilateral mini-hemilaminectomy and pediculectomy. Vet Comp Orthop Traumatol. 2009;22(5):422–6.

20. Trotter EJ, Brasmer TH, deLahunta A. Modified deep dorsal laminectomy in the dog. Cornell Vet. 1975 Jul;65(3):402–27.

21. Moissonnier P, Meheust P, Carozzo C. Thoracolumbar lateral corpectomy for treatment of chronic disk herniation: technique description and use in 15 dogs. Vet Surg. 2004 Nov–Dec;33(6):620–8.

22. Flegel T, Boettcher IC, Ludewig E, Kiefer I, Oechtering G, Bottcher P. Partial lateral corpectomy of the thoracolumbar spine in 51 dogs: assessment of slot morphometry and spinal cord decompression. Vet Surg. 2011 Jan;40(1):14–21.

32 Lumbosacral Disc Disease: Is Vertebral Stabilization Indicated?

Michael Farrell and Noel Fitzpatrick

Introduction

Canine lumbosacral (LS) disease is an umbrella term that refers to any condition causing compression of the cauda equina or its regional blood supply [1]. Although neoplasia, discospondylitis, sacral osteochondrosis, and trauma have been reported as possible causes of canine LS disease, the degenerative form is by far the most common [2]. Degenerative lumbosacral stenosis (DLSS) is a multifactorial disorder characterized by varying combinations of Hansen type II intervertebral disc (IVD) protrusion (or less commonly type I extrusion), hypertrophied soft tissue (ligamentous and synovial structures), articular facet joint osteophytosis, LS spondylosis, and instability [3, 4]. Clinical signs are a consequence of direct compression of the cauda equina, impingement of the spinal nerve roots as they exit their respective foramina, or a combination of both [5–7] (Figure 32.1A, B, and C).

Functional anatomy and clinical signs

The cauda equina lies within the LS canal and is composed of the seventh lumbar (L7), the sacral, and the caudal nerve roots [8]. The LS nerve roots and associated dorsal root ganglia exit through the lateral lumbar vertebral canal, which is divided into the entrance zone (lateral recess), middle zone, and exit zone [9]. Substantial epidural fat is normally present in the LS canal, and this may allow for a certain "anatomical reserve" of compression to occur before neurological deficits are seen [10]. When this reserve becomes exhausted, clinical signs relate either to sciatic neurapraxia (proprioceptive deficits, decreased hock flexion, patellar hyperreflexia, and sometimes flaccidity of the caudal thigh musculature) or to the pelvic, pudendal, or caudal nerves (urinary or fecal incontinence, motor or sensory deficits to the perineum or tail) [11]. It is noteworthy that in the authors' experience, pain only or pain and lameness are

Advances in Intervertebral Disc Disease in Dogs and Cats, First Edition. Edited by James M. Fingeroth and William B. Thomas.
© 2015 ACVS Foundation. Published 2015 by John Wiley & Sons, Inc.

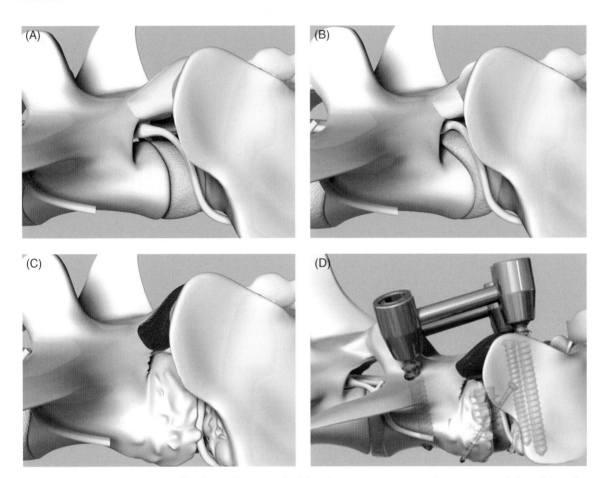

Figure 32.1   Schematic drawings of lumbosacral intervertebral disc degeneration. (A) Normal, (B) central and abaxial (lateral) intervertebral disc protrusion, (C) vertebral end-plate spondylosis and articular facet inflammation compressing the L7 nerve root in addition to disc protrusion, (D) placement of the Fitz Intervertebral Traction Screw (FITS) device through a dorsal laminectomy facilitates distraction of the end plates such that compression on the L7 nerve root(s) is alleviated. Stabilization is then provided using screws in the vertebral bodies of L7 and the sacrum connected by clamps and rods dorsally (Fitzateur). *Source*: Images by Tim Vojt, The Ohio State University. © Tom Vopjt.

often the only signs manifested. Pain may be elicited on physical examination by application of direct pressure over the lumbosacral junction, pressure application to the pathway of the sciatic nerve in the caudal recess of the thigh musculature, extension of the LS joint, or per rectal palpation of the sciatic nerve pathway (Figure 32.2).

Etiology

The etiology of DLSS remains controversial. Although neither the heritability nor the mechanism of inheritance for DLSS has been established to date, the high prevalence in German shepherd dogs (GSD) suggests a hereditary predisposition. The complex multifactorial pathogenesis supports a polygenic etiology with potentially important environmental influences. Previous studies have investigated the influence of anatomical variations peculiar to the GSD on the pathogenesis of DLSS, including a variant anatomy of the LS facet joints and a relatively high incidence of lumbar transitional vertebrae in this breed [12–15]. It has been hypothesized that these differences in vertebral morphology may alter motion of the LS discovertebral segment, resulting in excessive loading of the IVD, which ultimately leads to disc degeneration [13]. It is also possible that the high incidence of DLSS in military working dogs might indicate

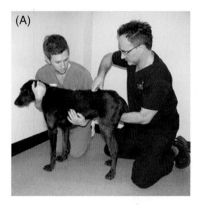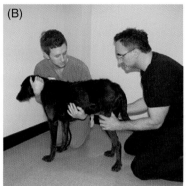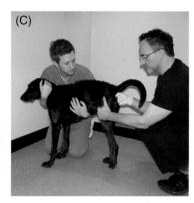

Figure 32.2 Clinical examination for lumbosacral-associated pain. (A) Application of digital pressure to the dorsal aspect of the lumbosacral spine. (B) Application of digital pressure to the pathway of the sciatic nerve in the groove between the semitendinosus/semimembranosus and the biceps femoris on the caudal aspect of the thigh. (C) Application of digital pressure per rectum to the sciatic nerve as it courses over the lesser ischiatic notch on the axial aspect of the pelvis.

that strenuous physical activity influences phenotypic expression of DLSS in genetically susceptible individuals [16].

Pathogenesis

Whether vertebral stabilization constitutes the most appropriate treatment option for DLSS depends in part on whether LS instability is the primary pathophysiological defect. It is thought that age-related degeneration of the nucleus pulposus through a progressive loss of its hydrodynamic properties is the most likely origin of lumbar spinal instability [17, 18]. The pathological consequences of this instability are degeneration of other stabilizing structures, including loss of pretension in the ligamentum flavum and longitudinal ligaments, laxity and inflammation of the facet joint capsule, and subluxation of the facet joint [18]. Other sequelae include thickening of the cartilaginous vertebral end plates and development of periarticular osseous proliferations, such as facet joint osteophytes and spondylosis [19]. This process further impairs the nutritional supply to the IVD, triggering a negative spiral leading to structural failure of the disc [20, 21] (Figures 32.1, 32.3, and 32.4). A pathophysiological hypothesis involving progressive instability is supported by MRI evidence of these compensatory changes in clinically affected dogs [10] and by *ex vivo* biomechanical [15] and *in vivo* kinematic [22] studies demonstrating significantly different

mobility of the LS spinal segment in dogs predisposed to DLSS because of their breed (GSD) or dogs affected by radiographic DLSS when compared with control populations of low-risk [15] or unaffected [22] dogs.

Some dogs affected by DLSS manifest disc-associated compression of the cauda equina or spinal nerve roots only when the LS spinal segment is fully extended [23]. This phenomenon is commonly termed "dynamic" LS IVD compression and is exemplified by the exaggerated pain response in some dogs during the lordosis test (which involves isolated hyperextension of the LS spine) and variable LS IVD protrusion noted during "dynamic" (flexion–extension) myelography or MRI [10, 24, 25] (Figure 32.5). MRI has rapidly become the gold standard diagnostic modality, and the authors have frequently observed lateral IVD protrusion, which can occur in the absence of central disc herniation (possibly similar to low lumbar disc disease seen in humans (see Chapter 3)). This is most common in highly active dogs such as those involved in agility or similar working/sport pursuits and can result in pain or unilateral lameness only. In some cases, the authors have observed that the cranial extent of the dorsal lamina of the sacrum may extend ventral to the caudal extent of the dorsal lamina of L7 and impinge the dorsal aspect of the cauda equina in hyperextension (Figures 32.6 and 32.7). This may be similar as well to the syndrome of spondylolisthesis reported in some human patients with LS disease (see Chapter 3).

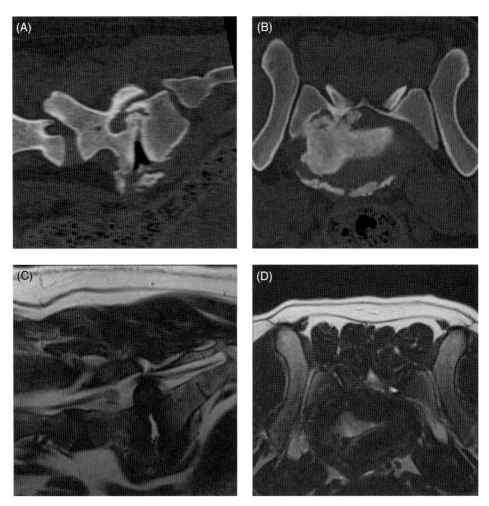

Figure 32.3 CT and MRI scans of the lumbosacral spine of a nine-and-a-half-year-old Rhodesian ridgeback dog. (A and B) CT scans in parasagittal and transverse planes illustrate dramatic spondylotic new bone formation encroaching the L7 neuroforamen on the right (left of picture). (C and D) T2-weighted MRI scans in sagittal and transverse planes illustrate severe intervertebral disc degeneration at the lumbosacral junction and very severe compression of the cauda equina and the abaxial nerve roots by protruding disc material and spondylotic new bone. The right L7 neuroforamen (left of picture) is most significantly compressed.

It is also important to recognize that any pathological LS instability is superimposed on an articulation that is already considered high motion. The healthy canine L7–S1 segment has a greater mobility in flexion and extension than the other lumbar segments [15, 25–27]. Although the most prominent motion direction is flexion and extension, lateral bending and torsion are also possible, and increased ranges of rotational and shear motion have also been reported within the normal LS discovertebral segment in comparison with the other lumbar spinal segments [18].

Treatment options

Surgical and nonsurgical options have been described for the treatment of canine DLSS. Objective measures of indication for treatment and outcome validation are lacking in current literature. Nonsurgical management has been recommended when pain is the only clinical sign [3, 28]. The results of treatment with prolonged rest and analgesic medication have only been documented in a few studies and with very limited numbers of dogs. Results are reported to

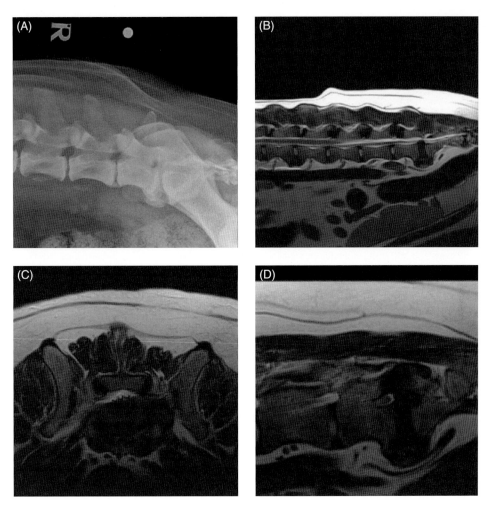

Figure 32.4 Radiographic and T2-weighted MR images of the lumbosacral spine of a 7-year-old German shepherd dog. (A) Radiography in lateral projection demonstrates ventral and abaxial spondylosis. (B) Midsagittal plane MRI demonstrates intervertebral disc degeneration at the lumbosacral junction associated with central protrusion and ventral spondylosis. (C and D) Transverse and parasagittal plane MR images demonstrate marked ventral spondylosis and marked abaxial encroachment of the left L7 neuroforamen (right on image) by protruding disc material and new bone formation. The right-sided neuroforamen is encroached to a lesser extent.

be mediocre and transient, lasting only as long as medication is administered, with signs recurring when normal activities are resumed [6, 29, 30]. Improved outcome in terms of the completeness and longevity of recovery was reported in a series of dogs treated using epidural infiltration of three sequential doses of methylprednisolone administered over 6 weeks [31]. In this series, all affected dogs had lameness, altered mobility, and pain prior to treatment, but no other neurological deficits. Success was defined as absence of clinical recurrence during a median follow-up duration of

approximately 4 years. When comparing outcome within and between groups of dogs managed nonsurgically or surgically, it is very important that variability between the study populations and outcome measures is considered. Prognosis varies widely depending on the presence or absence of preoperative neurological deficits and may depend on the type and degree of nerve root compression [11, 16, 32]. These factors should be clearly defined for any study. For example, decompressive laminectomy can be an effective treatment for DLSS, although dogs with urinary or fecal

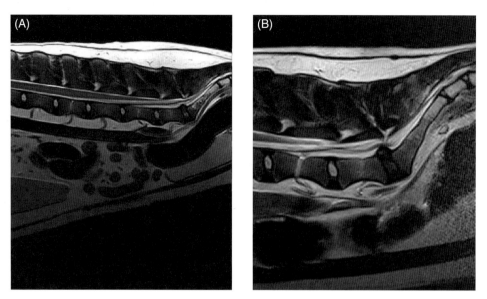

Figure 32.5 T2-weighted MRI scans of the lumbosacral spine in midsagittal plane of a five-and-a-half-year-old collie dog. (A) Neutral position MRI showing intervertebral disc degeneration at the lumbosacral junction and mild protrusion. (B) Hyperextended position MRI showing intervertebral disc degeneration at the lumbosacral junction and significant protrusion. This constitutes a dynamic intervertebral disc protrusion.

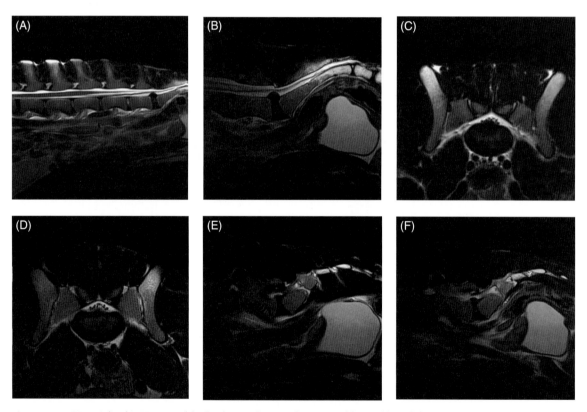

Figure 32.6 T2-weighted MRI scans of the lumbosacral spine of a 7-year-old mixed breed dog. (A) Neutral position midsagittal plane showing intervertebral disc degeneration at the lumbosacral junction and mild protrusion. (B) Hyperextended position midsagittal plane showing intervertebral disc degeneration at the lumbosacral junction and significant dynamic protrusion. (C and D) Transverse plane images of (A) and (B), respectively, showing central protrusion in neutral position and central plus abaxial protrusion in hyperextended position, with associated encroachment of the L7 neural pathways. (E and F) Parasagittal left and right images of the hyperextended position shown in (B) and (D) demonstrating encroachment of the L7 neuroforamina by disc annulus and migration of the dorsal lamina of S1 ventral to that of L7, creating an "hourglass" dorsal and ventral compression of the L7 nerve root.

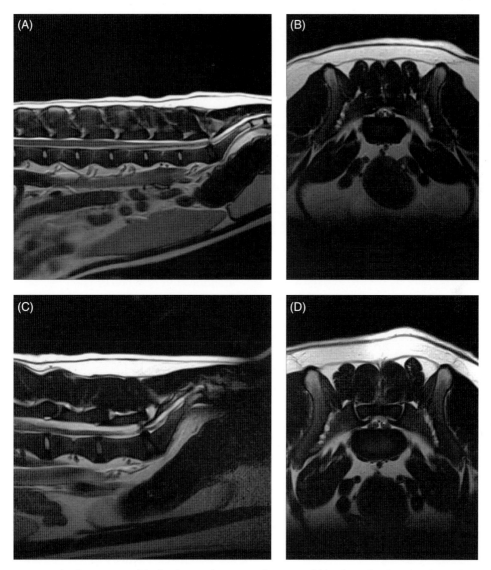

Figure 32.7 T2-weighted MRI scans of the lumbosacral junction of a 7-year-old border collie dog in midsagittal and transverse planes. (A and B) Neutral position showing a degenerated lumbosacral disc with mild protrusion centrally on sagittal images and abaxial protrusion, worse on one side, on transverse image. (C and D) Hyperextended position manifests greater protrusion of the degenerated lumbosacral disc and ventral migration of the dorsal lamina of the sacrum relative to L7, creating "hourglass" compression of the cauda equina and greater abaxial compression of the L7 neuroforamina.

incontinence have a worse prognosis than dogs that are continent before surgery and dogs with abaxial L7 nerve root impingement may fare badly with axial laminectomy alone [11, 16].

Surgical treatment is indicated when signs of pain are not alleviated by nonsurgical management or when there are motor or sensory deficits [30, 32, 33]. The available surgical techniques are dorsal laminectomy (with discectomy, foraminal decompression, or both), foramenotomy, and stabilization or distraction–stabilization [11, 19]. When selecting the optimal treatment, it is advisable to compile a pretreatment problem list and to define the preferred treatment outcome, for example, a return to long-term unrestricted active duty in a military working dog. The preoperative problem list includes any of the following abnormalities noted either in isolation or in combination: (i) static or dynamic disc-associated cauda equina compression, (ii) dorsal cauda equina compression (facet joint and ligamentum flavum hypertrophy), (iii) pathological LS instability, (iv) neuroforaminal impingement, and (v) neuroforaminal stenosis [19]. It is immediately obvious that marked variability exists between the available surgical procedures in their ability to simultaneously neutralize all of the preoperative problems.

Decompressive laminectomy

Surgical treatment based on bony decompression by dorsal laminectomy is limited to management of isolated dorsal impingement of the cauda equina. For this reason, dorsal laminectomy is almost always coupled with IVD fenestration or partial discectomy in order to concurrently address ventral cauda equina compression [16, 19, 32, 34]. Combined dorsal laminectomy and discectomy yields satisfactory medium-term results in most studies, with a reported overall postoperative improvement rate of approximately 70–90% [11, 16, 32, 34, 35]. However, detailed information on the long-term outcome of dorsal laminectomy and discectomy for DLSS is limited and the results have varied. Additionally, the nature and extent of neuroforaminal stenosis in such cases has not been clearly documented and it is intuitive that axial laminectomy will not treat abaxial neuroforaminal impingement. A potential conflict also exists when dorsal laminectomy is chosen to treat disc-associated compression in animals with pre-existing LS instability. Conventional dorsal laminectomy with or without discectomy was shown to possibly decease LS motion unit stiffness in a canine *ex vivo* study [36]. Although the reported reduction in stiffness was not statistically significant, this may have been a consequence of insufficient group size (type II error). Consequently, the ideal candidate for dorsal laminectomy and discectomy is probably a dog where the problem list excludes dynamic disc-associated cauda equina compression, LS instability, neuroforaminal impingement and/or neuroforaminal stenosis, for example, where Hansen type I IVD extrusion has been identified as an isolated abnormality or a central Hansen type II protrusion with no obvious instability.

LS foraminotomy

Although foraminal stenosis was described in the earliest veterinary literature describing canine LS disease [37], it is not until recently that increased availability of veterinary MRI has improved diagnostic recognition to the levels reported in humans [10, 38–41]. Unrecognized or recurrent foraminal stenosis is thought to be an important cause of "failed back surgery syndrome" in human neurosurgery [42] and might account, at least in part, for suboptimal results after conventional dorsal laminectomy in dogs. In canine studies, MRI evidence of nerve root compression is present in 68–90% of affected dogs [10, 43] (Figures 32.3 and 32.4). In such patients, we submit that the existing literature has been suboptimal with regard to identification of whether compression affects the entry, middle, or exit zones and that this is important as it may have a direct effect on the type and extent of surgical intervention.

In humans, foraminal impingement identified using MRI is often coupled with signs consistent with clinically important sciatic nerve compression [44]. Direct pressure applied to peripheral branches of the sciatic nerve can induce severe pain in affected individuals. Although the same phenomenon has not been reported in dogs to date, we have noticed that the majority of dogs affected by DLSS display a severe reproducible pain response during deep palpation of the sciatic nerve as it passes between the semimembranosus/semitendinosus and biceps femoris muscles. This finding may add clinical support to the MRI evidence documenting a high rate of L7 neuroforaminal impingement in dogs affected by DLSS (Figure 32.2).

Although in principle it is possible to relieve neuroforaminal impingement by lateral extension of a dorsal laminectomy to include unilateral or bilateral facetectomy [3, 25, 32, 37], partial or total facetectomy is contraindicated because of its potential to induce significant instability of the LS vertebral segment [37, 45]. LS foraminotomy does not suffer from this disadvantage [46], and it can also be performed from a dorsal approach either by dorsal fenestration of the IVD in a lateral direction or by ventrolateral extension of a standard laminectomy under the articular facet joint [32, 47]. However, whatever method is chosen for dorsal foraminotomy, inherent problems are associated with poor visibility, which increases the risk of iatrogenic trauma to the L7 nerve root [43]. Also, accurate decompression of the foraminal middle and exit zones is not possible with these approaches. Consequently, incomplete nerve root decompression may result in persistent postoperative deficits [43]. Attempts to compensate for these limitations by aggressive removal of the ventral portions of the articular facets risk exacerbation of instability and even facet fracture [45, 48]. Thus, in order to achieve complete decompression of all three neuroforaminal zones, dorsal foraminotomy must be combined with lateral foraminotomy, which addresses compressive lesions within the exit and middle zones [43]. This technique has been performed in humans with multiple-level foraminal stenosis [46]. In dogs, concerns exist regarding the practicality of multiple surgical approaches, the potential for exacerbation of instability or iatrogenic trauma, and the risk of latent osseous or soft tissue regrowth causing persistent foraminal stenosis [49].

Distraction–stabilization

Guidelines for lumbar fusion in human patients are still evolving. In human patients with lumbar disc herniation and radiculopathy, there is no convincing evidence to support the routine use of lumbar fusion at the time of a primary disc excision. Fusion in addition to discectomy may be beneficial for human patients with preoperative lumbar instability or recurrent disc herniation or in heavy laborers or athletes with back pain in addition to radiculopathy [50]. Lumbar fusion is recommended for patients with lumbar stenosis and associated degenerative spondylolisthesis who require decompression and in carefully selected patients with disabling low back pain due to degenerative disease without stenosis or spondylolisthesis [51, 52].

In dogs with degenerative LS stenosis, indications for the use of distraction–stabilization techniques in addition to partial discectomy are also unclear. However, this is the only technique that allows simultaneous neutralization of all abnormalities listed on the preoperative problem list. Stabilization techniques include transfacet screw fixation, cross-pin fixation, vertebral body fixation with a lag screw, and pedicle screw fixation

[53–55]. Concerns regarding the ability of the paired transfacet screws described by Slocum to resist the significant multidirectional forces acting across the LS articulation have prompted the evolution of more robust stabilization techniques [19, 36]. In the clinical veterinary literature, techniques have been reported whereby screws are inserted in the L7 and S1 pedicles with screw connection either by embedding the screw heads into a polymethyl-methacrylate (PMMA) cement bridge or by use of a human pedicle screw and rod fixation system [36]. In an experimental study in beagles that had spine destabilization followed by different spinal fusing techniques, dogs treated with pedicle screw and rod fixation had significantly lower neuropathologic spinal cord abnormalities than the dogs treated with sublaminar fixation with wires and rods [56].

Stabilization alone will not address static compressive elements of the neuroforamina, especially in the middle and exit zones, whether of annular or osseous origin (Figure 32.3). We submit that distraction–stabilization may be superior, and we have reported the application of a novel titanium intervertebral spacer device, the Fitz Intervertebral Traction Screw (FITS), inserted via dorsal laminectomy and annulectomy [57] (Figure 32.1D). This results in distraction of the vertebral end plates of L7 and S1 and reliable enlargement of all zones (entry, middle and exit) of the neuroforamina by stretching of the articular facets and distraction of abaxial spondylosis. We illustrated proof of principle in an *ex vivo* study using a plastic polymer surrogate of the FITS device and MRI measurement of neuroforaminal volume and end-plate distance (Figure 32.8A and B). Curettage of cartilage in the LS facets facilitates fusion and the device is coated in hydroxyapatite to encourage osseous ingrowth across the IVD. Dorsal stabilization in conjunction with the FITS device was provided in early cases using pins placed bilaterally in the body of L7 and in the alar wings of the sacrum linked with a bolus of PMMA cement dorsally [57] (Figure 32.8C and D) and in later cases by custom-designed pedicle screws in similar positions linked by dorsal clamps and rods (Fitzateur) [58] (Figure 32.9).

Some implant-associated complications were experienced with FITS–pin–PMMA constructs, but resolution of clinical signs was observed in a large cohort of clinical patients for up to 4 years.

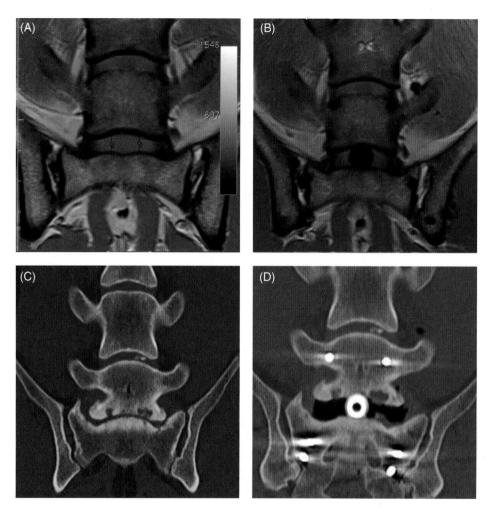

Figure 32.8 (A and B) T1-weighted MRI scans of the lumbosacral junction in dorsal plane acquisition from a pilot cadaver study using a polymeric surrogate intervertebral spacer of identical dimensions to the clinically Fitz Intervertebral Traction Screw (FITS) device. End-plate distance measured at four equidistant points and demonstration of proof-of-principle distraction separation of the caudal end plate of L7 from the cranial end plate of the sacrum. (C and D) Dorsal plane CT images of the lumbosacral spine of a 7-year-and-8-month-old Dogue de Bordeaux with distraction using a FITS device preoperatively and immediately postoperatively.

These complications have not been seen with the FITS–Fitzateur constructs, which have proven robust and reliable.

In a recent clinical study, 35 dogs affected by LS pain where cauda equina and neuroforaminal stenosis was identified were operated using FITS–Fitzateur constructs. According to owner assessment, clinical signs improved for 31 of the 35 dogs; according to veterinary assessment, lameness, musculature, and pain improved for all cases. Generally, there was early return to function and CT scan demonstrated maintenance of

distraction and stabilization at 6 months postoperatively. The technique allows immediate and indirect decompression of the neuroforamina without iatrogenic trauma to the nerve roots potentially associated with foraminotomy, and follow-up imaging supports that foraminal decompression is sustained.

In conclusion, the degenerative changes often associated with LS disc disease may cause clinical signs which prove recalcitrant to medical management and may not be possible to address or may be suboptimally addressed by existing

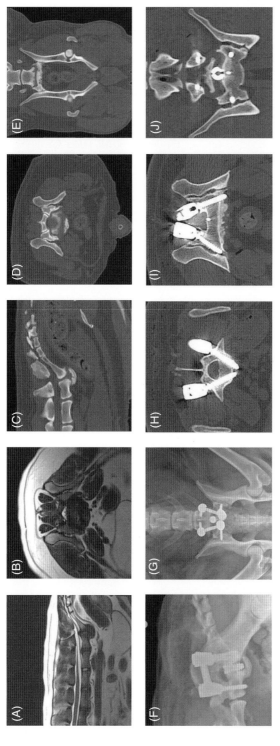

Figure 32.9 Images of the lumbosacral spine of a 9-year-old Labrador retriever dog. (A and B) T2-weighted MRI scans in sagittal and transverse planes illustrating intervertebral disc degeneration at L6–L7 and L7–S1 (and to a lesser extent L3–L4 and L4–L5). Disc protrusion at L7–S1 is producing moderate central cauda equina compression and significant abaxial encroachment of the L7 neuroforamina at the entry, middle, and exit zones. (C, D, and E) CT scans in midsagittal, transverse, and dorsal planes showing intervertebral disc degeneration and collapse at the lumbosacral junction, plus significant ventral and abaxial spondylotic new bone formation. Significant narrowing of the L7 nerve root pathways is noted. Degenerative changes are also noted affecting the vertebral end plates. (F and G) Radiography in lateral and flexed ventrodorsal projections demonstrates position of the Fitz Intervertebral Traction Screw (FITS) device producing distraction of the lumbosacral disc space. The screw is held in place with a 2.4 mm screw. The Fitzateur dorsally comprises two 4.5 mm screws on either side of the vertebral bodies of L7 and the sacrum. Each pair of screws is linked by a clamp and rod system bilaterally, facilitating multidirectional attachment. (H, I, and J) CT scans postoperatively illustrate screw position in the vertebral bodies of L7 and the sacrum in the transverse plane and also illustrate distraction of the end plates of the L7–S1 junction by the FITS device in the dorsal plane.

techniques. Therefore, vertebral stabilization is indicated in some cases of LS disc disease which are affected by instability, end-plate deformity, relative vertebral migration, and abaxial stenosis of the neuroforamina. Furthermore, recent studies have shown that distraction–stabilization may have salient advantages over stabilization alone and may provide an important surgical solution for debilitating pain, lameness, and neurogenic deficits associated with DLSS.

References

1. Smith MEH, Bebchuk TN, Shmon CL, Watson LG, Steinmetz H. An in vitro biomechanical study of the effects of surgical modification upon the canine lumbosacral spine. Vet Comp Orthop Traumatol 2004; 17: 17–24.
2. Seim HO III. Surgery of the lumbosacral spine. In Fossum T, ed. Small Animal Surgery. 2nd ed. Philadelphia: Mosby, 2002: 1302–1322.
3. Chambers JN. Degenerative lumbosacral stenosis in dogs. Vet Med Rep 1989; 1: 166–180.
4. Palmer RH, Chambers JN. Canine lumbosacral diseases. Part I. Anatomy, pathophysiology, and clinical presentation. Compend Contin Educ Pract Vet 1991; 13: 61–69.
5. Watt PR. Degenerative lumbosacral stenosis in 18 dogs. J Small Anim Pract 1991; 32: 125–134.
6. Ness MG. Degenerative lumbosacral stenosis in the dog: a review of 30 cases. J Small Anim Pract 1994; 35: 185–190.
7. De Risio L, Thomas WB, Sharp NJH. Degenerative lumbosacral stenosis. Vet Clin North Am Small Anim Pract 2000; 30: 111–132.
8. Fletcher TF. Spinal cord and meninges. In Evans H, Christiansen G, eds. Miller's Anatomy of the Dog. 3rd ed. Philadelphia: WB Saunders, 1993: 800–828.
9. Lee C, Rauschning W, Glenn W: Lateral lumbar spinal canal stenosis: classification, pathologic anatomy and surgical decompression. Spine 1988; 13: 313–320.
10. Mayhew PD, Kapatkin AS, Wortman JA, Vite CH. Association of cauda equina compression on magnetic resonance images and clinical signs in dogs with degenerative lumbosacral stenosis. J Am Anim Hosp Assoc 2002; 38: 555–562.
11. De Risio L, Sharp NJH, Olby NJ, Muñana KR, Thomas WB. Predictors of outcome after dorsal decompressive laminectomy for degenerative lumbosacral stenosis in dogs: 69 cases (1987–1997). J Am Vet Med Assoc 2001; 219: 624–628.
12. Morgan JP, Bahr A, Franti CE, Bailey CS. Lumbosacral transitional vertebrae as a predisposing cause of cauda equina syndrome in German Shepherd dogs:

161 cases (1987–1990). J Am Vet Med Assoc 1993; 202: 1877–1882.
13. Seiler G, Häni H, Busato AR, Lang J. Facet joint geometry and intervertebral disk degeneration in the L5–S1 region of the vertebral column in German Shepherd Dogs. Am J Vet Res 2002; 63: 86–90.
14. Rossi F, Seiler G, Busato A, Wacker C, Lang J. Magnetic resonance imaging of articular process joint geometry and intervertebral disk degeneration in the caudal lumbar spine (L5–S1) of dogs with clinical signs of cauda equina compression. Vet Radiol Ultr 2004; 45: 381–387.
15. Benninger MI, Seiler GS, Robinson LE, Ferguson SJ, Bonél HM, Busato AR, Lang J. Effects of anatomic conformation on three-dimensional motion of the caudal lumbar and lumbosacral portions of the vertebral column of dogs. Am J Vet Res 2006; 67: 43–50.
16. Linn LL, Bartels KE, Rochat MC, Payton ME, Moore GE. Lumbosacral stenosis in 29 military working dogs: epidemiologic findings and outcome after surgical interventions (1990–1999). Vet Surg 2003; 32: 21–29.
17. Stokes IA Wilder DG, Frymoyer JW, Pope MH. Volvo award in clinical sciences. Assessment of patients with low-back pain by biplanar radiographic measurement of intervertebral motion. Spine 1981; 6: 233–240.
18. Hediger KU, Ferguson SJ, Gedet P, Busatu A, Forterre F, Isler S, Barmettler R, Lang J. Biomechanical analysis of torsion and shear forces in lumbar and lumbosacral spine segments of nonchondrodystrophic dogs. Vet Surg 2009; 38: 874–880.
19. Meij BP, Bergknut N. Degenerative lumbosacral stenosis in dogs. Vet Clin North Am Small Anim Pract 2010; 40: 982–1009.
20. Raj PP. Intervertebral disc: anatomy-physiology-pathophysiology-treatment. Pain Pract 2008; 8: 18–44.
21. Colombini A, Lombardi G, Corsi MM, Banfi G. Pathophysiology of the human intervertebral disc. Int J Biochem Cell Biol 2008; 40: 837–842.
22. Gradner G, Bockstahler, Peham C, Henninger W, Podbregar I. Kinematic study of back movement in clinically sound Malinois dogs with consideration of the effect of radiographic changes in the lumbosacral junction. Vet Surg 2007; 36: 472–481.
23. Bagley R. Surgical stabilization of the lumbosacral joint. In Slatter D, ed. Textbook of Small Animal Surgery. 3rd ed. Philadelphia: Elsevier Science, 2003: 1238–1243.
24. Lang J. Flexion-extension myelography of the canine cauda equina. Vet Radiol 1988; 29: 242–257.
25. Sjöström L. L. Degenerative lumbosacral stenosis: surgical decompression. In Slatter D, ed. Textbook of Small Animal Surgery. 3rd ed. Philadelphia: Elsevier Science, 2003: 1227–1237.
26. Braundt KG, Taylor TK, Ghosh P, Sherwood AA. Spinal mobility in the dog. A study in chondrodystrophoid and non-chondrodystrophoid animals. Res Vet Sci 1977; 22: 78–82.

27. Benninger MI, Seiler GS, Robinson LE, Ferguson SJ, Bonél HM, Busato AR, Lang J. Three-dimensional motion pattern of the caudal lumbar and lumbosacral portions of the vertebral column of dogs. Am J Vet Res 2004; 65: 544–551.

28. Chambers JN, Barbara A, Selcer BA, Oliver JE. Results of treatment of degenerative lumbosacral stenosis in dogs by exploration and excision. Vet Comp Orthop Traumatol 1988; 3: 130–133.

29. Indrieri RJ. Lumbosacral stenosis and injury of the cauda equina. Vet Clin North Am Small Anim Pract 1988; 18: 697–710.

30. Wheeler SJ. Lumbosacral disc disease. Vet Clin North Am Small Anim Pract 1992; 22: 937–950.

31. Janssens L, Beosier Y, Daems R. Lumbosacral degenerative stenosis in the dog–the results of epidural infiltration with methylprednisolone acetate: a retrospective study. Vet Comp Orthop Traumatol 2009; 22: 486–491.

32. Danielsson F, Sjostrom L. Surgical treatment of degenerative lumbosacral stenosis. Vet Surg 1999; 28: 91–98.

33. Wheeler SJ, Sharp NJ. Lumbosacral disease. In Wheeler SJ, Sharp NJ, eds. Small Animal Spinal Disorders: Diagnosis And Surgery. London: Mosby Wolfe, 1994: 122–134.

34. Jones JC, Banfield CM, Ward DL. Association between postoperative outcome and results of magnetic resonance imaging and computed tomography in working dogs with degenerative lumbosacral stenosis. J Am Vet Med Assoc 2000; 216: 1769–1774.

35. Janssens F, Moens Y, Coppens P. Lumbosacral degenerative stenosis in the dog: the results of dorsal decompression with dorsal annulectomy and nuclectomy. Vet Comp Orthop Traumatol 2000; 13: 97–103.

36. Meij BP, Suwankong N, van der Veen, AJ, Hazewinkel HA. Biomechanical flexion-extension forces in normal canine lumbosacral cadaver specimens before and after dorsal laminectomy-discectomy and pedicle screw-rod fixation. Vet Surg 2007; 36: 742–751.

37. Tarvin G, Prata R. Lumbosacral stenosis in dogs. J Am Vet Med Assoc 1980; 177: 154–159.

38. Jones JC, Wilson ME, Bartels JE. A review of high resolution computed tomography and a proposed technique for regional examination of the canine lumbosacral spine. Vet Radiol Ultrasound 1994; 35: 339–346.

39. Jones JC, Sorjonen DC, Simpson ST, Simpson ST, Coates JR, Lenz SD, Hathcock JT, Agee MW, Bartels JE. Comparison between computed tomographic and surgical findings in nine large-breed dogs with lumbosacral stenosis. Vet Radiol Ultrasound 1996; 37: 247–256.

40. Jones JC, Shires PK, Inzana KD, Sponenberg P, Massicotte C, Renberg W, Giroux A. Evaluation of canine lumbosacral stenosis using intravenous contrast-enhanced computed tomography. Vet Radiol Ultrasound 1999; 40: 108–114.

41. Adams WH, Daniel GB, Pardo AD, Selcer RR. Magnetic resonance imaging of the caudal lumbar and lumbosacral spine in 13 dogs (1990–1993). Vet Radiol Ultrasound 1995; 36: 3–13.

42. Fritsch E, Heisel J, Rupp S. The failed back surgery syndrome: reasons, intraoperative findings and long term results (a report of 182 operative treatments). Spine 1996; 21: 626–633.

43. Gödde T, Steffen F. Surgical management of lumbosacral foraminal stenosis using a lateral approach in twenty dogs with degenerative lumbosacral stenosis. Vet Surg 2007; 36: 705–713.

44. Jenis L, An H. Spine update: lumbar foraminal stenosis. Spine 2000; 25: 389–394.

45. Thiel S, Steffen F, Gödde T. Articular Process Fractures following lumbosacral decompressive surgery (6 cases). In Proceedings of the 18th Annual Meeting of the ESVN, Munich, 2005: 39.

46. Osman S, Nibu K, Panjabi M, Marsolais EB, Chaudhary R. Transforaminal and posterior decompressions of the lumbar spine: a comparative study of stability and intervertebral foramen area. Spine 1997; 22: 1690–1695.

47. Chambers JN, Selcer BA, Sullivan SA, Coates JR. Diagnosis of lateralized lumbosacral disk herniation with magnetic resonance imaging. J Am Anim Hosp Assoc 1997;33:296–299.

48. Moens N, Runyon C. Fracture of L7 vertebral articular facets and pedicles following dorsal laminectomy in a dog. J Am Vet Med Assoc 2002; 221: 807–810.

49. Wood B, Lanz OI, Jones JC, Shires PK. Endoscope-assisted lumbosacral foraminotomy in the dog. Vet Surg 2004; 33: 221–231.

50. Resnick DK, Choudhri TF, Dailey AT, Groff MW, Khoo L, Matz Pg, Mummaneni P, Watters WC, Wang J, Walters BC, Hadley MN. Guidelines for the performance of fusion procedures for degenerative disease of the lumbar spine. Part 8: lumbar fusion for disc herniation and radiculopathy. J Neurosurg Spine 2005; 2: 673–678.

51. Resnick DK, Choudhri TF, Dailey AT, Grof MW, Khoo L, Matz Pg, Mummaneni P, Watters WC, Wang J, Walters BC, Hadley MN. Guidelines for the performance of fusion procedures for degenerative disease of the lumbar spine. Part 8: fusion in patients with stenosis and spondylolisthesis. J Neurosurg Spine 2005; 2: 679–685.

52. Resnick DK, Choudhri TF, Dailey AT, Grof MW, Khoo L, Matz Pg, Mummaneni P, Watters WC, Wang J, Walters BC, Hadley MN. Guidelines for the performance of fusion procedures for degenerative disease of the lumbar spine. Part 8: intractable low-back pain without stenosis or spondylolisthesis. J Neurosurg Spine 2005; 2: 670–672.

53. Slocum B, Devine T. L7–S1 fixation-fusion for treatment of cauda equina compression in the dog. J Am Vet Med Assoc 1986; 188: 31–35.

54. Slocum B, Devine T. Optimal treatment for degenerative lumbosacral stenosis. Traction, internal fixation, and fusion. Vet Med Report 1989; 1: 249–257.

55. Slocum B, Devine T. L7-S1 fixation-fusion technique for cauda equina syndrome. In Bojrab MJ, ed. Current Techniques in Small Animal Surgery. 5th ed. Philadelphia: Lea & Febiger, 1998; 861–864.

56. Zdeblick TA, Becker PS, McAfee PC, Sutterlin CE, Coe JD, Gurr KR. Neuropathologic changes with experimental spinal instrumentation: transpedicular versus sublaminar fixation. J Spinal Disord 1991; 4: 221–228.

57. Fitzpatrick N. Long-term follow-up of lumbosacral distraction-fusion using combined dorsal and ventral fixation including a novel intervertebral spacer device in 23 dogs. In ACVS Symposium, Chicago, IL, 2010.

58. Fitzpatrick N. Lumbosacral distraction-fusion using an intervertebral spacer and screw-rod fixation system for treatment of degenerative lumbosacral stenosis. In VOS-WVOC Congress, Breckenridge, CO, 2014.

33 The Rationale for Durotomy in Surgical Treatment of Intervertebral Disc Disease

Franck Forterre, Núria Vizcaíno Revés, and Natasha Olby

Introduction

Over the past 30 years and despite significant progress, intensive scientific and clinical research efforts have failed to develop convincingly efficient therapies to reverse the devastating paralysis of traumatic spinal cord injury [1]. The maintenance of adequate vascular perfusion and the decompression of the spinal cord are two important aspects of the clinical management of the acutely spinal cord injured patient. Both have received considerable attention in the past two decades, largely due to the belief that they have an influence on neurological recovery [2–4]. Durotomy, defined as an incision of the dura mater and in most cases of the arachnoid, has been described as an adjunctive method to relieve increased subdural pressure in case of intervertebral disc herniation. It had been suggested that the incision of the meninges decompresses the swollen spinal cord parenchyma, permits CSF drainage, and improves spinal cord perfusion pressure.

Effects of durotomy on outcome

The surgical role of durotomy in both spinal cord decompression and improvement of medullary blood flow dates back to the battlefields of the First World War and has always been a topic of controversy [4–7]. It is clear that for some specific lesions (i.e., subdural tumor, hemorrhage, and arachnoidal cyst), durotomy is mandatory to evaluate and treat the intradural and intramedullary lesions [8, 9]. However, in cases of spinal cord injury, the relative risks and benefits of durotomy are still unclear and controversial [9, 10]. After acute intervertebral disc herniation and spinal cord injury, focal swelling of the spinal cord may lead to a kind of "spinal compartment syndrome" due to the poor elasticity of the surrounding meningeal layers. An increase in intracranial pressure following head injury plays a central role in limiting brain perfusion and compounding secondary damage. CSF shunting and durotomy are both effective at controlling intracranial pressure and improving outcome [11, 12]. Accordingly, it would

Advances in Intervertebral Disc Disease in Dogs and Cats, First Edition. Edited by James M. Fingeroth and William B. Thomas.
© 2015 ACVS Foundation. Published 2015 by John Wiley & Sons, Inc.

be logical to think that performing a durotomy following spinal cord injury would decrease submeningeal pressure and restore normal spinal cord perfusion.

In a nonpublished study of the evolution of subdural pressure during surgical treatment of intervertebral disc herniation, subdural pressure at the site of herniation before decompression was constantly below 10 mm Hg in all dogs. A catheter was inserted through a small durotomy opening created one segment distal to the compression site. During measurement, CSF drainage occurring at the insertion site elicited a steady drop in subdural pressure in all patients, confirming the hypothesis of subdural pressure relief [13]. It has been hypothesized that CSF drainage might play a role in controlling intraspinal cord pressure in the same manner as intracranial pressure and might improve outcome after spinal cord injury by maintaining spinal cord perfusion [14, 15]. Indeed, a preliminary study in humans demonstrated the safety of the technique and the ability of CSF drainage to improve spinal cord perfusion in the postoperative period [14]. However, a recent study that assessed the effect of durotomy on spinal cord blood flow in dogs with intervertebral disc herniation failed to demonstrate an increase in spinal cord perfusion [16]. Directly after decompression and durotomy in dogs with incomplete spinal cord lesions, an increase in spinal cord blood flow at the site of herniation was seen. In these dogs, no spinal cord swelling was observed after durotomy. After 15 min, the spinal cord blood flow decreased again and returned to almost initial or even lower values in all dogs. In contrast, a study on the evolution of spinal cord blood flow in dogs with intervertebral disc herniation treated by hemilaminectomy without durotomy showed a steady increase in blood flow after decompression [17]. However, getting accurate measurements of spinal cord blood flow is difficult, and additional work needs to be done to confirm these observations.

From the clinical point of view, durotomy has been reported to improve functional recovery in dogs with spinal cord injury if performed immediately after impact trauma [6, 18]. These authors observed that a 2 h delay between trauma and durotomy reduced the difference in functional recovery between experimental and control dogs to an insignificant level. The clinical effect of durotomy has also been investigated retrospec-

tively in a recent study [4]. All clinical studies confirmed the results of the initial experimental studies and failed to demonstrate a positive clinical effect of durotomy if performed later than 2 h after injury. Neither durotomy nor myelotomy alter or interrupt the evolution of ascending/descending myelomalacia [5] (see Chapter 12). It is important to note that these studies were unlikely to have adequate statistical power to draw absolute conclusions. However, the negative findings could simply be a result of the difficulty in producing a long enough durotomy to truly decompress the severely injured spinal cord in which swelling is detected over multiple segments. One could argue that the durotomy should result in free flow of CSF in order to be effective, but in practice, in patients with paraplegia and loss of deep pain perception that might benefit from such an intervention, the spinal cord frequently swells into the durotomy, obstructing CSF flow. Thus, while the concept may be sound, the practical application is impossible. In summary, neither positive therapeutic effects of durotomy on spinal cord blood flow nor on surgical outcome could be established in dogs with thoracolumbar disc herniation. Therefore, durotomy is not recommended as a therapeutic procedure in patients with intervertebral disc disease.

Durotomy to assess prognosis

Controversy remains about the diagnostic and prognostic value of durotomy in cases of myelomalacia in patients lacking deep pain perception [4, 19, 20]. Durotomy allows direct visualization of the spinal cord to evaluate the presence of edema, hemorrhages, and myelomalacia, and it is performed as a diagnostic aid to determine spinal cord structural integrity [4]. Euthanasia has been recommended if spinal cord liquefaction is observed following durotomy. However, euthanasia of dogs based on finding focal spinal cord malacia certainly leads to death of some dogs that would otherwise recover [9, 21]. Local necrosis of gray matter over one or two spinal segments is common after severe injury, and it is not unusual for this material to ooze out after durotomy [9]. Furthermore, focal myelomalacia does not preclude neurological recovery [19]. As few as 10% of axons surviving in the lesion after spinal cord injury appear to allow functional recovery. This would be impossible to identify at the time of durotomy because of the lateral approach (hemilaminectomy) and limited spinal cord exposure [9, 21].

Risks of durotomy

The potential negative aspect of durotomy is the risk of iatrogenic spinal cord trauma because of associated manipulation of the injured spinal cord [5]. This risk has been suggested in early studies [7]. In normal dogs, durotomy resulted in mild temporary neurological deficits [6]. However, a more recent study has shown that it did not affect postoperative recovery in patients without deep pain perception that underwent hemilaminectomy and durotomy compared with those that underwent hemilaminectomy alone [4]. In another clinical study evaluating spinal cord blood flow after hemilaminectomy and durotomy in dogs with intervertebral disc herniation and intact deep pain perception, recovery times were similar to that in dogs treated with hemilaminectomy without durotomy [16]. These observations however should not lead the surgeon to overlook the inherent risks associated with performing a durotomy. Excessive or inappropriate manipulation of the injured spinal cord may result in further structural injury or hemorrhage from the pial vessels. In the severely injured spinal cord, durotomy may lead to spinal cord herniation and encroachment of the spinal cord through the incision site [9]. Accordingly, durotomy should be performed by experienced surgeons confident with spinal cord anatomy.

Even when intervertebral disc patients recover and return to a normal neurological state, possible long-term complications may occur related to the durotomy itself. These are associated with the healing of the durotomy site that occurs within 16 weeks. The edges of the incision rejoin but they often adhere to the spinal cord, potentially disturbing CSF flow that might result in development of arachnoid pseudocysts or syringomyelia [7]. In an MRI study following the evolution of epidural and intradural scarring after hemilaminectomy and durotomy, distortion of the spinal cord developed in all dogs due to tethering of the cord to the healing dura mater [22].

In conclusion, it can be stated that nowadays there are neither real valuable arguments nor scientific findings justifying the use of a durotomy in the treatment protocol of dogs with intervertebral disc herniation. However, lumbar CSF drainage as a safe, less invasive modification of the durotomy might become an option in the future if adequately controlled trials show a benefit [14, 15].

References

1. Donovan WH. Spinal cord injury—past, present, and future. J Spinal Cord Med. 2007;30(2):85–100.
2. Fehlings MG, Perrin RG. The timing of surgical intervention in the treatment of spinal cord injury: a systematic review of recent clinical evidence. Spine. 2006;31(11S):S28–S35.
3. Hadley MN, Walters BC, Grabb PA, Oyesiku NM, Przybylski GJ, Resnick DK, et al. Guidelines for the management of acute cervical spine and spinal cord injuries. Clin Neurosurg. 2002;49:407–98.
4. Loughin CA, Dewey CW, Ringwood PB, Pettigrew RW, Kent M, Budsberg SC. Effect of durotomy on functional outcome of dogs with type I thoracolumbar disc extrusion and absent deep pain perception. Vet Comp Orthop Traumatol. 2005;18(3):141–6.
5. Fingeroth JM. Treatment of canine intervertebral disk disease. Recommendations and controversies. In: Bonagura JD, editor. Kirk's current veterinary therapy XII. Philadelphia: Saunders; 1995. pp. 1146–53.
6. Parker AJ, Smith CW. Functional recovery from spinal cord trauma following delayed incision of spinal meninges in dogs. Res Vet Sci. 1975 Jan;18(1):110–2.
7. Trevor PB, Martin RA, Saunders GK, Trotter EJ. Healing characteristics of free and pedicle fat grafts after dorsal laminectomy and durotomy in dogs. Vet Surg. 1991 Sep–Oct;20(5):282–90.
8. Jeffery ND, Phillips SM. Surgical treatment of intramedullary spinal cord neoplasia in two dogs. J Small Anim Pract. 1995 Dec;36(12):553–7.
9. Sharp NJH, Wheeler SJ. Small animal spinal disorders: diagnosis and surgery. 2nd ed. Edinburgh: Elsevier; 2005.
10. Perkins PG, Deane RH. Long-term follow-up of six patients with acute spinal injury following dural decompression. Injury. 1988 Nov;19(6):397–401.
11. Bullock MR, Chesnut R, Ghajar J, Gordon D, Hartl R, Newell DW, et al. Surgical management of traumatic parenchymal lesions. Neurosurgery. 2006 Mar;58(Suppl 3):S25–46; discussion Si–iv.
12. Bagley RS, Harrington ML, Pluhar GE, Keegan RD, Greene SA, Moore MP, et al. Effect of craniectomy/durotomy alone and in combination with hyperventilation, diuretics, and corticosteroids on intracranial

pressure in clinically normal dogs. Am J Vet Res. 1996 Jan;57(1):116–9.

13. Kunz RE, Rohrbach H, Gorgas D, Henke D, Forterre F. Assessment of intrathecal pressure in chondrodystrophic dogs with acute thoracolumbar disk disease. Vet Surg. 2014, in press.

14. Kwon BK, Curt A, Belanger LM, Bernardo A, Chan D, Markez JA, et al. Intrathecal pressure monitoring and cerebrospinal fluid drainage in acute spinal cord injury: a prospective randomized trial. J Neurosurg Spine. 2009 Mar;10(3):181–93.

15. Olby N. The pathogenesis and treatment of acute spinal cord injuries in dogs. Vet Clin North Am Small Anim Pract. 2010 Sep;40(5):791–807.

16. Blaser A, Lang J, Henke D, Doherr MG, Adami C, Forterre F. Influence of durotomy on laser-Doppler measurement of spinal cord blood flow in chondrodystrophic dogs with thoracolumbar disk extrusion. Vet Surg. 2012 Feb;41(2):221–7.

17. Malik Y, Spreng D, Konar M, Doherr MG, Jaggy A, Howard J, et al. Laser-Doppler measurements of spinal cord blood flow changes during hemilaminectomy in chondrodystrophic dogs with disk extrusion. Vet Surg. 2009 Jun;38(4):457–62.

18. Parker AJ, Smith CW. Functional recovery from spinal cord trauma following incision of spinal meninges in dogs. Res Vet Sci. 1974 May; 16(3):276–9.

19. Brisson BA. Intervertebral disc disease in dogs. Vet Clin North Am Small Anim Pract. 2010 Sep;40(5):829–58.

20. Parker AJ. Durotomy and saline perfusion in spinal cord trauma. J Am Anim Hosp Assoc. 1975;11:412–3.

21. Olby N, Levine J, Harris T, Munana K, Skeen T, Sharp N. Long-term functional outcome of dogs with severe injuries of the thoracolumbar spinal cord: 87 cases (1996–2001). J Am Vet Med Assoc. 2003 Mar 15;222(6):762–9.

22. Olby NJ, Lim JH. Epidural and intradural scarring post laminectomy and durotomy: a comparison of gelfoam and sentrx film. Montreal: ACVIM Forum; 2009. p. 740.

34 What Should Cover the Bone Defect after Laminectomy/ Hemilaminectomy?

William B. Thomas and James M. Fingeroth

Laminectomy defects heal in a fashion that is similar to that which occurs in long-bone fractures: organization of a hematoma that fills the defect and formation of a fibrous callus or scar with a varying extent of metaplasia of this callus into the cartilage and bone. This normal consequence of vertebral healing is called a "laminectomy membrane," "epidural fibrosis," or "postlaminectomy scar."

In human patients, perineural fibrosis developing after laminectomy for lumbar disc disease is a common cause of postoperative pain or neurological deficits [1]. In dogs, the potential for postoperative compression of the spinal cord is the major limiting factor for the extent of bone removal during laminectomy. A variety of methods for preventing epidural fibrosis have been studied, including free or pedicle fat grafts, absorbable gelatin films and sponges, and cellulose products. Despite numerous studies, there is no clear consensus on which technique consistently reduces epidural fibrosis in dogs and human patients. This chapter reviews the formation of laminectomy membrane and discusses

some of the materials used to cover the laminectomy after thoracolumbar disc surgery. We also address the topical use of analgesics in conjunction with disc surgery.

Healing of laminectomies

Healing of a laminectomy starts with the formation of a hematoma that completely fills the laminectomy defect and is in contact with the adjacent epaxial muscles. By 1 week after surgery, the hematoma organizes by infiltration of fibroblasts from the adjacent epaxial muscles. A thick fibrous scar gradually forms, starting from the epaxial muscles and extending over the dura mater and nerve roots. By 2 weeks, this fibrous connective tissue completely bridges the defect, resulting in a dense, tough membrane called the laminectomy membrane [2]. Woven bone starts forming at the cut surfaces of the vertebral bone, and by 4 weeks, most of the woven bone has been replaced by lamellar bone. Between 8 and 16 weeks, there is further maturation of connective tissue, and bony

Advances in Intervertebral Disc Disease in Dogs and Cats, First Edition. Edited by James M. Fingeroth and William B. Thomas.
© 2015 ACVS Foundation. Published 2015 by John Wiley & Sons, Inc.

proliferation varies from minimal to completely bridging the defect [3].

It is important to realize that all laminectomies heal by the formation of a laminectomy membrane. Three factors are responsible for the extent of laminectomy membrane: the destruction of epidural fat, epidural hematoma, and the invasion of muscle fibers from the epaxial muscles into the defect. The extent of peridural fibrosis is directly proportional to the size of the laminectomy defect [2]. Whether the laminectomy membrane compresses the spinal cord is related to the location and degree of bone removal. For example, with an extensive laminectomy called a Funkquist type A laminectomy, the lamina, articular facets, and pedicles are removed bilaterally down to a level at the middle of the spinal cord. With the Funkquist type A laminectomy, the spinal cord often becomes compressed by the laminectomy membrane. This complication is prevented by a Funkquist type B laminectomy, which preserves the facets and lamina/pedicles to a level dorsal to the cord. This prevents late spinal cord compression but severely limits exposure [3]. A modification to the type B laminectomy has been described where the inner cortical bone of the pedicles and medial articular facet are removed, thus still preventing secondary compression from laminectomy membrane but improving exposure and room to manipulate surgical instruments in the vertebral canal [4]. Neural compression due to laminectomy membrane is uncommon with hemilaminectomy or similar procedures such as pediculectomy [5]. Brown et al. found that 3 of 187 (1.6%) dogs with thoracolumbar disc surgery developed spinal cord compression from a laminectomy membrane after hemilaminectomy and 3/3 had resolution of signs with removal of the laminectomy membrane [6]. However, the precise incidence of this complication is unknown because many dogs with persistent deficits after surgery do not undergo follow-up imaging to document the presence or causes of persistent or recurrent spinal cord compression.

Materials used to cover the laminectomy

Gelatin foams

Gelatin foam is manufactured from porcine skin gelatin whipped and baked into its sponge form. It is nonantigenic and has a neutral pH. Gelatin foam is available as Gelfilm (Gelfilm, absorbable gelatin film. Pharmacia and Upjohn Company, Kalamazoo, MI, USA) and GelFoam (Gelfoam, absorbable gelatin compressed sponge. Pharmacia and Upjohn Company, Kalamazoo, MI, USA). Gelfilm is a thin film that when dry has the appearance and consistency of cellophane. When wet, it assumes a soft, rubber-like consistency. When placed over a laminectomy, it is gradually absorbed over several months. One study found that using Gelfilm to cover the laminectomy in dogs caused more attenuation of neural elements compared to GelFoam [3].

GelFoam is a porous, nonelastic material that is easily cut and absorbs up to 45 times its weight of blood or other fluids. GelFoam has hemostatic properties and hastens clot formation by providing a mechanical scaffold for the forming clot [7]. After implanting GelFoam, the interstices of the foam initially fill with the cellular components of blood. By 3 days, the GelFoam begins to fragment and becomes infiltrated with leukocytes. By 3 weeks, there is considerable lysis of the GelFoam and the material is completely resorbed by 6 weeks [2].

Results of using GelFoam over the laminectomy vary. LaRocca and Macnab were the first to study GelFoam in dogs with laminectomy and found that resorption of this substance was not associated with invasion of granulation tissue into the vertebral canal and the nerve roots were mobile and free of adhesions [2]. However, subsequent investigators found scar formation to be worse than in control groups. For example, Pospiech et al. found results varying from limited scar formation with no dura mater or nerve root incorporation to extensive scar formation surrounding and infiltrating the neural structures [1].

Cellulose products

Cellulose mesh was introduced with the idea of reducing the epidural hematoma by more complete hemostasis. However, it was found to cause extensive scar tissue invading the vertebral canal and adhering to the dura mater and the nerve roots. It must be regarded as unsuitable to cover the laminectomy [1].

Da Costa et al. studied a cellulose membrane implant in laboratory dogs undergoing dorsal laminectomy [8]. This biosynthetic product is 50 μm thick and resembles paper film with a smooth surface (F biosynthetic cellulose membrane. Fibrocell

Produtos Biotecnologicos, Ibiporã, Paraná, Brazil). During healing, there was a lymphocytic–plasmacytic infiltrate but the cellulose membrane isolated the dura mater from the fibrosis in most cases. In a few cases, the cellulose membrane became unwoven causing a local increase in inflammatory cells. Currently there are no clinical studies evaluating this product in dogs with intervertebral disc surgery.

Other products

Because of the significance of laminectomy scar to potentially cause compression or stretching of neural structures in humans after back surgery, a variety of materials beyond those above and below have been investigated for prevention. Two of these, ADCON-L (Adcon-L, anti-adhesion barrier gel. Gliatech Inc., Cleveland, OH, USA), a bioresorbable carbohydrate polymer gel composed of a polyglycan ester and porcine-derived gelatin, and Seprafilm adhesion barrier® (Seprafilm adhesion barrier, Genzyme Biosurgery, Framingham, MA, USA), a bioresorbable membrane composed of two anionic polysaccharides, sodium hyaluronate, and carboxymethylcellulose, have been studied in rat laminectomy models with promising results [9]. Their clinical use in humans undergoing laminectomy or in dogs has not been reported to our knowledge. Another study evaluated the use of human-derived amniotic membrane stripped from placentas on laminectomy defects in experimental dogs [10]. It was unclear whether this material would be clinically advantageous when compared to fat grafts (see the following section).

Fat grafts

Autologous fat, either as a free fat graft or as a pedicle fat graft, is commonly used to cover the laminectomy. A free fat graft is usually harvested from the subcutaneous tissue dorsal to the deep fascia that overlies the epaxial muscles at the site of the surgical incision. The graft is trimmed to a thickness of approximately 5 mm and of a sufficient width and length to cover the laminectomy. Some studies found that free autologous fat grafts are associated with less hematoma and with less scar tissue formation when compared to GelFoam [1].

However, other studies found that although free autologous fat grafts were effective at decreasing scar formation, there could be substantial compression of the spinal cord [7]. Neurological deficits started 6 to 12 h after surgery and improved over 3–10 days after surgery, but mild deficits persisted over the period of observation in most dogs [8].

A pedicle fat graft is created by sharply detaching subcutaneous fat along the margin of the incision, leaving the base attached cranially or caudally. The graft is trimmed to a thickness of approximately 5 mm with the length of the graft approximately three times the width of the base. To avoid vascular compromise, the epaxial fascia adjacent to penetration of the graft is not closed tightly around the graft after the graft has been transferred to the laminectomy defect.

There is no clear advantage to the use of pedicle grafts when compared to free grafts, and the processes of healing are similar with both graft types [11]. By 2 weeks, there is an infiltration of leukocytes, fat cell degeneration, and fibrosis that reach a peak at week 8. By 16 weeks, the inflammation resolves, leaving a viable fat graft approximately 50% the original dimensions in size. In dogs with dorsal laminectomy, there is early compression of the spinal cord severe enough to cause neurologic deficits. This compression resolves by 2–8 weeks [8, 11].

Epidural analgesics

Topical epidural analgesics applied at surgery have been used to provide additional pain relief. One protocol is to apply morphine (0.1 mg/kg) over the dura mater before closure. The morphine is diluted in 0.9% saline, so the total volume instilled ranges from 0.4 to 0.8 ml [12]. Another protocol is to cut a piece of GelFoam to fit over the laminectomy and soak the GelFoam in morphine (0.1 mg/kg) and dexmedetomidine (2.5 µg/kg) [9]. Both techniques reduce but do not eliminate postoperative analgesic requirements [12, 13].

Recommendations

Currently available techniques are only moderately successful in inhibiting epidural fibrosis, scar formation, and dural adhesion. And no method appears to be clearly superior. In fact, one study found fewer complications with leaving the laminectomy uncovered compared to using either fat or cellulose membrane, bringing into question the use of any implant [8]. The best strategy seems to be using a hemilaminectomy or pediculectomy whenever possible and making the bony defect only as large as necessary to adequately remove the extruded disc material. If an implant is used, a free fat graft or GelFoam provides comparable results. The use of epidural analgesics may be an effective component of pain control in the perioperative phase.

References

1. Pospiech J, Pajonk F, Stolke D. Epidural scar tissue formation after spinal surgery: an experimental study. Eur Spine J. 1995;4(4):213–9.
2. LaRocca H, Macnab I. The laminectomy membrane. J Bone Joint Surg. 1974;56B:545–50.
3. Trotter EJ, Crissman J, Robson D, Babish J. Influence of nonbiologic implants on laminectomy membrane formation in dogs. Am J Vet Res. 1988 May;49(5):634–43.
4. Trotter EJ, Brasmer TH, deLahunta A. Modified deep dorsal laminectomy in the dog. Cornell Vet. 1975 Jul;65(3):402–27.
5. Gage ED, Hoerlein BF. Hemilaminectomy and dorsal laminectomy for relieving compressions of the spinal cord in the dog. J Am Vet Med Assoc. 1968 Feb 15;152(4):351–9.
6. Brown NO, Helphrey ML, Prata RG. Thoracolumbar disk disease in the dog: a retrospective analysis of 187 cases. J Am Anim Hosp Assoc. 1977;13:665–72.
7. Achneck HE, Sileshi B, Jamiolkowski RM, Albala DM, Shapiro ML, Lawson JH. A comprehensive review of topical hemostatic agents: efficacy and recommendations for use. Ann Surg. 2010 Feb;251(2):217–28.
8. da Costa RC, Pippi NL, Graca DL, Fialho SA, Alves A, Groff AC, et al. The effects of free fat graft or cellulose membrane implants on laminectomy membrane formation in dogs. Vet J. 2006 May; 171(3):491–9.
9. Kasimcan MO, Bakar B, Aktas S, Alhan A, Yilmaz M. Effectiveness of the biophysical barriers on the peridural fibrosis of a postlaminectomy rat model: an experimental research. Injury. 2011;42(8):778–81.
10. Tao H, Fan H. Implantation of amniotic membrane to reduce postlaminectomy epidural adhesions. Eur Spine J. 2009;18(8):1202–12.
11. Trevor PB, Martin RA, Saunders GK, Trotter EJ. Healing characteristics of free and pedicle fat grafts after dorsal laminectomy and durotomy in dogs. Vet Surg. 1991 Sep–Oct;20(5):282–90.
12. Aprea F, Cherubini GB, Palus V, Vettorato E, Corletto F. Effect of extradurally administered morphine on postoperative analgesia in dogs undergoing surgery for thoracolumbar intervertebral disk extrusion. J Am Vet Med Assoc. 2012 Sep 15;241(6):754–9.
13. Barker JR, Clark-Price SC, Gordon-Evans WJ. Evaluation of topical epidural analgesia delivered in gelfoam for postoperative hemilaminectomy pain control. Vet Surg. 2013;42(1):79–84.

Pros and Cons of Prophylactic Fenestration: Arguments in Favor

Brigitte A. Brisson

Intervertebral disc (IVD) fenestration was initially described as a treatment modality for disc extrusion [1–3], but its therapeutic efficacy was soon questioned on the basis that fenestration or discectomy alone does not achieve effective decompression of the spinal cord in patients with disc herniation [4–6]. Patients presenting with neurologic deficits that were treated with fenestration alone reportedly had prolonged recovery times similar to those of patients treated conservatively [4, 7] and were less likely to recover than if treated by decompressive surgery [3, 7]. In contrast, a more recent study that described a technique for partial percutaneous discectomy reported an 88.8% recovery rate for patients that still had deep pain perception with a mean time for first improvement of 8.3 days, a rate similar to those reported after decompressive surgery [8]. Of clinical interest is the fact that neurological deterioration has been documented following discectomy and was associated with the displacement or herniation of additional disc material into the vertebral canal during the discectomy procedure [9, 10]. Supporting this, a more recent study

assessing the usefulness of percutaneous disc fenestration to treat cervical and thoracolumbar disc extrusion causing mild neurological deficits also reported deterioration of neurological signs in 3 of 32 cases and recurrence of signs in 5 of 32 patients [11]. Overall, a poor success rate is reported for dogs without deep pain perception that are treated with percutaneous discectomy alone [8]; disc fenestration as the sole therapeutic procedure for dogs with paralysis or loss of deep nociception is therefore not recommended [5, 7, 12].

IVD fenestration involves the mechanical removal of the nucleus pulposus (NP) through a window (fenestra) created in the lateral annulus fibrosus (AF) using an air drill and burr (power-assisted fenestration) or a scalpel blade (blade fenestration) [13, 14] (Figure 35.1). The simple creation of a window within the lateral AF does not result in a path for any remaining disc material to herniate in the future [14–16]. In fact, studies assessing the fate of the NP following surgical disc fenestration have failed to document the significant inflammatory reaction that had been postulated as a mechanism for further disc dissolution. Nor has

Advances in Intervertebral Disc Disease in Dogs and Cats, First Edition. Edited by James M. Fingeroth and William B. Thomas.
© 2015 ACVS Foundation. Published 2015 by John Wiley & Sons, Inc.

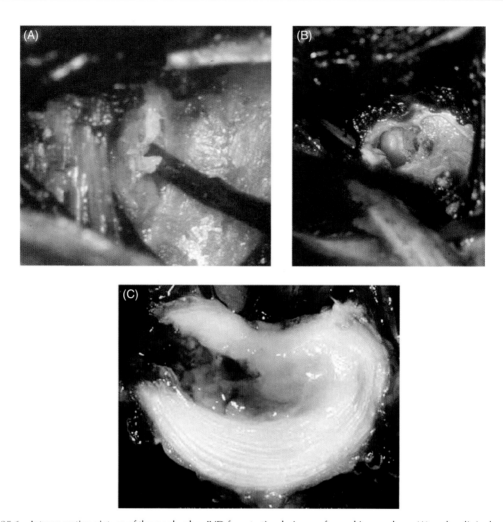

Figure 35.1 Intraoperative picture of thoracolumbar IVD fenestration being performed in a cadaver (A) and a clinical patient (B). Saggital section through a thoracolumbar IVD after fenestration demonstrating the incomplete removal of the nucleus pulposus and the remaining nucleus pulposus mostly located on the contralateral side of the spine (C).

it been confirmed that the window remains open and offers an alternate path for future disc extrusion, since fibrocartilage fills the void created by fenestration soon after surgery [15, 17]. Rather, the effectiveness of fenestration is thought to be governed by the amount of NP removed at the time of surgery [15]. In addition, complete removal of the remaining NP is not expected when performing fenestration [14]. This is supported by a recent study that found some residual disc material in all fenestrated discs even after power-assisted fenestration through a lateral approach [18]. A cadaver study comparing blade and power-assisted fenestration documented that power-assisted fenestra-

tion removed on average 65% of the NP compared with approximately 41% of the NP being removed with blade fenestration [14]. Despite these results, this author believes that either technique can remove large amounts of disc material as long as the surgeon is comfortable with the technique and understands that there is no latent or residual effect that will result in further NP dissolution after surgery.

A study evaluating the effect of surgical approach to the spine determined that using the lateral approach for IVD fenestration may increase the efficiency of the procedure compared with the dorsal or dorsolateral surgical approaches by providing a better angle and working depth for fenestration [19]. Despite the increased efficiency obtained through a lateral approach, it is likely to result in removal of more NP from the ipsilateral side and less from the contralateral side of the IVD being fenestrated [20] (Figure 35.1C). It is also likely that the residual, nonherniated NP still present within the affected disc space is located on the contralateral side to a lateralized extrusion and will be difficult to remove from the side approached for decompressive surgery.

The benefit of fenestration should increase with increasing amounts of degenerative nucleus material remaining within the disc after the initial extrusion [16, 18]. The amount of nucleus remaining within the disc space and its exact location cannot be determined using imaging or be anticipated based on how much extruded disc material is retrieved from the surgical site [18]. However, radiographic evidence of mineralization at the herniated IVD space is thought to be indicative of residual degenerated nucleus material and to support fenestration of the affected disc space at the time of decompressive surgery [16]. In one study, preoperative disc mineralization of the affected IVD was identified in all three of the dogs that developed early recurrence of herniation. One of the three dogs in this report had reportedly been fenestrated through a dorsal approach but still went on to develop recurrence [16]. Although one study reported that disc extrusion occurs as frequently in discs that have radiographic evidence of calcification as those that do not [21], this is inconsistent with another study that reported none of the 24 dogs with first-time disc herniation had radiographic evidence of disc mineralization at the affected disc space [22].

Potential complications associated with fenestration include increased anesthetic and surgical times [23], displacement of disc material into the vertebral canal and/or spinal cord trauma causing worsening of neurologic deficits [10, 24–26], hemorrhage [27, 28], pneumothorax [24, 28], soft tissue and nerve root trauma leading to postoperative pain, scoliosis and abdominal wall weakness [24, 27, 29], discospondylitis [4, 30], difficulty identifying one or more disc spaces for fenestration [26–28], and vertebral subluxation and instability weeks to months after hemilaminectomy and prophylactic fenestration [26]. Most reported

complications are minor and have no long-term negative effects [24, 26–29]. Increased cost associated with longer surgical and anesthetic times, increased surgical incision length, and possibly postoperative morbidity related to additional tissue dissection and trauma should however also be considered.

At this time, therapeutic disc fenestration of the cervical and thoracolumbar spine is clearly *not* recommended as an alternative to decompressive procedures that allow the physical removal of the compressive disc material. A possible exception to this would be a patient in which advanced imaging has failed to identify a compressive disc but where discogenic pain is highly suspected [5] (see Chapter 14). Fenestration of the decompressed disc space at the time of surgery *is* highly recommended to prevent further herniation through the ruptured AF, which could result in early or late recurrence at that site. Prophylactic fenestration of adjacent, unaffected disc spaces at the time of decompressive surgery in the thoracolumbar region has been shown to significantly reduce the rate of recurrent disc herniation at a new disc space regardless of the fact that some discs remain intact. However, the increased surgical time, tissue dissection, possible complications, and surgeon comfort with the prophylactic fenestration procedure must be weighed against its benefits. Dachshunds have been shown to be 10 times more likely to develop recurrence than other dogs, and disc mineralization at the time of first surgery has been associated with recurrence [27, 28, 31, 32]. Since recurrence has also been shown to occur most frequently at a disc space immediately adjacent to or one disc space away from the initial herniation, it seems reasonable to recommend that adjacent, mineralized disc spaces in the dachshund breed be fenestrated prophylactically at the time of decompressive surgery.

References

1. Olsson S-E. Observations concerning disc fenestration in dogs. Acta Orthop. 1951;20(4):349–56.
2. Olsson SE. Surgical treatment with special reference to the value of disc fenestration. Acta Orthop Scand Suppl. 1951;8:51–70.
3. Flo GL, Brinker WO. Lateral fenestration of thoracolumbar discs. J Am Anim Hosp Assoc. 1975;11:619–26.

4. Funkquist B. Investigations of the therapeutic and prophylactic effects of disc evacuation in cases of thoraco-lumbar herniated discs in dogs. Acta Vet Scand. 1978;19(3):441–57.

5. Fingeroth JM. Fenestration. Pros and cons. Probl Vet Med. 1989;1:445–66.

6. Hoerlein B. The status of the various intervertebral disc surgeries for the dog in 1978. J Am Anim Hosp Assoc. 1978;14:563–70.

7. Butterworth SJ, Denny HR. Follow-up study of 100 cases with thoracolumbar disc protrusions treated by lateral fenestration. J Small Anim Pract. 1991; 32:443–7.

8. Kinzel S, Wolff M, Buecker A, Krombach G, Stopinski T, Afify M, et al. Partial percutaneous discectomy for treatment of thoracolumbar disc protrusion: retrospective study of 331 dogs. J Small Anim Pract. 2005;46(10):479–84.

9. Lincoln JD, Pettit GD. Evaluation of fenestration for treatment of degenerative disc disease in the caudal cervical region of large dogs. Vet Surg. 1985;14(3):240–6.

10. Tomlinson J. Tetraparesis following cervical disk fenestration in two dogs. J Am Vet Med Assoc. 1985;187(1):76.

11. Sterna J, Burzykowski T. Assessment of the usefulness of the fenestration method in cases of disc extrusion in the cervical and thoraco-lumbar spine in chondrodystrophic dogs. Pol J Vet Sci. 2008; 11(1):55–62.

12. Knapp D, Pope E, Hewett J, Bojrab M. A retrospective study of thoracolumbar disk fenestration in dogs using a ventral approach: 160 cases (1976 to 1986). J Am Anim Hosp Assoc. 1990;26(5):543–9.

13. Sharp NJH, Wheeler SJ. Small Animal Spinal Disorders: Diagnosis and Surgery. 2nd ed. Edinburgh: Elsevier; 2005.

14. Holmberg D, Palmer N, VanPelt D, Willan A. A comparison of manual and power-assisted thoracolumbar disc fenestration in dogs. Vet Surg. 1990; 19(5):323–7.

15. Shores A, Cechner P, Cantwell H, Wheaton L, Carlton W. Structural changes in thoracolumbar disks following lateral fenestration: a study of the radiographic, histologic, and histochemical changes in the chondrodystrophoid dog. Vet Surg. 1985; 14(2):117–23.

16. Stigen Ø, Ottesen N, Jäderlund KH. Early recurrence of thoracolumbar intervertebral disc extrusion after surgical decompression: a report of three cases. Acta Vet Scand. 2010;52(1):10.

17. Wagner SD, Ferguson HR, Leipold H, Guffy MM, Butler HC. Radiographic and histologic changes after thoracolumbar disc curettage. Vet Surg. 1987; 16(1):65–9.

18. Forterre F, Konar M, Spreng D, Jaggy A, Lang J. Influence of intervertebral disc fenestration at the herniation site in association with hemilaminectomy on recurrence in chondrodystrophic dogs with thoracolumbar disc disease: a prospective MRI study. Vet Surg. 2008;37(4):399–405.

19. Morelius M, Bergadano A, Spreng D, Schawalder P, Doherr M, Forterre F. Influence of surgical approach on the efficacy of the intervertebral disk fenestration: a cadaveric study. J Small Anim Pract. 2007; 48(2):87–92.

20. Forterre F, Dickomeit M, Senn D, Gorgas D, Spreng D. Microfenestration using the CUSA excel ultrasonic aspiration system in chondrodystrophic dogs with thoracolumbar disk extrusion: a descriptive cadaveric and clinical study. Vet Surg. 2011; 40(1):34–9.

21. Rohdin C, Jeserevic J, Viitmaa R, Cizinauskas S. Prevalence of radiographic detectable intervertebral disc calcifications in Dachshunds surgically treated for disc extrusion. Acta Vet Scand. 2010;52(1):24.

22. Bos AS, Brisson BA, Nykamp SG, Poma R, Foster RA. Accuracy, intermethod agreement, and inter-reviewer agreement for use of magnetic resonance imaging and myelography in small-breed dogs with naturally occurring first-time intervertebral disk extrusion. J Am Vet Med Assoc. 2012;240(8):969–77.

23. Scott HW. Hemilaminectomy for the treatment of thoracolumbar disc disease in the dog: a follow-up study of 40 cases. J Small Anim Pract. 1997 Nov; 38(11):488–94.

24. Bartels K, Creed J, Yturraspe D. Complications associated with the dorsolateral muscle-separating approach for thoracolumbar disk fenestration in the dog. J Am Vet Med Assoc. 1983;183(10):1081.

25. Sterna J, Burzykowski T. Assessment of the usefulness of the fenestration method in cases of disc extrusion in the cervical and thoraco-lumbar spine in chondrodystrophic dogs. Pol J Vet Sci. 2008;11(1):55.

26. Aikawa T, Fujita H, Shibata M, Takahashi T. Recurrent thoracolumbar intervertebral disc extrusion after hemilaminectomy and concomitant prophylactic fenestration in 662 chondrodystrophic dogs. Vet Surg. 2012 Apr;41(3):381–90.

27. Brisson BA, Holmberg DL, Parent J, Sears WC, Wick SE. Comparison of the effect of single-site and multiple-site disk fenestration on the rate of recurrence of thoracolumbar intervertebral disk herniation in dogs. J Am Vet Med Assoc. 2011 Jun 15;238(12):1593–600.

28. Brisson BA, Moffatt SL, Swayne SL, Parent JM. Recurrence of thoracolumbar intervertebral disk extrusion in chondrodystrophic dogs after surgical decompression with or without prophylactic fenestration: 265 cases (1995–1999). J Am Vet Med Assoc. 2004 Jun 1;224(11):1808–14.

29. Black A. Lateral spinal decompression in the dog: a review of 39 cases. J Small Anim Pract. 1988; 29(9):581–8.

30. Hoerlein BF. The treatment of intervertebral disc protrusion in the dog. Proceedings of the American Veterinary Medical Association. Atlantic City, NJ, USA. 1952; pp. 206–12.

31. Dhupa S, Glickman N, Waters DJ. Reoperative neurosurgery in dogs with thoracolumbar disc disease. Vet Surg. 1999;28(6):421–8.

32. Mayhew PD, McLear RC, Ziemer LS, Culp WT, Russell KN, Shofer FS, et al. Risk factors for recurrence of clinical signs associated with thoracolumbar intervertebral disk herniation in dogs: 229 cases (1994–2000). J Am Vet Med Assoc. 2004;225(8):1231–6.

36 Pros and Cons of Prophylactic Fenestration: The Potential Arguments Against

Franck Forterre and James M. Fingeroth

Fenestration is a well-known method to attempt prevention of recurrent disc extrusion in small-breed dogs and thus possibly avoid morbidity, costs, and potential choice of euthanasia for dogs affected a second or more time after initial decompressive surgery. The decreased rate of recurrence after prophylactic fenestration shown in recent studies seems to justify its consideration as an adjunctive treatment of first-time intervertebral disc extrusion [1]. However, there are some factors that the veterinary surgeon has to consider when contemplating adding fenestration of remote discs concomitant with decompression of a herniated disc.

Nonherniated intervertebral discs should not only be considered as potential sites of future extrusions but also as important spinal stabilizers. Fenestration of healthy discs not only accelerates degeneration within the fenestrated discs but also affects the spinal biomechanics (see Chapter 2). There are already some controversies as to whether stabilization should be considered after conventional decompressive surgery for disc herniation, and this deserves even more consideration if

multiple adjacent levels of the vertebral column undergo fenestration and discectomy [2–4]. Although serious, clinically apparent repercussions have rarely been described after fenestration, the main goal of surgery should be to preserve function of healthy structures. Therefore, one should consider whether to routinely fenestrate **all** discs within a certain zone cranial and caudal to the site of decompression or selectively fenestrate only those discs that have imaging characteristics suggestive of degeneration *and* high potential for clinically significant herniation in the future. In this regard, the most documented risk appears to be with nonherniated discs where the nucleus pulposus is densely mineralized but there has not yet been any disc space narrowing [5] (Figure 36.1). These "plump" discs do seem more likely to become herniated at a subsequent point than those discs that have degenerated with mineralization, disc space collapse, and noncompressive herniation. The latter discs, although often the most common finding on plain radiographs, may have already reached a stage of degeneration that is less prone to future displacement of disc material into

Advances in Intervertebral Disc Disease in Dogs and Cats, First Edition. Edited by James M. Fingeroth and William B. Thomas.
© 2015 ACVS Foundation. Published 2015 by John Wiley & Sons, Inc.

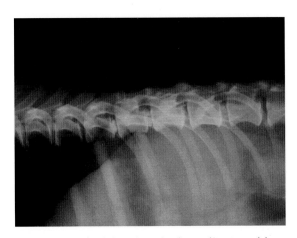

Figure 36.1 Coned-down lateral radiographic view of the thoracolumbar junction region of a chondrodystrophic dog's spine. Note the mineralization of the nucleus pulposus of the intervertebral discs at T10–T11, T11–T12, and T13–L1 and the absence of associated disc space collapse. None of these discs are currently herniated (verified with advanced imaging), reinforcing the importance of distinguishing disc *disease/degeneration* from disc *herniation*. Note also that there is collapse of the disc space at T12–T13, with absent mineralization. On advanced imaging, this was confirmed to be the site of clinically relevant herniation. However, in the dachshund breed in particular (and less well documented in other chondrodystrophic breeds), the mineralized discs without collapse represent a risk for subsequent herniation (as compared with mineralized discs where disc space narrowing has already occurred), and images such as this would justify consideration of prophylactic treatment of the nonherniated discs in conjunction with therapeutic decompressive surgery at the herniated level.

the vertebral canal. Fenestration of these discs may have less prophylactic value than anticipated.

The risk of recurrence is also different between canine breeds, and the definition of recurrence varies in the literature. In some publications, recurrence is defined as any new signs of neck or back pain (with or without neurologic deficits and with or without proving a disc-based cause), while in others it might include only patients with neurologic deficits but without documentation of compressive lesions [6–11]. It is also important to remember that recurrent signs in dogs that have not previously undergone decompressive surgery do not imply that each episode of clinical signs is due to a new disc level. More common, in our opinion, is recurrence of signs associated with the *same* disc undergoing sequential episodes of herniation. The most meaningful statistic for helping

decide the value of fenestration is the number of dogs with documented new compression at a level not previously treated with decompression surgery, and for which decompressive surgery would be recommended again based on associated signs. Very few studies address this key question. If we had more reliable statistics concerning the rate of recurrent surgical lesions and about recurrence rates after prophylactic fenestration, it would be possible to use formal decision analysis to determine the cost–benefit ratio of fenestration versus not fenestrating in dogs with first-time decompression surgery. Based on published studies, it appears that fenestration can be justified for adjacent degenerated discs in dachshunds, which appear to have an increased risk for recurrence (10 times higher than in other breeds) [12, 13], but might be considered as overtreatment in breeds only sparsely affected by intervertebral disc extrusion or chondrodystrophoid breeds in which the recurrence rate is much lower than in dachshunds. An important concept to bear in mind is the ratio of *degenerated* discs to *herniated* discs, and of the latter, the number that produce signs that warrant surgical decompression. Studies in chondrodystrophoid dogs reveal extensive and early onset disc degeneration throughout the vertebral column (see Chapters 1, 5, and 18). If one multiplied the number of degenerated discs at typical vulnerable levels in the neck and back in these dogs by the number of dogs in these breeds, it is clear that there are many, many more vulnerable and degenerated discs than there are patients who ultimately are presented to veterinarians because of signs related to disc herniation. Hence, even though we easily conjure "breeds at risk," it is apparent that in actuality, very few of the individual members of any particular breed ever require medical or surgical treatment for intervertebral disc disease. This raises the question of whether dogs with a prior documented disc herniation that required treatment are at a higher risk for subsequent discs herniating, and necessitating treatment. It also raises the question of whether clinical disc herniation is a familial problem more than a breed problem. If individual or closely related dogs had a higher risk than all dogs within a particular breed, it would be greater justification for considering prophylactic fenestration not only in a dog undergoing decompression but also possibly for as yet asymptomatic close relatives (see Chapter 37). However, absent knowledge about whether an affected individual or close relatives have an increased risk, the routine use of fenestration, especially in nondachshunds, means that many more discs and dogs are being subjected to additional surgery than were ever going to have a clinically significant problem with those discs. The philosophical question for the surgeon is whether to subject, say, 100 dogs to a surgery (fenestration) that might only be helpful in perhaps 5 of those dogs, knowing too that in those 5 dogs fenestration may yet not be 100% effective in preventing a future herniation and recommendation for surgery. On the other hand, the argument favoring fenestration would counter that the implications of recurrence can be devastating (both because of neurologic consequences as well as client unwillingness or inability to pursue a second major disc operation), and so, if fenestration can be done without significant added morbidity and cost for the 95% of dogs in whom it was not going to be helpful, and it perhaps saves a few dogs from a second, potentially catastrophic recurrence, it is reasonable to do it in all dogs deemed at risk.

The number of discs to be fenestrated will affect the dimensions of the surgical approach and will subsequently lead to increased soft tissue trauma. In a time where keyhole and minimally invasive surgery becomes more and more trendy, it might be considered paradoxical to enlarge a surgical incision and perform more extensive dissection to get access to discs that might or might not extrude. Is the greater amount of soft tissue injury caused in balance with the potential advantages brought by fenestration? Here again, we lack some of the key statistics that would permit mathematical analysis of the pros and cons. Even after extended fenestrations, a recurrence risk still exists, albeit lower [1, 3]. As no operation is foolproof, it is inherent that some fenestrated discs may yet still suffer herniation requiring treatment and also that nonfenestrated discs beyond the sites of fenestration may develop an increased risk for herniation, owing to altered biomechanical forces after fenestration of multiple levels cranial to them. It has been demonstrated that fenestration is seldom complete and that parts of the nucleus pulposus will remain in place [14, 15]. Further if a disc extrusion occurred in the thoracolumbar region, a recurrence is always possible either in the cervical

and/or in the lumbar spine caudal to L3, since these sites are not routinely fenestrated in conjunction with a thoracolumbar decompressive procedure. Recently, some efforts have been made to reduce the soft tissue injury associated with fenestration using minimally invasive techniques (see Chapters 37 and 39). However, these soft tissue sparing methods are not widely available at the present time, and a conventional approach remains the rule in most cases.

Fenestration of intervertebral discs prolongs surgery and anesthesia duration. This potentially leads to increased treatment costs and also to an increased risk of complications. It is well established that prolonged anesthesia associated with extended soft tissue injury is a common predisposing factor for the development of postsurgical infections. Discospondylitis following fenestration described in early reports [6, 16] is still seen on occasion (Fingeroth, personal observation) and may confirm this theory. At each fenestration site, the spinal nerve and radicular artery are located close to the surgical site and thus are vulnerable to iatrogenic injury. In the thoracolumbar area, these iatrogenic lesions could remain occult, without visible deleterious clinical consequences except muscle atrophy of the multifidus muscle in some cases, and/or flaccidity of the abdominal wall. However, in the lumbar area caudal to L3, a persistent lameness or paresis might result from nerve root trauma. In the caudal thoracic region, inadvertent opening of the thoracic cavity during fenestration might lead to pneumothorax. There is also some potential risk to the great vessels (aorta and caudal vena cava) from overly aggressive or inadvertent manipulations with instruments during fenestration. While most of these complications are rare, they nonetheless have to be considered, and thus, it has to be remembered that fenestration is not always an innocuous procedure with no potential downsides.

References

1. Brisson BA, Holmberg DL, Parent J, Sears WC, Wick SE. Comparison of the effect of single-site and multiple-site disk fenestration on the rate of recurrence of thoracolumbar intervertebral disk herniation in dogs. J Am Vet Med Assoc. 2011 Jun 15;238(12):1593–600.
2. Shires P, Waldron D, Hedlund C, Blass C, Massoudi L. A biomechanical study of rotational instability in

unaltered and surgically altered canine thoracolumbar vertebral motion units. Prog Vet Neurol. 1991;2:16–14.

3. Aikawa T, Fujita H, Shibata M, Takahashi T. Recurrent thoracolumbar intervertebral disc extrusion after hemilaminectomy and concomitant prophylactic fenestration in 662 chondrodystrophic dogs. Vet Surg. 2012;41(3):381–90.

4. Aikawa T, Shibata M, Sadahiro S. Hemilaminectomy and vertebral stabilization for thoracolumbar intervertebral disc associated dynamic compression in 11 dogs. Vet Comp Orthop Traumatol 2013; 26:498–504.

5. Mayhew PD, McLear RC, Ziemer LS, Culp WT, Russell KN, Shofer FS, *et al.* Risk factors for recurrence of clinical signs associated with thoracolumbar intervertebral disk herniation in dogs: 229 cases (1994–2000). J Am Vet Med Assoc. 2004;225(8):1231–6.

6. Funkquist B. Investigations of the therapeutic and prophylactic effects of disc evacuation in cases of thoraco-lumbar herniated discs in dogs. Acta Vet Scand. 1978;19(3):441–57.

7. Knapp D, Pope E, Hewett J, Bojrab M. A retrospective study of thoracolumbar disk fenestration in dogs using a ventral approach: 160 cases (1976 to 1986). J Am Anim Hosp Assoc. 1990;26(5):543–9.

8. Levine S, Caywood D. Recurrence of neurological deficits in dogs treated for thoracolumbar disk disease. J Am Anim Hosp Assoc. 1984;20:889–94.

9. Davies J, Sharp N. A comparison of conservative treatment and fenestration for thoracolumbar intervertebral disc disease in the dog. J Small Anim Pract. 1983;24(12):721–9.

10. Funkquist B. Decompressive laminectomy in thoraco-lumbar disc protrusion with paraplegia in the dog. J Small Anim Pract. 1970;11(7):445–51.

11. Black A. Lateral spinal decompression in the dog: a review of 39 cases. J Small Anim Pract. 1988;29(9):581–8.

12. Brisson BA, Moffatt SL, Swayne SL, Parent JM. Recurrence of thoracolumbar intervertebral disk extrusion in chondrodystrophic dogs after surgical decompression with or without prophylactic fenestration: 265 cases (1995–1999). J Am Vet Med Assoc. 2004 Jun 1;224(11):1808–14.

13. Dhupa S, Glickman N, Waters DJ. Reoperative neurosurgery in dogs with thoracolumbar disc disease. Vet Surg. 1999;28(6):421–8.

14. Holmberg D, Palmer N, VanPelt D, Willan A. A comparison of manual and power-assisted thoracolumbar disc fenestration in dogs. Vet Surg. 1990;19(5):323–7.

15. Morelius M, Bergadano A, Spreng D, Schawalder P, Doherr M, Forterre F. Influence of surgical approach on the efficacy of the intervertebral disk fenestration: a cadaveric study. J Small Anim Pract. 2007;48(2):87–92.

16. Hoerlein BF. The treatment of intervertebral disc protrusion in the dog. Proceedings of the American Veterinary Medical Association. 1952. pp. 206–12.

37 Use of Lasers in Veterinary Surgery and Percutaneous Laser Disc Ablation

Kenneth Bartels

Introduction

Lasers for neurosurgery include both high-power surgical lasers for incisional/ablative procedures (i.e., carbon dioxide ($CO_2 - \lambda = 10.6\,\mu m$)), neodymium–yttrium aluminum garnet (Nd:YAG $- \lambda = 1.064\,\mu m$), diode ($\lambda = .805/.980\,\mu m$), holmium–yttrium aluminum garnet (Ho:YAG $- \lambda = 2.1\,\mu m$), as well as low-level lasers for rehabilitative therapy. Carbon dioxide lasers, used for soft tissue surgical approaches to the spine, have the advantages of decreasing hemorrhage by photocoagulating small blood vessels and decreasing pain and inflammation by photothermal coagulation/sealing of nerves and lymphatics. Concurrently, when used correctly considering wavelength and laser–tissue interaction, the CO_2 laser can potentially provide exquisite control for dissection and photoablation of tissue. Control of laser energy has also enabled the application of photothermal tissue welding using various organic solders that enhance weld strength of both blood vessels and peripheral nerves [1].

Fiber-delivered high-power lasers, including the Nd:YAG, diode, and Ho:YAG lasers, are used for tissue ablation/photocoagulation as well as for endoscopic or stereotactic applications [1]. Minimally invasive procedures include percutaneous laser ablation of the nucleus pulposus of intervertebral discs [2, 3].

Photodynamic therapy (PDT) utilizes laser energy of varying low-level power and wavelengths (visible to near infrared), as well as broader-band light sources such as light-emitting diodes (LEDs), to initiate a photochemotherapeutic action. A photosensitizer, such as a porphyrin compound, is coupled with the light source and specifically targets pathologic tissue using systemic or intralesional injections to release singlet oxygen as a toxic substance, especially for intracranial tumors in human patients.

This chapter will concentrate on the use of the Ho:YAG for intervertebral disc ablation and attempt to outline efficacy as well as results of the current protocol. There will also be a brief

Advances in Intervertebral Disc Disease in Dogs and Cats, First Edition. Edited by James M. Fingeroth and William B. Thomas.
© 2015 ACVS Foundation. Published 2015 by John Wiley & Sons, Inc.

discussion regarding the use of low-level lasers for rehabilitation of the neurologic patient.

Percutaneous laser disc ablation

Appropriate and accurate neurologic evaluation coupled with proper treatment, both medical and surgical, for intervertebral disc herniation has been well described [4]. The use of disc fenestration as a definitive therapeutic procedure for disc displacement cannot be recommended [5–7] (see Chapters 18 and 35). Most veterinarians recognize that fenestration deserves a very restricted role in neurosurgical management of dogs with acute neurological signs. Some surgeons are reluctant to perform prophylactic fenestration, either simultaneously with decompression or at a later date as a separate surgical procedure, since a prolonged or additional surgical procedure presents opportunity for potential postoperative complications [8] (see Chapter 36). Another question that must be answered is the effectiveness of fenestration in preventing recurrence of disc displacement. In evaluating literature and establishing evidence-based conclusions, it is apparent that efficacy will continue to be questioned until objective effectiveness is established involving prospective evaluation to determine whether fenestration is truly successful in preventing future disc displacement [9] (see Chapters 35 and 36). Although prophylactic fenestration was reported to be successful in preventing future disc extrusions at fenestrated sites, the presumption that there could be an increase in disc displacement at adjacent, non-fenestrated sites was also considered possible. It was also concluded that multiple-site disc fenestration decreased the rate of recurrent intervertebral disc disease (IVDD) in small-breed dogs when compared to use of single-site fenestration [9]. With increased emphasis toward minimally invasive techniques that may reduce costs, decrease operative time, and improve patient care, minimally invasive prophylactic percutaneous laser discectomy at multiple disc sites is an alternative to surgical fenestration. The procedure has the potential for reduced complications associated with open surgery and to reduce recurrence for future disc displacement in the thoracolumbar (TL) area (T10–T11 to L4–L5) [2, 3]. A percutaneous approach for photothermal ablation or vaporization

of the nucleus pulposus in lumbar discs by use of laser energy has been reported as a treatment of IVDD in human patients since 1975 [10–13]. The U.S. Food and Drug Administration has approved the Nd:YAG ($\lambda = 1064\,\mu m$), frequency-doubled Nd:YAG (KTP/potassium titanyl phosphate – $\lambda = 0.532\,\mu m$), and Ho:YAG ($\lambda = 2.1\,\mu m$) lasers for use in intervertebral disc surgery [10–13]. Erbium–yttrium aluminum garnet (Er:YAG – $\lambda = 2.8\,\mu m$) and carbon dioxide lasers ($\lambda = 10.6\,\mu m$) have also been used experimentally, but with difficulty since transmission of the respective wavelengths through optical fibers is not possible or extremely restricted because of technologic limitations. Excimer laser ($\lambda = 0.308\,\mu m$) has also been evaluated experimentally for use in laser discectomy [14]. The diode laser (($\lambda = 805\,nm$) coupled with indocyanine green (ICG) as a wavelength-specific chromophore has also been advocated as a method for percutaneous laser disc ablation (PLDA) in the canine model [15].

The Ho:YAG laser has advantages over other approved lasers [16–18]. The Ho:YAG wavelength is strongly absorbed by water, so depth of tissue penetration is limited, and zones of necrosis and collateral thermal effects are minimized because of the high water content of the nucleus pulposus. The Ho:YAG laser is also a pulsed laser (5–12 Hz), which allows cooling of tissue between pulses, potentially limiting tissue damage through a thermorelaxation phenomenon [19]. However, since the Ho:YAG laser operated at ambient room temperature is a pulsed laser, energy delivery elicits a photoacoustic or photomechanical effect which is problematic in potentially forcing additional disc material dorsally through the annulus fibrosus into the vertebral canal [20]. Finally, due to the solid state construction, portability, ruggedness, and ease of operation of most Ho:YAG laser systems, they become attractive for clinical application.

As mentioned previously, studies using laser for discectomy in human patients focused on minimally invasive techniques that avoid damage to surrounding structures but still achieved ablation of the nucleus pulposus. Proponents of laser discectomy claim positive results in human patients that are related to a decrease in intradiscal pressure caused by a decrease in volume of the nucleus pulposus after ablation [21]. Further disc extrusion can also be prevented, although disc ablation is not effective for sequestered disc fragments [22].

Using the dog as a model, investigators have reported that acute and chronic histopathologic effects of PLDA on neighboring tissue are minimal [23]. In a more recent study, depending on the total energy applied during disc ablation, extensive photothermal damage can occur to cells of the nucleus pulposus which would be irreversible, but with lower energy/fluency levels based on *in vitro* studies, proteoglycan matrix synthesis may be promoted sufficiently to activate self-repair ability of the tissues [24]. Moreover, to improve accuracy and safety of needle placement, endoscopy, fluoroscopy, computerized tomography, and magnetic resonance imaging have been used to assess the precise location of laser fibers during percutaneous placement, which potentially minimizes intraoperative trauma [25, 26].

Technique for PLDA in dogs

PLDA was initiated at Oklahoma State in 1992, using the canine model for determining potential adverse effects of the procedure when applied to human patients. Successful completion of the preliminary research project illustrated that percutaneous placement was possible in the TL area via a left dorsolateral approach in the dog [2, 3, 27]. Initially, a uniplanar fluoroscopic interventional radiology technique was employed. Later, a portable C-arm unit was used for percutaneous needle placement, which allowed the procedure to be performed aseptically in a surgery suite. This modification also allowed PLDA concurrently with a decompressive surgical procedure when indicated.

Dogs are currently included in the Oklahoma State clinical protocol when they have a documented history of TL disc herniation and have recovered from either medical or surgical treatment. That is, they exhibit no neurologic abnormalities including lumbar pain, and ambulate normally. If a dog is presented with only lumbar pain and confirmed to have TL disc herniation through physical/neurologic and radiographic examination, usually confirmed with myelographic evaluation or computerized tomography (CT), it is treated conservatively for at least 2 weeks prior to laser disc ablation. If at any time the patient deteriorates neurologically, decompression and removal of the extruded disc are performed on an emergent basis after definitive localization of the lesion. Dogs included in the PLDA protocol are not administered oral or parenteral glucocorticoids for a minimum of 2 weeks prior to disc ablation.

Acceptable candidates for PLDA undergo a presurgical evaluation that includes general physical and neurologic examinations, hematologic and serum biochemical analyses, and urinalysis. The dog is anesthetized and the hair on the left TL area is clipped from the caudal dorsocervical to the lumbosacral areas, and it is then aseptically prepared for surgery (Figure 37.1). Initially, the patient is placed in right lateral recumbency and fluoroscopic images from the portable C-arm are obtained. No repositioning of the dog is required when using the C-arm, which expedites the procedure in contrast to using the uniplanar technique on a radiology table (Figure 37.2). Lateral and dorsoventral views are obtained prior to and after needle insertion to ascertain potential anatomic variability of the spine and ascertain if there are any calcified intervertebral discs.

Using sterile technique, eight needles (20 gauge, 2.5 inch or 3.5 inch spinal needles) are placed percutaneously through the skin and epaxial musculature using a left dorsolateral approach. The spinal needle, with stylet in place, is carefully positioned through the annulus toward the nucleus of eight disc spaces (T10–T11 to L4–L5). Repeated 1–2 s, fluoroscopic images are taken to check position of the needle as it is advanced toward the disc. Palpation of the needle against bone and soft tissue is used to ascertain when the needle encounters the vertebral body or disc space. A characteristic soft, granular feel of the needle tip entering the annulus fibrosus is usually

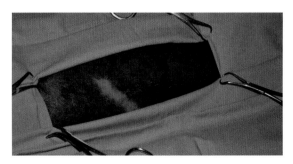

Figure 37.1 Percutaneous laser disc ablation myelographic needle insertion site (dorsolateral aspect) of left epaxial area aseptically prepared for minimally invasive approach.

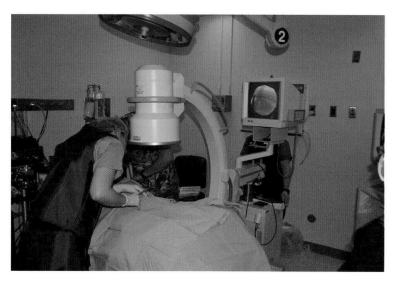

Figure 37.2   Surgery suite is prepared for use of C-arm fluoroscopic imaging of percutaneous placement of myelographic needles.

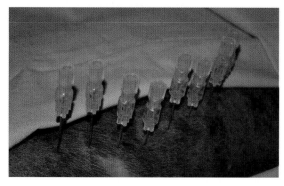

Figure 37.3   Eight 2.5 in. ×20 gauge myelographic needles have been inserted into intervertebral disc spaces T10–T11 to L4–L5 (8 total spaces).

detected, and the needle is advanced carefully into the peripheral border of the nucleus pulposus. Entry of the needle into the nucleus often is accompanied by a slight extrusion of the needle stylet, attributable presumably to intradiscal pressure. Needles are placed sequentially into each disc from T10–T11 through L4–L5 (Figure 37.3). When needles are placed, the bevel of each tip is positioned, so it faces the center of the disc rather than the vertebral end plate. Insertion of spinal needles is often aided by use of a needle holder and digital manipulation to stabilize the needle near the hub. Both lateral and dorsoventral fluoroscopic images are examined and the image is recorded to ensure and document proper needle placement. That is,

the tip of the needle enters the lateral aspect of the annulus fibrosus and penetrates no further than the approximate peripheral one-third of the nucleus pulposus. Considering that the laser fiber extends no further than 1–2 mm beyond the beveled needle tip, precise needle placement permits a more defined ablation site with less concern for potential collateral photothermal tissue damage.

A reusable, sterile, cleaved 320 μm low-OH quartz optical fiber[1] is used for laser ablation of the nucleus pulposus. Prior to packaging and sterilization of the fiber using hydrogen peroxide gas plasma technology (Sterrad®), it is measured by placing it through the lumen of a similar spinal needle, and then the outside rubber cladding is removed using a fiber-optic stripper, so 2–3 mm of bare fiber extends beyond the end of the spinal needle; the remainder of the cladding encasing the fiber acts as a "stop" at the needle hub which ensures entry through the annulus and into the nucleus but prevents complete penetration of the disc space. The same fiber is used for the entire procedure, unless it is determined between applications that energy transmission is blocked due to fiber degradation/carbonization. Fiber viability is determined by viewing the spot size of the aiming beam (from the integral .632 μm helium–neon (He:Ne) laser) before each exposure. Between each insertion, the laser fiber is gently wiped with a

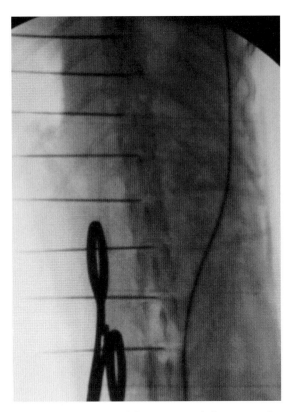

Figure 37.4 Dorsoventral fluoroscopic/radiologic view of eight disc spaces with correct placement of myelographic needles. Tips of needles are inserted through the annulus fibrosus and into the nucleus pulposus.

sterile, moistened gauze sponge to remove any carbonized tissue adhering to the fiber. If the He:Ne aiming beam is not visible or appears dim, or the fiber tip appears degraded (carbonized or broken), that fiber is replaced with another pre-packaged sterile fiber of proper length before proceeding to another disc site. The manufacturer's dedicated SMA fiber adapter is securely connected to the Ho:YAG laser.[2] The cleaved end of the laser fiber is inserted into each needle hub beginning at T10–T11. The precise position of each needle is rechecked fluoroscopically in both lateral and dorsoventral views prior to removal of the stylet and insertion of the laser fiber (Figure 37.4). The fiber is inserted and the Ho:YAG laser is activated for 40 s at 2 W of power and a 12 Hz repetition rate, resulting in a total energy dose of 80 J and a fluency of 10^5 J/cm^2 at the fiber tip (Figures 37.5 and 37.6).

After treatment at each site, needles are removed sequentially (Figure 37.7). Dogs are recovered from general anesthesia and observed for 24 h in the hospital. Discharge instructions include a recommendation of restricted activity for 2 weeks. It is recommended that animals be examined by the referring veterinarian if any postoperative complications develop including persistent lumbar pain or recurrent neurologic signs. Examination is performed on an emergent basis if the dog exhibits severe lumbar pain or paresis/paralysis of the pelvic limbs. Appropriate

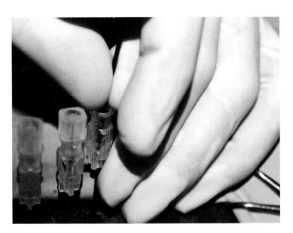

Figure 37.5 Ho:YAG laser fiber (320 μm diameter) is inserted through 20 gauge myelographic needle and annulus fibrosus so the fiber tip is located within 1–2 mm of center of nucleus pulposus. Laser fiber cladding trimmed to appropriate length acts as fiber "stop" at needle hub to prevent further fiber penetration beyond center of nucleus.

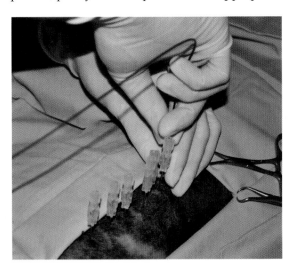

Figure 37.6 View of dorsolateral area of canine spinal area with multiple needle placement and laser fiber in place (T10–T11) for sequential ablation of nucleus pulposus of each disc (T10–T11 to L4–L5).

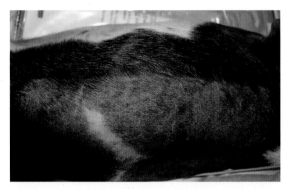

Figure 37.7   Immediate postoperative postablative view of percutaneous laser ablation sites.

surgical or medical treatment should immediately be considered based on neurologic signs.

Discussion of PLDA

To reiterate, TL laser disc ablation is not recommended as a therapeutic procedure for dogs suffering from acute, severe disc herniation. If attenuation of the spinal cord is confirmed with a myelogram, CT or MRI, a hemilaminectomy is recommended, depending on history, severity of clinical signs, and owner's decision. For dogs with less severe neurologic signs and treated by medical therapy alone, PLDA is not performed for a period of at least 2 weeks. The Ho:YAG laser used for this procedure is a pulsed laser (12 Hz) which produces a photomechanical effect that could potentially push more nuclear material through the dorsal annulus into the spinal canal, causing severe attenuation of the spinal cord. Allowing a period for fibrotic stabilization and decrease in inflammation is deemed appropriate based on previous clinical experience. In addition, glucocorticoid administration during the 2-week preoperative period is contraindicated since the potential for increased movement by ambulatory dogs is considered a risk for further disc herniation. Dogs that undergo decompressive surgery are disqualified as candidates for PLDA until a later date; usually until they are neurologically normal. Due to the severity of the neurologic signs that warrant a decompressive surgery, clinical impression has been to expedite the decompressive procedure and not to increase operative time by performing a PLDA, although PLDA operative time has

averaged approximately 30 min once the clinician is comfortable with the technique. Disc sites previously having undergone a hemilaminectomy are ablated in the same manner as nonoperated disc sites after the operative incision has healed and the dog has regained either normal neurologic status or is neurologically stable (no worse than minimal persistent proprioceptive deficits) for a period of approximately 4–6 months.

To date, only two "stand-alone" independent prophylactic PLDA procedures have been performed on dogs that have not had a previous history of TL intervertebral disc problems. These two patients were from the same litter of eight dachshund puppies in which six littermates had TL disc herniation requiring surgery. Although not statistically significant, to date (6 years post-PLDA), these two patients have not exhibited clinical signs attributable to TL disc herniation. The use of a totally prophylactic PLDA on potentially susceptible dogs (chondrodystrophic breeds with familial histories of disc herniation) could be reconsidered in the future *if* prospective studies prove the unequivocal efficacy of the procedure.

Preoperative imaging of the TL spine is performed to document any herniated calcified disc material and to provide retrospective information on recurrence rates of extrusion/protrusion of calcified discs. Previous retrospective studies revealed that recurrence rates of displaced discs associated with PLDA were related to disc calcification [3]. The efficiency of ablation varies from disc to disc due to differences in laser–tissue interaction. Different effects relating to laser–tissue interaction can result from interaction of laser wavelength and energy parameters coupled with the optical absorption characteristics of the disc material. A calcified nucleus pulposus could require different energy parameters compared to a noncalcified disc.

Initial fluency/power values (2 W/40 s/12 Hz, 320 μm fiber) were extrapolated from early *in vitro* work using a clear gelatin mixed with a pulverized calcium carbonate powder contained within a 15 × 60 mm culture plate to mimic an *in vitro* calcified disc as far as laser–tissue interaction. An ablative "lesion" was formed in the gelatin mold using various laser power settings, pulse lengths, and exposure times to minimize temperature change as well as lesion diameter (1–2 cm diameter). Once a baseline of parameters was established, a sequence of studies using thermocouples placed in the periphery of the annulus, on the floor of the vertebral canal, and in the spinal cord was initiated in a small group of dogs that included cadavers obtained from a pound and IACUC procedure approved animals evaluated using a terminal exploratory approach to the disc sites. This was done to ensure safety of the ablative procedure as well as verify grossly and histologically if the nucleus pulposus was either vaporized or photothermally coagulated without harming the periphery of the annulus pulposus and most certainly the spinal cord itself [23]. Even with over 500 PLDA procedures performed to date and a recurrence rate of approximately 4%, adequate ablation of the nucleus pulposus is still questioned, especially with discs that have undergone significant chondroid metaplasia.

Considering this presumption, current work involving an *in vitro* needle-based single-fiber spectroscopy to probe scattering changes associated with mineralization in canine intervertebral discs prior to disc ablation is being finalized. This evaluation will occur immediately prior to PLDA to ascertain potential changes in laser energy/fluency in order to effect a more complete and effective laser ablation technique for calcified discs. The procedure will be performed on a real-time basis using the same size percutaneously placed needle and a laser spectroscopy fiber identical in size/diameter to the fiber used for PLDA. Accordingly, after determination of water content (objective evaluation of disc calcification), Ho:YAG laser settings (power, time of exposure, total delivered energy) can be modified in the future to more effectively ablate calcified intervertebral discs [28].

Initially, intervertebral discs selected for PLDA were similar to those selected for surgical fenestration as originally described, except for the L4–L5 disc [29]. This site was not included in the initial clinical protocol because it was not included in the preliminary investigation designed to prove safety and efficacy of the procedure. Prevalence of disc herniation at L4–L5 is also reported to be lower, and a surgical approach to this disc space was initially thought to potentially cause postoperative complications due to iatrogenic trauma to the femoral nerve. As technical experience for needle placement occurred as well as the ease of the procedure using a C-arm for imaging, a protocol that includes the L4–L5 disc has been

implemented. Therefore, a total of eight discs (T10–T11 to L4–L5) now undergo PLDA. Retrospectively, no postoperative complications have occurred involving additional disc ablation of the L4–L5 disc.

PLDA can potentially be technically difficult to perform. A "learning curve" is expected, even when experienced interventional radiologists and surgeons perform the procedure. Prior to introduction of this procedure into a clinical setting, needle insertion and laser ablation should be performed progressing from cadavers to laboratory dogs. Discs at T10–T11 through T13–L1 may also be more difficult to approach due to the close proximity of the ribs. If any of the disc spaces designated for PLDA cannot be approached due to anatomic or technical difficulties, extrusion/protrusion of the unoperated disc can occur in the future. To date, however, with PLDA, there has not been an increased incidence of herniation of unoperated, adjacent discs [30–32]. Based on postablation imaging, an immobile or fused spine has not resulted from the PLDA procedure. Although the nucleus pulposus is targeted for ablation, the minimally invasive nature of PLDA from inserting a 20 gauge spinal needle through the annulus fibrosus reduces traumatic insult that potentially results from a more aggressive approach using a scalpel or other cutting instruments.

As mentioned, when needles are placed through the annulus and enter the nucleus pulposus, the bevel of each tip is positioned so it faces the center of the disc rather than the vertebral end plate. A report in the literature regarding PLDA in a human patient revealed that an improperly placed laser fiber allowed a photothermal change in the vertebral end plate [33]. This potential complication was also documented in the dog during an earlier study, but the associated subchondral changes were not associated with clinical abnormalities in either the human or canine patients [3].

Finally, as an isolated observation, PLDA performed in very small dogs (<2kg) with smaller intervertebral discs should be considered with care since the recommended laser fluency parameters is based on initial studies based on animals weighing more than 2kg. It will take additional work (thermal studies at the ablative sites) to determine if fluency settings need to be decreased in very small patients to ensure no potential collateral photothermal injury.

Clinical relevance of PLDA

Percutaneous Ho:YAG laser disc ablation is a minimally invasive technique developed to photothermally vaporize or coagulate the nucleus pulposus of intervertebral discs. With few complications, this technique potentially reduces the recurrence of disc herniation at ablated sites in at-risk dogs by preventing further herniation of nucleus pulposus from a partially herniated disc and reducing the chance of subsequent herniation of other discs at eight significant locations in the TL area (T10–T11 to L4–L5). PLDA is a minimally invasive technique that can be considered a positive extension of current therapeutic interventions to prevent catastrophic neurologic complications from extrusion/protrusion of the nucleus pulposus from ablated TL discs. Continued work is being performed to review additional cases on a retrospective basis. Results of this study are pending. PLDA of cervical discs has also been performed on a limited basis with satisfactory results.

Use of lasers in rehabilitation of the canine IVDD patient

Low-level laser devices are being advertised and used in multiple clinical settings as primary and secondary rehabilitative treatment modalities [34, 35]. Concern should be directed for use of low-level laser therapy (LLLT) as a means to treat acutely paralyzed dogs in lieu of conventional and proven surgical intervention with removal of the extruded disc. However, secondary spinal cord injury caused by biochemically ischemic related events could potentially be partially alleviated by adjunctive, safe, protocols that include appropriate pharmacologic treatment. Based mostly on anecdotal reports, nonpharmacologic methods including LLLT are being utilized for pain control, wound healing, and neuronal regeneration [34, 35]. LLLT has been studied for years in both Europe and the Pacific Rim and has received extensive attention in the United States when one application of LLLT was approved by the FDA (510(k) Number K012580: *"Lamp, Non-Heating, for Adjunctive Use in Pain Therapy,"* 2002). Since that time, many low-level laser devices (ANSI Z136.3 Classes 2–4/varying wavelengths and power) have been approved for limited use in human and veterinary

medicine. Their use has expanded tremendously in veterinary medicine for applications involving wound healing, pain amelioration, and nerve regeneration, as well as other less documented applications such as potential antibacterial effects [36–38]. A multitude of *in vitro* tissue culture as well as *in vivo* laboratory animal applications have been published, but very few projects have objectively targeted veterinary cases in clinical evaluations [34, 35]. LLLT is considered by most objective observers as an alternative therapy similar to acupuncture which is certainly accepted more and more by mainstream medicine as positive modes of therapy for specific applications.

Effects of LLLT as a treatment for IVDD are aimed at relief of acute and chronic pain by theoretically causing a reversible blockade of fast axonal flow and mitochondrial transport along nociceptive axons [39]. Long-term effects are attributed to neuromodulation of ascending and descending pain-associated pathways within the spinal cord [39]. Other studies cite laser therapy as a procedure preventing further degeneration of motor neurons, inciting higher metabolism within nerve cells, promoting myelination of nerves, and increasing axonal regeneration [40].

Current objective studies taking place in university veterinary hospitals (Colorado State University, Robinson *et al.*; Animal Medical Center, Shumway; University of Florida, Schubert *et al.*) [34, 35, 41] are directed toward clinical applications using LLLT as adjunctive rehabilitative therapy for dogs after TL decompressive procedures. Subjective results are reported to be positive.[3] It still must be realized that mechanisms of action for LLLT are mostly theoretical and need to be further investigated to maximize effectiveness. Selection of proper wavelengths and therapeutic parameters must be based on solid research and documented clinical observations.

Success for LLLT as adjunctive treatment for TL disc problems will be difficult to objectively assess since the different laser manufacturers have provided multiple ANSI classes of laser that include different laser wavelengths in their respective devices, varying pulse or continuous-wave modes of emission, and power/energy delivery differences (i.e., ANSI Z136.1 devices: Class 2a, Class 2, Class 2 M, Class 3a, Class 3R, Class 3B, Class 4). Each device is sold on the basis of being the most scientifically sound in theoretical application but there is still much objective work to be performed to recommend one particular device. It is essential that veterinarians using any laser device be cognizant of the safety requirements for both high-power and low-power lasers and follow guidelines delineated in the ANSI Z136.3 (2011): American National Standard for Safe Use of Lasers in Health Care [42]. The safety of their patients, technicians, and themselves depends on that understanding. The main objectives of any laser safety program, no matter what type or class of laser used, are to (i) establish a laser-safe operating area posted with proper warning signage; (ii) use protective eye wear appropriate for the specified laser wavelength for the operator, technician, and patient; and (iii) assure proper respiratory protection and evacuation of laser-generated airborne contaminants from the target area in the event that occurs with a Class 4 laser.

Conclusion

The use of lasers in neurosurgery is based on development of objective clinical techniques that enhance the veterinarian's ability to safely approach and control light energy, namely, monochromatic laser light. Understanding laser tissue interaction based on a device's wavelength, absorption characteristics, total available energy, mode of action and delivery, as well as safety can complement our profession or provide impediments to those just looking for a tool in search of another medical application to enhance income. The economics of any technology will always influence acceptance into veterinary medicine. This has been the case for advanced imaging, specialty surgical procedures, as well as the expense for advanced training. The use of laser for exquisitely controlled incisions and minimally invasive procedures such as PLDA can not only enhance patient care but augment income, especially if the procedure can be more thoroughly documented for efficacious treatment of cervical disc displacement as well as potentially used as adjunctive therapy for disc herniation in the lumbosacral area. Finally, more prospective work as well as additional advances in LLLT for neurologic rehabilitation and continued work

using PDT for tumors of the CNS will continue to aid in specifically targeting pathology when coupled with advances in diagnostic imaging.

Notes

1. Ho:YAG laser fiber: model H320R/Part # 9400-0310, 320 micron diameter silica core fiber jacketed with ethylene tetrafluoroethylene; SMA 905 connector.
2. Ho:YAG laser: model NS 1500, $\lambda = 2.1\,\mu m$, 12 W, New Star Lasers, 9085 Foothills Blvd., Roseville, CA, 95747.
3. Editor's comment: moreover, it cannot be ignored that many of the investigators of these and other "alternative" modalities are often biased themselves and approach their investigations not as skeptics, but often as *a priori* believers.

References

1. Krishnamurthy, S.; Powers, K.P. 1994. Lasers in neurosurgery. *Lasers Surg Med*, 15:126–167.
2. Dickey, D.T.; Bartels, K.E.; Henry, G.A.; Stair, E.L.; Schafer, S.A.; Fry, T.R.; Nordquist, R.E. 1996. Use of holmium yttrium aluminum garnet laser for percutaneous thoracolumbar intervertebral disk ablation in dogs. *JAVMA*, 208(8), April 15:1263–1267.
3. Bartels, K.E.; Higbee, R.G.; Bahr, R.J.; Galloway; D.S.; Healey, T.S.; Arnold, C. 2003. Outcome of and complications associated with prophylactic percutaneous laser disk ablation in dogs with thoracolumbar disk disease: 277 cases (1992–2001). *JAVMA*, 222(12), June 15:1733–1739.
4. Fingeroth, J.M. 1985. Fenestration – pros and cons. *Problems in Vet Med*, 1:445–465.
5. Brown, N.O.; Helphrey M.L.; Prata, R.G. 1977. Thoracolumbar disc disease in the dog: A retrospective analysis of 187 cases. *JAAHA*, 13:665–672.
6. Harrari, J.; Marks, S.L. 1985. Surgical treatments for intervertebral disc disease. *Vet Clin N Am*, 22: 899–915.
7. Prata, R.G. 1981. Neurosurgical treatment of thoracolumbar discs; The rationale and value of laminectomy and concomitant disc removal. *JAAHA*, 17:17–25.
8. Bartels, K.E.; Creed J.E.; Yturraspe, D.J. 1983. Complications associated with the dorsolateral muscle separating approach for thoracolumbar disk fenestration in the dog. *JAVMA*, 183:1081–1083.
9. Brisson, B.A.; Moffat, S.L.; Swayne, S.L.; Parent, J.M. 2004. Recurrence of thoracolumbar intervertebral disk extrusion in chondrodystrophic dogs after surgical decompression with or without prophylactic fenestration: 265 cases (1995–1999). *JAVMA*, 224(11), June 1:1808–1814.

10. Choy, D.S.L.; Ascher, P.W.; Ranu, H.S. 1992. Percutaneous laser disc decompression: A new therapeutic modality. *Spine*, 17:949–956.

11. Choy, D.S.J.; Case, R.B.; Fielding, W.; Hughes, J.; 1987. Percutaneous laser nucleolysis of lumbar discs. *N Engl J Med*, 317:771–772.

12. Choy, D.S.J.; Tassi, G.P.; Hellinger, J.; Hellinger, S.; Lee, S. 2009. Twenty-three years of percutaneous laser disc decompression (PLDD)—State of the art and future prospects. *Med Laser Applications*, 24: 147–157.

13. Sherk, H.H.; Black J.D.; Prodoehl, J.A. 1993. Laser diskectomy. *Orthopedics*, 16:573–576.

14. Wolgin, M.; Finkenberg, J.; Papaioannu, T. 1992. Excimer ablation of human intervertebral discs at 808 nm. *Lasers Surg Med*, 9:124–131.

15. Sato, M.; Ishihara, M.; Tsunenori, A.; Asazuma, T.; Kikuchi,T.; Hayashi, T.; Yamada, T.; Kikuchi, M.; Fujikawa, K. 2001. Use of a new ICG-dye-enhanced diode laser for percutaneous laser disc decompression. *Lasers Surg Med*, 29:282–287.

16. Dillingham, M.F.; Price, J.M.; Fanton, G.S. 1993. Holmium laser surgery. *Orthopedics*, 16:563–566.

17. Quigley, M.R.; Maroon, J.C. 1994. Laser discectomy: a review. *Spine*, 19: 53–56.

18. Mayer, H.M.; Brock, M.; Berlien, H.P. 1992. Percutaneous endoscopic laser discectomy (PELD): A new surgical technique for nonsequestered lumbar discs. *Acta Neurochir Suppl (Wien)*, 54, 53–58.

19. Jacques, S.L. 1992. Laser-tissue interactions: Photochemical, photothermal, and photomechanical. *Surg Clin N Am*, 72:531–558.

20. Spindel, M.L.; Moslem, A.; Bhatia, K.S. 1992. Comparison of holmium and flashlamp pumped dye lasers for use is lithotripsy of biliary calculi. *Lasers Surg Med*, 12:482–489.

21. Choy, D.S.L.; Altman P.; Liebler, W.A. 1992. Laser ablation of nucleus pulposus results in a marked fall of intradiscal pressure. *Am J Arthroscopy*, 11:15.

22. Mayer, H.M.; Brock, M. 1993. Percutaneous endoscopic discectomy: Surgical technique and preliminary results compared to microsurgical discectomy. *J Neurosurg*, 78:216–225.

23. Fry, T.R.; Bartels, K.E.; Henry, G.A. 1994. Holmium:YAG laser discectomy in dogs: A pilot study. *Biomed Opt*, 2128:42–48.

24. Sato, M.; Ishirhara, M.; Kiluchi, M.; Mochida, J. 2011. The influence of Ho:YAG laser radiation on intervertebral disc cells. *Lasers Surg Med*, 43:921–926.

25. Phillips, J.J.; Kopchock, G.E.; Peng, S. 1993. MR imaging of Ho:YAG laser diskectomy with histologic correlation. *JMRI*, 3:515–519.

26. Besalti, O.; Pekcan, Z.; Sirin, Y.; Sinan, E.G. 2006. Magnetic resonance imaging findings in dogs with thoracolumbar intervertebral disk disease: 69 cases (1997–2005). *JAVMA*, 228(6), March 15: 902–908.

27. Yturraspe, D.J.; Lumb, W.V. 1973. A dorsolateral approach for thoracolumbar intervertebral disk fenestration in the dog. *JAVMA*, 162:1037–1040.

28. Jiang, Y.; McKiernan, K; Piao, D.; Bartels, K.E. 2011. Feasibility of minimally invasive fiber based evaluation of chondrodystrophoid canine intervertebral discs by light absorption and scattering spectroscopy., *Proc. SPIE*, 7895, Optical Biopsy IX 789505.

29. Creed, J.E.; Yturraspe, D.J. 1983. Intervertebral disk fenestration. In: Bojrab, M.J. (ed.) *Current Techniques in Small Animal Surgery*. 2nd ed., 1983: 556–562. Philadelphia: Lea & Febiger.

30. Hill, T.P.; Lubbe, A.M., Guthrie, A.J. 2000. Lumbar spine stability following hemilaminectomy, pediculectomy, and fenestration. *Vet Comp Ortho Traumatol*, 13:165–171.

31. Brisson, B.A.; Holmberg, D.L.; Parent, J.; Sears, W.C; Wick, S.E. 2011. Comparison of the effect of single site and multiple-site disk fenestration on the rate of recurrence of thoracolumbar intervertebral disk herniation in dogs. *JAVMA*, 238(12), June 15:1593–1600.

32. Mayhew, P.D.; McLear, R.C.; Ziemer, L.S.; Culp, W.T.N.; Russell, K.N.; Schofer, F.S.; Kapatkin, A.S., Smith, G.S. 2004. Risk factors for recurrence of clinical signs associated with thoracolumbar intervertebral disk herniation in dogs: 229 cases (1994–2000). *JAVMA*, 225(8), Oct. 15:1231–1236.

33. Cvitanic, O.A.; Schimandle, J.; Casper, G.D.; Tirman, P.F. 2000. Subchondral marrow changes after laser discectomy in the lumbar spine: MR imaging findings and clinical correlation. *Am J Roentgenol*, 174(5), May:1363–1369.

34. Robinson, Narda G. Laser therapy may work on TL IVDD. *Veterinary Practice News*, March 2010.

35. Robinson, Narda G. Evidence based medicine: Non-surgical options for IVDD? Keeping hope, and dogs alive. *Veterinary Practice News*, June 2011.

36. Moges, H.; Wu, X.; McCoy, J.; Vasconcelos, O.; Olavo, M.; Bryant, H.; Grunberg, N.E.; Sanders, J.J. 2011. Effect of 810 nm light on nerve regeneration after autograft repair of severely injured rat median nerve. *Lasers Med Surg*, 43:901–906.

37. Silveira, P.C.L.; Streck, E.L.; Pinho, R.A. 2007. Evaluation of mitochondrial respiratory chain activity in wound healing by low level laser therapy. *J Photochem Photobiol*, 86:279–282.

38. Posten, W.; Wrone, D.A.; Dover, J.S.; Arndt, K.A.; Silapunt, S.; Alam, M.; 2005. Low-level laser therapy for wound healing: Mechanism and Efficacy. *Dermatol Surg*, 31:334–340.

39. Chow, R.T.; David, M.A.; Armati, P.J. 2007. 830 nm laser irradiation induces varicosity formation, reduces mitochondrial membrane potential and blocks fast axonal flow in small and medium diameter rat dorsal root ganglion neurons: implications for the analgesic effects of 830 nm laser. *J Peripheral Nervous System*, 12:28–39.

40. Rochkind, S.; Vogler, I.; Barr-Nea, L. 1990. Spinal cord response to laser treatment of injured peripheral nerve. *Spine*, 15(1):6–10.

41. Shumway, R. 2007. Rehabilitation in the first 48 hours after surgery. *Clin Tech Small Anim Pract*, 22(4), Nov:166–170.

42. American National Standard ANSI Z136.3 – 2011. *American National Standard for Safe Use of Lasers in Health Care*. Laser Institute of America 13501 Ingenuity Drive, Suite 128, Orlando, FL, 32826.

38 Physical Rehabilitation for the Paralyzed Patient

Rick Wall

Introduction

The discipline of physical rehabilitation is one of the recent additions to therapeutic protocol of the intervertebral disc disease patient. However, the paucity of veterinary literature combined with the absence of controlled scientific studies sometimes hampers its universal or widespread acceptance. Anecdotal observations and conclusions by experienced rehabilitation practitioners are currently the largest source of both information and therapeutic recommendations.

Primary care veterinarians and specialists accept that in adult dogs intervertebral disc herniation is considered to be one of the most common causes of spinal cord injury and subsequent neurologic deficits [1]. Education of veterinary professionals regarding rehabilitation will enhance their consideration for including formal physical therapy as part of the management of conservative nonsurgical and postoperative intervertebral disc herniation patients.

This chapter aims to assist veterinarians with understanding rehabilitation assessment of the intervertebral disc herniation patient, establishment of prognosis and goals, development of a patient rehabilitation program, and assessment of patient progress and outcome. This knowledge will assist the practitioner with the ability to promote rehabilitation services to their clients, with the possibility of improved patient outcomes.

Patient evaluation and establishment of a prognosis

Initial physical evaluation and a review of the clinical history are required to accurately suggest a prognosis and develop a specific rehabilitation program. The physical evaluation should involve a neurologic assessment, including urogenital function, evaluation for concomitant orthopedic problems, examination for general medical conditions, and an evaluation of patient discomfort.

Advances in Intervertebral Disc Disease in Dogs and Cats, First Edition. Edited by James M. Fingeroth and William B. Thomas.
© 2015 ACVS Foundation. Published 2015 by John Wiley & Sons, Inc.

Clinical history

In both conservatively managed and postoperative intervertebral disc herniation patients, the most important component of the clinical history used to shape prognosis is the subjective observation by the owner and/or referring veterinarian of changes in neurologic dysfunction since the onset of signs or since surgical intervention. Perceived improvements in ambulation, musculoskeletal strength, or voluntary motor activity of impaired limbs are considered very positive for the prognosis.

Neurologic examination

Voluntary motor activity or gait assessment if the patient is able to walk, proprioceptive positioning, and nociception are of importance in determining neurologic status. The Texas Spinal Cord Injury Score for dogs can be used to numerically score each limb (Table 38.1) [2]. The scale reflects the typical sequence after spinal cord injury of functional loss and recovery in gait, proprioceptive positioning, and nociception [3]. Video recordings of neurologic examination and ambulation can serve as a baseline reference of initial presenting status for comparison to future evaluations.

Table 38.1   Texas Spinal Cord Injury Score (TSCIS) for dogs

Gait
0 = no voluntary movement seen when supported
1 = intact limb protraction with no ground clearance
2 = intact limb protraction with inconsistent ground clearance
3 = intact limb protraction with consistent ground clearance (>75%)
4 = ambulatory, consistent ground clearance with moderate paresis–ataxia (will fall occasionally)
5 = ambulatory, consistent ground clearance with mild paresis–ataxia (does not fall, even on slick surfaces)
6 = normal gait

Proprioceptive positioning
0 = absent response
1 = delayed response
2 = normal response

Nociception
0 = no deep nociception
1 = intact deep nociception, no superficial nociception
2 = nociception present

Source: Levine *et al.* [2]. © Elsevier.

It must be understood, regardless of the severity of the spinal cord injury, that a diagnosis of intervertebral disc herniation is tentative and the prognosis may be guarded without further diagnostic information in those patients where only conservative treatment is being utilized.

Micturition

Micturition disorders are common in intervertebral disc herniation patients with spinal cord injury. These disorders are discussed elsewhere in this text (see Chapters 10, 22, and 27).

Pain examination

Discomfort in the intervertebral disc herniation patient is often a complex combination of injury to the spinal cord or nerve roots (referred to as neuropathic pain), myalgia, surgically induced trauma, and exacerbation of preexisting conditions such as osteoarthritis. Clinical history and careful examination to identify pain generators are necessary to develop a patient specific pain management protocol. This complex pain may not be controllable with any single pharmaceutical or modality. Therefore, a multimodal approach is preferred (see Chapter 24).

The use of gabapentin in combination with an opioid, nonsteroidal anti-inflammatory drug, or antidepressant has shown positive responses in the treatment of neuropathic pain in people [4]. Others reported a dramatic improvement in three dogs with presumed neuropathic pain treated with gabapentin or amitriptyline [5].

Goals of rehabilitation therapy

Establishment of realistic goals in the impaired intervertebral disc herniation patient provides the veterinary client with both a definition of success and an awareness of a potential therapeutic endpoint. Goals should focus on the reestablishment of ambulation and a level of musculoskeletal strength sufficient to provide a minimum level quality of life. This minimum level can be defined as the restoration of the patient's ability without assistance to secure nourishment (drink and eat) and complete eliminations (urination and defecation). When these minimum goals cannot be met, the patient will require prolonged or lifetime nursing care. A particular nursing task acceptable to some veterinary clients may, however, be impossible to maintain by others.

Development of a rehabilitation program

Following patient assessment and establishment of treatment goals, a rehabilitation therapy program should be designed. Therapy is focused on addressing neurologic dysfunction due to the spinal cord injury. The primary components include (i) passive and active range of motion exercise to maintain or improve proper joint and spinal range of motion; (ii) neurologic therapeutic exercises to increase both proprioceptive and kinesthetic awareness; (iii) therapeutic exercises to improve musculoskeletal strength, limit disuse atrophy, and strengthen core muscles; (iv) exercise to maintain or improve cardiovascular fitness; and (v) gait retraining.

Range of motion and stretching exercises

Range of motion and stretching exercises are defined as either passive (movement of the limb by the therapist) or active (movement of the limb by the patient with or without therapist assistance). Range of motion exercise takes a joint to its end range and/or patient awareness, and usually involves only flexion and extension. Stretching takes a joint to its end range and applying gentle pressure to hold the limb at that position. Both range of motion and stretching are usually performed with the patient in lateral recumbency in a quiet setting to promote relaxation. Spinal flexion and extension are more often performed with patient standing. An exception to this is in the quadriplegic patient.

In the early phase of care (immediately following an acute onset of signs in the conservatively managed patient or in the immediate postoperative period for surgically managed patients), only gentle passive range of motion exercise should be performed to limit pain induction. Stretching should not begin until acute pain begins to subside, usually several days following the acute onset of signs or surgery. In the distal aspects of

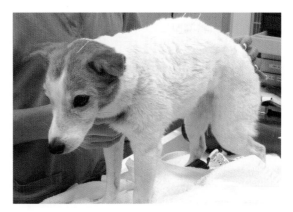

Figure 38.1 Kyphosis due to contracture of ventral paraspinal muscles.

the limbs, flexors overpower the extensors, and stretching becomes imperative in preventing contracture. It is best to perform 10–20 repetitions 2–3 times daily. Clients can easily be educated to perform these exercises.

Passive spinal stretching is critical in the postoperative thoracolumbar intervertebral disc herniation patient. Laminectomy traumatizes the dorsal paraspinal musculature and disturbs the structural integrity of the vertebral canal while leaving the antagonistic ventral paraspinal musculature largely unharmed. Pain and/or a nonambulatory status prevents normal active stretching of the ventral paraspinal musculature, often resulting in extreme contracture of these muscles and production of a kyphotic posture (Figure 38.1). This posture can become permanent if intervention does not begin early.

Passive spinal stretching is accomplished by placement of one hand between the pelvic limbs, ventral to pelvis, with the other hand on the dorsal thoracolumbar spine. Gentle downward pressure is applied on the spine, while upward pressure is applied on the pelvis (Figure 38.2). This stretch should be done carefully so as to never produce discomfort.

Therapeutic exercises

Many therapeutic exercises serve to address both neurologic dysfunction and musculoskeletal strength and therefore will be discussed together. Most of these exercises may be performed daily;

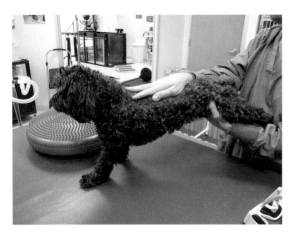

Figure 38.2   Spinal stretching by hyperextension of the spine combined with extension of coxofemoral joints to insure stretch of iliopsoas.

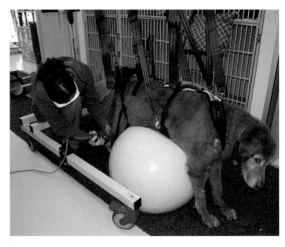

Figure 38.3   Body weight-supporting slings for the severe spinal cord injury.

however, the patient should be closely monitored for signs of fatigue.

Assisted standing exercises

Assistance can be partial to complete based on the severity of the clinical signs. Periods of standing assist in strengthening, stimulate proprioceptive awareness, improve circulation and respiration, provide an opportunity for elimination, and enhance the patient's psychological well-being [6]. Body slings can assist with standing and provide support to assist in maintenance of the position (Figures 38.3 and 38.4). Slings also serve to assist with stability as the patient begins to ambulate. All assisted standing exercise can be performed in water and benefit from the buoyancy and support of the water medium.

Proprioceptive awareness exercises

This group of exercises stimulates awareness of limb and body position. Movement of a portion or all of the body stimulates a counter or corrective movement. Proprioceptive receptors exist throughout the body in joints and muscles. Deficits in the distal aspects of the limb are often not reflective of more proximal areas. Therapeutic proprioceptive exercises may enhance the awareness of one area to compensate for the deficiency of a more distal area. These exercises may consist of simple weight shifting during assisted standing

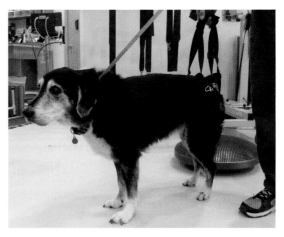

Figure 38.4   Pelvic limb slings to assist with ambulation in patients with pelvic limb paraparesis.

and the use of appliances such as balance boards (Figure 38.5) and balance cushions[1] (Figure 38.6).

Musculoskeletal maintenance and strengthening

Spinal cord injury resulting in lower motor neuron signs will result in rapid neurogenic atrophy of the muscles served by the affected spinal cord segment(s) and nerve root(s), and therapeutic exercises are of little benefit in reversing this. Neuromuscular electrical stimulation must be employed to limit muscular atrophy as much as possible in these

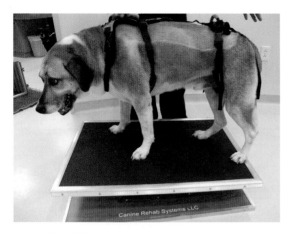

Figure 38.5   Balance board encourages muscle contraction and stimulates proprioceptive awareness.

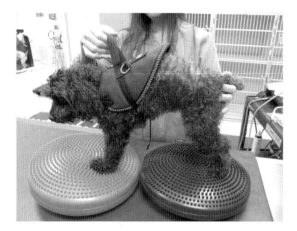

Figure 38.6   DynaDisc (air-filled disc) can be used to stimulate proprioceptive awareness and to strengthen core body muscles.

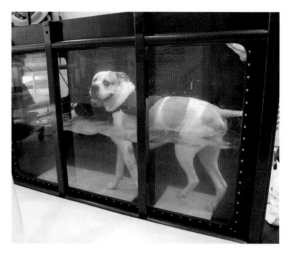

Figure 38.7   Buoyancy in underwater treadmill can allow the impaired patient to ambulate, providing exercise.

patients. Proper application of neuromuscular electrical stimulation requires advanced training to understand proper use of this modality.

Upper motor neuron paresis or paralysis results in less debilitating effects on the muscles. However, some of these patients have diminished voluntary musculoskeletal activity. Many of the same therapeutic exercises used to improve proprioceptive awareness also stimulate muscle activity and limit disuse atrophy. Musculoskeletal strength and muscle size are maintained or improved by exercises and/or manual stimulation that result in muscle contraction.

Activation of reflex activity can serve as therapy for muscles. Pinching of toes to stimulate the flexor withdrawal of the limb is an example. With improvement in neurologic function, more active exercises such as assisted walking and walking in the underwater treadmill result in improved strength.

Gait retraining

Gait retraining, a commonly used term in veterinary rehabilitation, is really just an extension of assisted walking. Communication limitations with the veterinary patient limit directing focus on the proper movement of the limb or body. The veterinary therapist must create an environment and provide assistance to promote as normal an ambulation as possible. Conversely, abnormal ambulation such as allowing the patient to move through its environment by dragging the pelvic limbs can be counterproductive and should be prevented.

An underwater treadmill promotes active exercise in a semicontrolled water medium (Figure 38.7). The buoyancy of the water counters diminished musculoskeletal strength and the warm water environment produces more proprioceptive awareness for the limbs and trunk. Water also slows movement allowing the impaired patient longer to make kinesthetic adjustments. Water level and treadmill speed can be adjusted to achieve optimum gait patterns. The underwater treadmill can allow the impaired patient to perform movement against gravity earlier in the course of therapy.

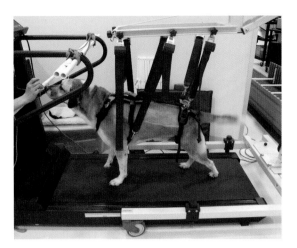

Figure 38.8   Body weight-supported treadmill provides a more controlled setting for the severely impaired patient.

A body weight-supported treadmill provides more control of gait, but does not provide as much proprioceptive stimulation as the underwater treadmill (Figure 38.8). The body weight-supported treadmill consists of a land treadmill capable of very slow speed (e.g., 0.1 mile/h) and a multiadjustable body sling attached to a hoist system. Body sling adjustments alter weight bearing allowing focused activity on thoracic or pelvic limbs, and treadmill speed is controlled for improved gait pattern. The therapist can assist in passive placement of the impaired limbs creating a patterning process.

As neurologic function improves, provide less assistance and challenge the patient with obstacles and varied terrain. This is always under the control of a leash attached to a harness system rather than a simple collar. Minimal holding of the tail will provide stability and improve gait if assistance is needed.

Assessment of patient outcome

Periodically assess the patient to document improvement. Neurologic examination, video assessment, and functional grading using the Texas Spinal Cord Injury Scale should be included in all reevaluations. The standard neurologic examination is perhaps the least accurate tool in determining progress. The absence of proprioception in the distal aspect of the limb does not account for the adaptation by other areas of the body to compensate for neurologic deficits. Comparison of voluntary motor activity and ambulation by video analysis, combined with individual limb scores derived from the Texas Spinal Cord Injury Scale, are more useful in assessing progress. Improvements based on the aforementioned serve to upgrade the prognosis and suggest recommendations for further rehabilitation therapy.

Carts

Several models of mobility carts ("wheelchairs") are available for dogs and cats. Most common are rear-wheel carts that utilize two wheels to support the pelvic limbs and are used for patients with paraparesis or paraplegia and strong thoracic limbs. Four-wheel carts support most of the patient's weight and are used for tetraparetic patients. The least commonly used design is a front-wheel cart that supports only the thoracic limbs and are used for patients with paresis or paralysis of the thoracic limbs and normal strength in the pelvic limbs. Benefits of carts are increased mobility and a sense of independence, urination and defecation in an upright posture, exercise of unaffected limbs and the cardiovascular system, and decreased risk of pressure sores from recumbency. Carts also allow proprioceptive feedback that aids gait retraining.

The most common indication for a cart is a patient with thoracolumbar disc extrusion resulting in long-term or permanent paraplegia. A cart is not used until the patient recovers from the acute phase of injury during which time it is important to restrict activity and minimize stress to the spine in order to minimize spinal pain, reduce the risk of further disc extrusion, and allow soft tissue healing in postoperative patients. It is also important to allow adequate time to determine if the patient will recover the ability to walk relatively soon; this avoids having the client purchase a cart only to find it is not necessary. Usually, a 6- to 8-week period is sufficient for initial recovery and assessment of long-term prognosis.

Proper fit and adjustment of the cart is essential to provide correct weight bearing and minimize risk of sores from ill-fitting supports. Initially, have the pet spend only a short period of time in the cart to allow the patient to become accustomed to the cart and develop endurance. With time, the patient is allowed to spend more time in the cart. However, the client must understand that the pet should always be supervised while in the cart because it is possible for the wheels to become caught on obstacles, the cart can tip over on uneven ground, and the pet may not be able to lie down to rest while in the cart. Also, the patient will need assistance to go over certain obstacles such as stairs or curbs.

Summary

Spinal cord injury due to intervertebral disc herniation is an all too common problem in the veterinary patient. Prior to the advent of veterinary rehabilitation therapy little hope was given when a rapid reversal in deficits induced by spinal cord injury did not occur spontaneously or in response to decompressive surgery. These patients were often euthanized or destined for a life in a cart. Veterinary rehabilitation now offers some of these patients more hope for recovery and return to a level of function that provides a better quality of life for them and for their owners.

Note

1. DynaDisc balance cushion, Physical Enterprise, Petaluma, CA, United States.

References

1. Sharp NJH, Wheeler SJ. Small Animal Spinal Disorders: Diagnosis and Surgery. 2nd ed. Edinburgh: Elsevier; 2005.
2. Levine GJ, Levine JM, Budke CM, Budke CM, Kerwin SC, Au J, *et al.* Description and repeatability of a newly developed spinal cord injury scale for dogs. Prev Vet Med. 2009;89:121–7.
3. Sharp NJ, Wheeler SJ. Functional anatomy. In: Sharp NJ, Wheeler SJ, editors. Small Animal Spinal Disorders. Philadelphia: Elsevier Mosby; 2005. pp. 1–17.
4. Vorobeychik Y, Gordin V, Mao J, Chen L. Combination therapy for neuropathic pain: a review of current evidence. CNS drugs. 2011 Dec 1;25(12):1023–34.
5. Cashmore RG, Harcourt-Brown TR, Freeman PM, Jeffery ND, Granger N. Clinical diagnosis and treatment of suspected neuropathic pain in three dogs. Aust Vet J. 2009 Jan–Feb;87(1):45–50.
6. Millis DL, Levine D. Canine Rehabilitation and Physical Therapy. 2nd ed. Philadelphia: Elsevier; 2013.

Section VI

Future Directions

In this final section, we look at some of the emerging technologies that may play a larger role in disc disease treatment in the future. It should be noted that neither here nor elsewhere in this text have we included discussions of so-called alternative therapies, ranging from acupuncture to chiropractic, from homeopathy to herbal medications, or any of the myriad other extant or developing interventions promulgated on both human and veterinary patients. While we realize that both our clientele and not a few of our colleagues have become enamored of such therapies, it is our duty to acknowledge that, despite years of research and great fortunes expended, none of these paradigms of therapy have been scientifically validated to provide benefit beyond either chance or placebo effect. And while we freely acknowledge that not all of the therapeutic interventions we *have* discussed in this text have climbed the pinnacle of evidence-based medicine validation, they at least have a solid scientific underpinning and *willingness to be refuted* by accepted scientific methods that evaluate their efficacy. Should future *valid* studies reveal a useful role for any of the abovementioned alternative disciplines, we will be delighted to include them in subsequent editions. In the meantime, we are guided by the words of Dr. Paul Offit at the Children's Hospital of Philadelphia, offering the benediction to those of us "who have dared proclaim that the emperors of pseudoscience have no clothes," and Dr. Joe Schwartz at McGill University, who observed, "There's a name for alternative medicines that work. It's called medicine."

39 Minimally Invasive Techniques for Spinal Cord and Nerve Root Decompression

Michael J. Higginbotham, Otto I. Lanz, and Claude Carozzo

Introduction

Innovation is an ongoing and evolving process in the field of surgery. Experience allows for more accurate incision placement, more precise dissection, and more skilled tissue manipulation. Accompanying this, the need for *wide* exposure diminishes. Minimally invasive techniques are widely accepted and routinely practiced in human neurosurgery. The trend toward less or minimally invasive surgery (MIS) has already been applied to several areas of veterinary surgery, including fracture repair, arthroscopy, thoracoscopy, and laparoscopy [1]. There have also been several MIS techniques recently described for veterinary neurosurgery.

We do not recommend complete abandonment of traditional, "open" surgical procedures as treatment for canine or feline disc herniation. It is much too premature to know whether these MIS techniques are necessarily better than traditional techniques. In this chapter, we will discuss the principles of MIS, introduce the concept of performing these, and review currently used MIS procedures employed in human and veterinary neurosurgery.

Principles of MIS

The ultimate goal of an MIS procedure is to accomplish the same surgical result as with traditional approaches but with better optical detail, less tissue trauma, and a smaller incision. As with any technique, there are indications and contraindications, as well as advantages and disadvantages.

There are few absolute indications for choosing MIS. However, severe dermatitis or the presence of other structural hindrances (e.g., tumor, scar tissue) may warrant a less invasive approach. Conversely, there are several, more straightforward, contraindications to MIS that must be considered. Hemodynamic instability, sepsis, coagulopathy, and inability to convert to an open procedure are all contraindications to proceeding with MIS [2].

The most commonly purported benefits to any MIS procedure include smaller incisions and less tissue dissection (and, therefore, presumably, less pain and inflammation), less perioperative bleeding, reduced need for postoperative analgesia, quicker and more complete recovery of

Advances in Intervertebral Disc Disease in Dogs and Cats, First Edition. Edited by James M. Fingeroth and William B. Thomas.
© 2015 ACVS Foundation. Published 2015 by John Wiley & Sons, Inc.

normal function, decreased infection rate, shorter hospitalization, less reliance on ancillary support services (e.g., physical rehabilitation), and improved cosmesis [3–5]. Objective data are somewhat limited and only available for some of the aforementioned benefits. Other benefits appear to be subjective or anecdotal in nature, and some benefits may only be apropos in humans.

While magnifying loupes or operating microscopes are sometimes used, most MIS procedures are "video assisted." This implies that an endoscope is used to provide visualization. Use of the video endoscope has several benefits. Besides the ease and speed of manipulation, technological advancements have led to stronger magnification, higher image quality, and stronger, more efficient illumination [6]. With endoscopy, the surgical site is viewed from a much closer perspective than that of the operating microscope. This eliminates the possibility of the surgeon's hands obscuring the surgical field. Also, use of a surgical microscope has the disadvantage of requiring the surgeon (or assistant) to make multiple, fine adjustments to the microscope during the procedure in order to explore the surgical field. Endoscopy does not require constant refocusing.

While there are many advantages to MIS, there are also equally important disadvantages to this form of surgery that must be considered. First, the smaller overall field of view can result in failure to protect vital structures or to recognize abnormalities that are not directly within the field. Second, there is inherent difficulty in translating the three-dimensional surgical field familiar to all surgeons into a two-dimensional surgical field viewed on a video monitor. Third, absence or alteration in traditional feedback signals is also an important drawback to MIS [7]. Surgeons constantly utilize information (e.g., tissue texture, consistency, adhesion, etc.) from the surgical environment to make continuous adjustments to their performance. These tactile sensations are lost or changed in the process of using longer and smaller instruments while watching on a viewing monitor.

Learning to perform MIS procedures

Several important points must be considered when determining when and how to learn to perform MIS procedures. First, we must consider when to implement this training. If these procedures are to be taught and practiced during a residency training program, care must be taken that adequate training in non-MIS surgery is not compromised [8]. Alternatively, if these procedures are to be taught as part of a postresidency continuing education program or in a "short-course" environment, adequate prerequisite skill and standardization of training must be ensured [7, 9].

While a detailed discussion of learning MIS is beyond the scope of this chapter, a few key points should be recognized. The skill needed to properly perform an MIS procedure requires a proper understanding of image formation, three-dimensional orientation, and instrument manipulation, as well as a thorough knowledge of the regional anatomy. Learning and becoming proficient at MIS requires proper mentoring, continual practice, self-motivation and criticism, and dedication to self-improvement. It has also been suggested that the more traditional learning sequence of observation and incremental skill acquisition may not translate well to MIS [10].

It is generally accepted that adopting new surgical techniques results in an initial rise in the rate of complications. The frequency and severity of the complications associated with this "learning curve" vary depending on the skill of the operator and the nature of the procedure [8]. Oftentimes, the initial complication rates of an MIS procedure are reported to be similar to those of the traditional technique, although this may falsely reflect the expertise of those individuals developing or describing the technique [7].

Minimally invasive procedures commonly performed in human neurosurgery

In human neurosurgery, significant postoperative pain, muscle weakness, instability, and spinal deformity (e.g., kyphosis) associated with traditional approaches are major forces driving the development of minimally invasive approaches [4]. There are many MIS techniques published in the human literature to accomplish decompression of the spinal nerve roots and/or the spinal cord in the cervical, thoracolumbar, and lumbar spine regions [11]. Cervical radiculopathy secondary to either foraminal stenosis or disc herniation is a common cause of morbidity in people [11].

Microendoscopic discectomy and foraminotomy are described from either a posterior or posterolateral approach [4, 12]. Similar techniques are used for discectomy and tumor removal in the thoracic spine [13, 14]. While lumbar stenosis and disc herniation are treated in many ways, direct decompression, microdiscectomy, foraminotomy, and spinal fusion are all described as MIS procedures [15–17].

Minimally invasive procedures performed in veterinary neurosurgery

While MIS has thrived in human neurosurgery over the past two decades, little work is being done in veterinary neurosurgery to implement MIS techniques with regard to spinal cord and nerve root decompression. In part, this may reflect the tremendous size difference between even the largest dogs and human patients, as well as the morphology of the vertebrae and the intervertebral foramina. That being said, there may be a place for these MIS procedures as evidenced by several recent studies.

Lumbosacral disease is a common cause for morbidity and chronic neurologic dysfunction in dogs. Several pathologic processes are often identified that contribute to the clinical signs seen. Degenerative lumbosacral stenosis (DLSS) is a common component of this syndrome and is surgically treated by various methods [18–20]. In a recent, prospective, experimental study, endoscopy-assisted lumbosacral foraminotomy was performed on six dogs through small, midline incisions [21]. While being viewed through a video arthroscope, foraminotomy was performed using curettes and laminectomy rongeurs (Figures 39.1 and 39.2). Results from this study found that widening of the foramen could be successfully accomplished with this technique. Since then, the authors have used this technique to treat other cases of lumbosacral foraminal stenosis with nerve root entrapment (Otto Lanz, unpublished data).

Intervertebral disc protrusion/extrusion with subsequent spinal cord compression is a common cause of myelopathy in the dog. In particular, chronic disc protrusion poses a significant challenge as the herniated material can be hard and encapsulated and is often adhered to the dura mater and internal vertebral venous plexus. These

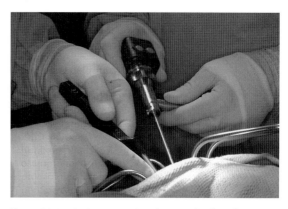

Figure 39.1 An intraoperative photograph of a video endoscope-assisted lumbosacral foraminotomy. The video endoscope is being held by the surgeon on the right side of the photograph, while the surgeon to the left performs the foraminotomy using a cervical microdiscectomy curette.

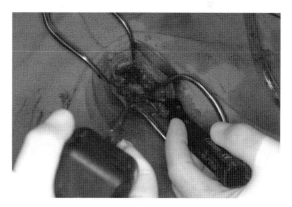

Figure 39.2 Intraoperative photograph of the foraminotomy showing the surgical site. Note the relatively small incision utilized in this procedure.

factors make removal technically difficult while increasing the risk of iatrogenic spinal cord injury and hemorrhage from the venous sinus. Partial lateral corpectomy provides one way to facilitate removal of chronic, herniated disc material along with any remaining disc material left in the interspace all while reducing spinal cord manipulation and allowing for nerve root inspection [22–24]. In a cadaveric study, the open procedure was modified to be minimally invasive using endoscopic assistance [25] (Figure 39.3). Using blunt muscle dissection and self-retaining retractors through a 2 cm skin incision, the surgeons were able to laterally approach the vertebral column (both thoracic and lumbar) using long burrs in a

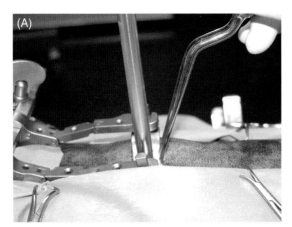
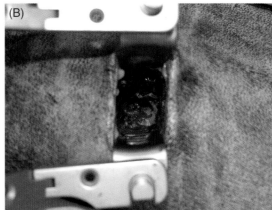

Figure 39.3 (A) Intraoperative photograph of a muscle-splitting lateral approach to the thoracolumbar spine. A Caspar cervical retractor is in place to allow for the introduction of instrumentation. (B) View of the surgical site through the minimally invasive approach. The lateral margin of the corpectomy can be seen to the right of the surgical site.

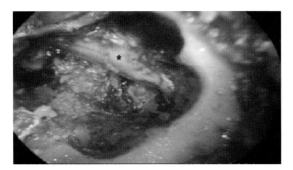

Figure 39.4 Endoscopic view of the completed lateral corpectomy. The bony margins of the corpectomy can be seen in the near field, and the spinal cord (*) is adequately decompressed.

standard pneumatic drill to perform corpectomy and achieve spinal cord decompression [25] (Figure 39.4). A recent retrospective study of 23 dogs proved the viability of this technique [26].

Conclusions

The modern era in human medicine continuously influences and popularizes the demand for and development of MIS procedures. Much of this same demand is simultaneously translated into the field of veterinary surgery. However, it will be through continued accumulation of data obtained by proper experimental studies that it will be ultimately determined where these MIS procedures should be placed in the veterinary neurosurgeon's

armamentarium. As noted earlier, veterinary MIS techniques are already developed (at least in preliminary studies) for lumbosacral foraminotomy as well as thoracic and lumbar partial lateral corpectomy. Further refinement of these techniques and large, prospective studies are warranted to validate the safety and efficacy of these procedures. It is also unknown at this time what role MIS might play in treatment of acute disc herniation in dogs and cats. However, as both technique and instrumentation become more refined in the future, it is possible that MIS may become an alternative or even preferred means for treating acute intervertebral disc herniation in veterinary patients.

References

1. Tams TR, Rawlings CA. Small Animal Endoscopy. 3rd ed. St. Louis: Elsevier; 2011.
2. Bowers SP, Hunter JG. Contraindications to laparoscopy. In: Whelan RL, Fleshman J, Fowler DL, editors. The SAGES Manual of Perioperative Care in Minimally Invasive Surgery. New York: Springer 2006. pp. 25–32.
3. Huang TJ, Hsu RW, Li YY, Cheng CC. Less systemic cytokine response in patients following microendoscopic versus open lumbar discectomy. J Orthop Res. 2005 Mar;23(2):406–11.
4. O'Toole JE, Eichholz KM, Fessler RG. Surgical site infection rates after minimally invasive spinal surgery. J Neurosurg Spine. 2009 Oct;11(4):471–6.

5. Shih P, Wong AP, Smith TR, Lee AI, Fessler RG. Complications of open compared to minimally invasive lumbar spine decompression. J Clin Neurosci. 2011 Oct;18(10):1360–4.

6. Liu CY, Wang MY, Apuzzo ML. The physics of image formation in the neuroendoscope. Childs Nerv Syst. 2004 Nov;20(11–12):777–82.

7. Rosenberg AG. What is minimally invasive surgery and how do you learn it? In: Scuderi GR, Tria AJ, editors. Minimally Invasive Surgery in Orthopedics. New York: Springer; 2010. pp. 3–10.

8. McCormick PH, Tanner WA, Keane FB, Tierney S. Minimally invasive techniques in common surgical procedures: implications for training. Irish J Med Sci. 2003 Jan–Mar;172(1):27–9.

9. Rogers DA. Ethical and educational considerations in minimally invasive surgery training for practicing surgeons. Semin Laparosc Surg. 2002 Dec;9(4):206–11.

10. Rosser JC, Jr., Rosser LE, Savalgi RS. Objective evaluation of a laparoscopic surgical skill program for residents and senior surgeons. Arch Surg. 1998 Jun;133(6):657–61.

11. Fessler RG, O'Toole JE, Eichholz KM, Perez-Cruet MJ. The development of minimally invasive spine surgery. Neurosurg Clin N Am. 2006 Oct;17(4):401–9.

12. Adamson TE. Microendoscopic posterior cervical laminoforaminotomy for unilateral radiculopathy: results of a new technique in 100 cases. J Neurosurg. 2001 Jul;95(Suppl 1):51–7.

13. Perez-Cruet MJ, Kim BS, Sandhu F, Samartzis D, Fessler RG. Thoracic microendoscopic discectomy. J Neurosurg Spine. 2004 Jul;1(1):58–63.

14. Tredway TL, Santiago P, Hrubes MR, Song JK, Christie SD, Fessler RG. Minimally invasive resection of intradural-extramedullary spinal neoplasms. Neurosurgery. 2006 Feb;58(Suppl 1):ONS52–8; discussion ONS-8.

15. Lee MC, Fox K, Fessler RG. Minimally Invasive Spinal Surgery: Evidence-Based Review of the Literature. In: Scuderi GR, Tria AJ, editors. Minimally Invasive Surgery in Orthopedics. New York: Springer; 2010. pp. 529–33.

16. Armin SS, Holly LT, Khoo LT. Minimally invasive decompression for lumbar stenosis and disc herniation. Neurosurg Focus. 2008;25(2):E11.

17. Knight M. Endoscopic foraminoplasty: key to understanding the sources of back pain and sciatica and their treatment. In: Scuderi GR, Tria AJ, editors. Minimally Invasive Surgery in Orthopedics. New York: Springer; 2010. pp. 535–53.

18. Danielsson F, Sjostrom L. Surgical treatment of degenerative lumbosacral stenosis in dogs. Vet Surg. 1999 Mar–Apr;28(2):91–8.

19. Godde T, Steffen F. Surgical treatment of lumbosacral foraminal stenosis using a lateral approach in twenty dogs with degenerative lumbosacral stenosis. Vet Surg. 2007 Oct;36(7):705–13.

20. Meij BP, Bergknut N. Degenerative lumbosacral stenosis in dogs. Vet Clin North Am Small Anim Pract. 2010 Sep;40(5):983–1009.

21. Wood BC, Lanz OI, Jones JC, Shires PK. Endoscopic-assisted lumbosacral foraminotomy in the dog. Vet Surg. 2004 May–Jun;33(3):221–31.

22. Moissonnier P, Meheust P, Carozzo C. Thoracolumbar lateral corpectomy for treatment of chronic disk herniation: technique description and use in 15 dogs. Vet Surg. 2004 Nov–Dec;33(6):620–8.

23. Sharp NJH, Wheeler SJ. Small Animal Spinal Disorders: Diagnosis and Surgery. 2nd ed. Edinburgh: Elsevier; 2005.

24. Flegel T, Boettcher IC, Ludewig E, Kiefer I, Oechtering G, Bottcher P. Partial lateral corpectomy of the thoracolumbar spine in 51 dogs: assessment of slot morphometry and spinal cord decompression. Vet Surg. 2011 Jan;40(1):14–21.

25. Carozzo C, Maitre P, Genevois JP, Gabanou PA, Fau D, Viguier E. Endoscope-assisted thoracolumbar lateral corpectomy. Vet Surg. 2011 Aug;40(6):738–42.

26. Maitre P, Gabanou PA, Viguier E, Carozzo C. Endoscopic-assisted thoracolumbar lateral corpectomy: retrospective study on 23 dogs. 19th Annual Scientific Meeting ECVS, Helsinki, Finland, 2010.

40 Will There be a Role for Disc Prostheses in Small Animals?

Filippo Adamo and Franck Forterre

Introduction

Spinal arthroplasty offers an exciting alternative to fusion for the treatment of degenerative disc disease. Currently, the main indication for disc prosthesis in small animals is the treatment of disc-associated cervical spondylomyelopathy in dogs, also known as disc-associated wobbler syndrome (DAWS) (see Chapter 7). Another potential indication is the treatment of disc-associated lumbosacral stenosis (see Chapter 32). DAWS in dogs shares many similarities with cervical spondylotic myelopathy in people, and the Doberman breed has been proposed as a natural model to study the disease in humans [1].

The knowledge gained over the last 15 years in people with disc arthroplasty can be applied in veterinary medicine for the treatment of DAWS. However, this information should be interpreted cautiously by veterinarians because of biomechanical differences in dogs such as greater axial forces and greater amount of coupled motions in dogs compared to people [2, 3].

The goal of cervical arthroplasty is to preserve intervertebral mobility while providing distraction,

stability, and neural decompression [4–6]. Cervical disc arthroplasty involves discectomy, spinal cord decompression, milling of the vertebral end plates, and placement of a device to maintain distraction and preserve intervertebral mobility at the treated space [4–11]. Maintenance of motion at a decompressed interspace may result in improved load transfer and reduced stress on the adjacent intervertebral discs and dorsal elements, although this has not yet been demonstrated conclusively in the canine spine.

Comparison of DAWS in people and in dogs

In people with cervical myelopathy and radiculopathy secondary to degenerative disc disease, anterior cervical discectomy and fusion (ACDF) is a reliable surgical treatment with a satisfactory outcome in 90–95% of patients [12]. However, there is a significant incidence of disc disease at adjacent sites causing recurrence of neurologic symptoms, termed domino effect [12–14]. Within 5 years of surgery, 92% of patients have radiographic

Advances in Intervertebral Disc Disease in Dogs and Cats, First Edition. Edited by James M. Fingeroth and William B. Thomas.
© 2015 ACVS Foundation. Published 2015 by John Wiley & Sons, Inc.

evidence of degenerative disc disease at adjacent segments, and by 10 years, about 25% of people require a second surgery for the same problem at an adjacent space [12, 14]. The cause of this subsequent disc degeneration remains unknown. One suggested factor is an increase in intradiscal pressure at adjacent discs after fusion [15–18]. This increased pressure blocks the diffusion of nutrients from the end plate and is the most significant cause of disc degeneration [19].

Clinical studies using dynamic radiography show increased motion at adjacent segments above and below the level of cervical fusion, and this is also a factor associated with deterioration [20, 21]. After arthroplasty, the range of motion is increased or maintained in the surgically treated segment and mildly decreased at adjacent levels. However, this reduction is compensated by the movement of the artificial disc itself [22].

An interesting dilemma regarding domino lesions is whether such lesions are the natural progress of an underlying similar process at the adjacent vertebral motion units or if they are an accelerated degenerative process influenced by the biomechanical effect of fusion [21–23]. Motion preservation at the surgery site may reduce the rate of adjacent-level cervical disc disease [24–28].

Cervical disc prosthesis in people

The use of a cervical disc prosthesis in human patients was first reported by Ferstron in 1966 [29]. Over the last decade, clinical experience with many different types of artificial discs has been reported, including Cummins artificial cervical joint [30] (which evolved into Prestige [31], ProDisc-C [32], Bryan Cervical Disc [33], Discover [34, 35]), and several clinical trials are currently underway [28].

Classification of artificial discs

Currently, artificial discs are classified into three types: non-, uni-, and biarticulating. The implant may consist of a metal-on-metal design, metal-on-polymer (ultrahigh-molecular-weight polyethylene), and less commonly ceramic-on-polymer or a ceramic-on-ceramic design [36]. The disc is either modular (having replaceable components) or nonmodular (without replaceable components) and

some are used in conjunction with supplemental vertebral body screw fixation [36]. Certain designs promote biological bone ingrowth at the disc-end-plate interface. In terms of motion, artificial discs may be constrained, semiconstrained, or unconstrained [36]. Devices are considered constrained in certain planes if they restrict motion to less than that seen physiologically. Devices are considered semiconstrained in certain planes if they allow motion similar to that seen physiologically. Devices are considered nonconstrained in certain planes of motion if there is no mechanical stop to the motion and if they are reliant on the perispinal soft tissue and the inherent compression across the disc space to provide restraint to extremes of motion [37].

The distribution of force and subsidence is possibly the most important biomechanical consideration for an artificial disc. The idea is to distribute the forces involved as uniformly as possible over a large area [37].

Intradiscal replacement of the nucleus pulposus represents an alternative to total disc replacement and spinal fusion procedures. The aim is to reconstruct the nucleus pulposus primarily while preserving the biomechanics of the annulus fibrosus and cartilaginous end plate. Nucleus pulposus implants are designed to provide stable motion, increase disc space width, relieve or lessen transmission of shear forces on the remaining annulus, and stabilize ligaments [38]. Nucleus pulposus replacement devices can be categorized into two groups: the intradiscal implants and *in situ* curable polymers. Intradiscal implants are biomechanically more similar to the native nucleus pulposus, whereas *in situ* curable polymers consist of compounds that harden after implantation. These implants are currently at different stages of preclinical and clinical investigations in veterinary medicine [39; F. Forterre, personal communication].

Cervical disc prosthesis in dogs

The first cervical prosthesis specifically for the canine cervical spine[1] was designed and biomechanically tested *in vivo* in 2007 [7]. This prosthesis is made of a titanium alloy (Ti-6AI-4V-ELI) and consists of two end plates, with a range of movement of 30° between the plates (Figure 40.1). Titanium alloy was selected because it is resistant, is relatively inexpensive, has a good corrosion

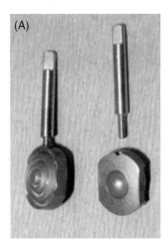
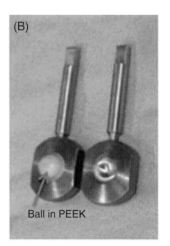
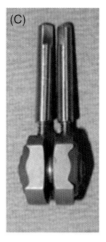
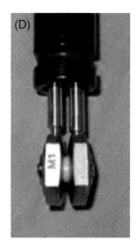

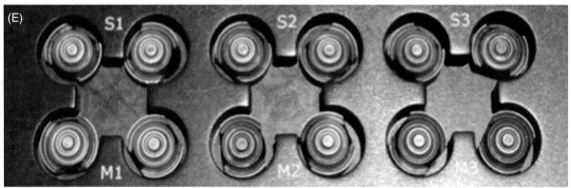

Figure 40.1 Adamo spinal disc®. US Patent # 8,496,707 B2. The prosthesis is made of a titanium alloy, and the concavity and convexity of the central aspects of the end-plate surfaces result in a ball-and-socket type of connection between the end plates. The external surface of each end plate is convex, resembling the concavity of the caudal end plate of the most caudal cervical vertebrae. The outer surface of each end plate has concentric grooves to allow bone ingrowth into the implant and is pretreated with a dual acid etch bath to promote bone ingrowth into the prosthesis (A). The convexity of the central aspect of the end-plate surface is made of polyether ether ketone (PEEK) (B). Two end-threaded stainless steel pins screwed into each piece of the implant and a barrel holder are used to hold together the two pieces of the implant during placement within the disc space (C and D). Six standard sizes of prosthesis are available, labeled S1, S2, and S3 and M1, M2, and M3. However, since each male piece of the prosthesis has to be assembled with a separate female piece, this makes a total of 12 different sizes when the disc is assembled in all possible combinations (E).

resistance compared to other materials, and is ideal for follow-up MRI studies in the event of postsurgical worsening and to evaluate domino lesions. This prosthesis is rotationally unconstrained, following the ball-and-socket principle, and does not require supplemental fixation. Unconstrained cervical prostheses designed for people usually allow about 11° of freedom [24]. The higher degree of freedom in this prosthesis was arbitrarily chosen considering that heterotopic ossification at the treated site observed in people significantly decreases the range of motion at the site of

implantation over time. The outer surface of each end plate is convex to avoid prosthesis migration and has concentric grooves to allow bone ingrowth into the prosthesis. In the *in vitro* study, it was concluded that cervical spine specimens with the implanted prosthesis have biomechanical behaviors more similar to an intact spine compared to spinal specimens with ventral slot and PMMA fusion [7]. This was the prerequisite for the subsequent clinical investigation [8–10].

A pilot long-term clinical study using this prosthesis in two dogs affected by DAWS showed that cervical arthroplasty was well tolerated with excellent outcome in both dogs. Mobility at the treated site was lost and distraction decreased over time in both dogs, without affecting the clinical outcome. Furthermore, the presence of the prosthesis did not affect the ability to reassess the area via MRI at a follow-up 18 months later, and domino lesions were not observed in either dog [9].

A multicenter study evaluating the short and intermediate clinical and radiological results (average 15 months) using the same prosthesis in 12 dogs with single- and multilevel lesions has been reported [10]. In this study, the external surface of the prosthesis was treated with dual acid bath etch [40, 41] to promote bone–implant incorporation at the implant–vertebral end-plate interface, and dedicated surgical tools were created to facilitate implantation (Figure 40.2). To improve visual assessment, a high-powered headlamp , magnification loupes, and a Caspar cervical distractor were used as in the previous study (Figure 40.3). All 12 dogs had immediate postoperative recovery with good degree of distraction in the immediate postoperative radiographs (Figure 40.4). All dogs in this

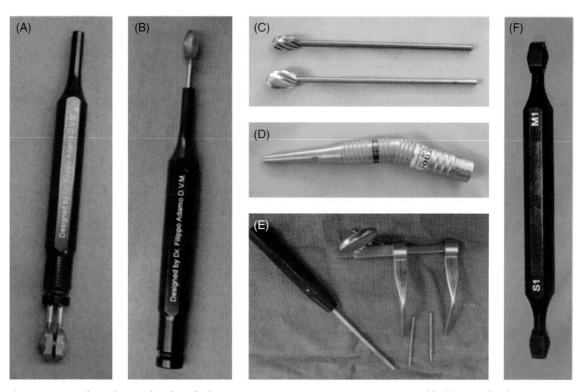

Figure 40.2 Dedicated surgical tools and other accessories. US Patent # 8,491,655 B2. Barrel holder. (A) After the two pieces of the implant are assembled, the two pins are inserted into the barrel holder. (B) The barrel holder has the double function of holding the prosthesis assembled with one extremity and to unscrew the end-threaded pins after the prosthesis is placed in the slot with the other extremity. Custom-made burrs. (C) Two dedicated custom-made burrs are used. The small burr head is used to enlarge the discectomy and to create enough space for the insertion of larger burr. The large head burr resembles the external convexity of the implant, and it is used for the final burring to create the specular concavity to accommodate the implant into the disc space. Twenty degree angle attachment. (D) A 20° angle attachment for the high-speed air drill is used to facilitate burring at an angle parallel to the disc space. Caspar cervical distractor. (E) This instrument is used to distract the two cervical vertebrae at the affected disc space. It allows better visualization of the dorsal aspect of the discectomy, facilitates the removal of the bulging disc, improves visualization of the dorsal longitudinal ligament, and facilitates the inspection of the vertebral canal for adequate spinal cord decompression. Sizing probe. (F) This instrument resembles at each extremity the shape of the S or M disc size, respectively. It is used to probe the discectomy between burring (in place of the implant), and to assess the congruity of the discectomy to the implant. This instrument shortens the total surgery time by avoiding multiple times of checking of the discectomy with the actual implant, and it also facilitates proper selection of the size of the implant after the discectomy is completed.

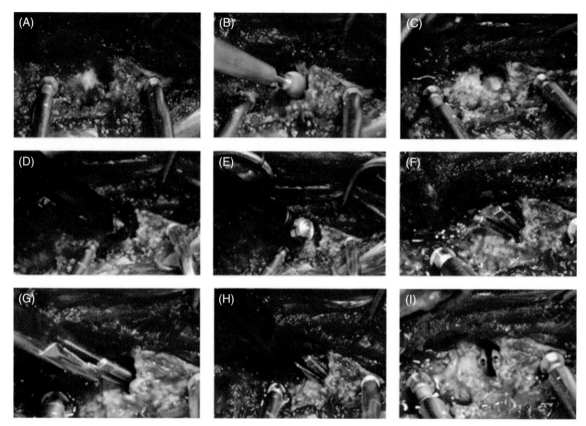

Figure 40.3   Surgical technique. After routine surgical preparation, the ventral aspect of the affected vertebral bodies is accessed via a standard approach as for a ventral slot procedure. A discectomy is performed across the intervertebral space. The self-retaining Caspar distractor is placed and maintained distracted (A) to allow the final cleaning of the disc space and the subsequent burring with the two dedicated burrs (B). Burring is done following the direction of the intervertebral space, which is facilitated by the 20° angle attachment. Burring should be kept on the midline of the disc space and the widest part of the burr should be centered at a depth of approximately 50% of the total disc space depth. Burring of the end plate of the cranial vertebra is minimal and limited to the removal of the final debris of the annulus fibrosus. The cranial end plate does not require excessive burring because it already has a natural concavity, which accommodates the convexity of the implant. Burring of the end plate of the caudal vertebra is limited in the central surface. Burring is also extended to the lateral edge of the discectomy as needed to allow the insertion of the sizing probe and later of the prosthesis. If the MRI study is suggestive of static spinal cord compression, the dorsal longitudinal ligament should be incised to visualize the spinal cord and explore the vertebral canal (C). In between burring, the sizing probe (which simulates the prosthesis) is used for pretesting how the actual prosthesis will be firmly seated in place (D). The prosthesis is inserted while maintaining the Caspar distractor in maximal distraction. Gentle pressure is applied to force the implant into the slot, and an audible click is usually heard when the convex area of the implant slips past the edge of the slot (E). To ensure that the implant is seated as much as possible on the midline, the barrel holder is rotated until the fissure of its proximal end is aligned with the long axis of the vertebrae. After implantation, the distraction is released, allowing the two vertebral end plates to collapse on the prosthesis (F). After assessing that the prosthesis is correctly seated in position, in order to ensure that the implant is firmly in position, the two pins still screwed in the prosthesis are grasped with a needle holder, and upward traction is applied in an attempt to dislocate the prosthesis from the slot (G). Once the surgeon is satisfied that the prosthesis is held snuggly between the vertebrae, the two pins are unscrewed from the two prosthetic end plates (H), and the two Caspar distractor pins are removed from the vertebral bodies (I). Bone wax or gel foam is placed to stop the bleeding that might occur at the holes created by the two Caspar distractor pins. The longus colli, sternohyoideus, and sternocephalicus muscles and subcutaneous and subcuticular tissues are then closed in a routine manner.

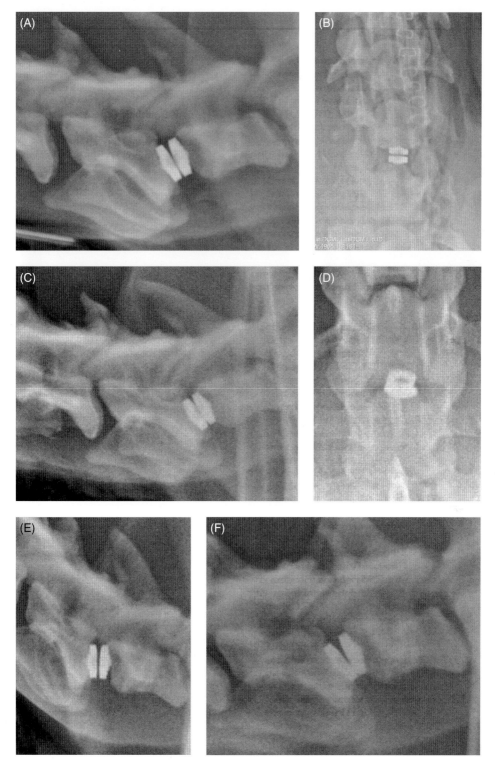

Figure 40.4 Postoperative radiographs. Immediate postoperative radiographs. German shepherd, 9 years old. Correct positioning of the implant on the lateral (A) and ventrodorsal projection (B) at the level of C5–C6. The implant used is M1, which provides adequate distraction. Two weeks post-op (same dog). The lateral (C) and ventrodorsal (D) views show that the implant is still well in place providing distraction at the treated site. The extension (E) and the flexion (F) views are performed to evaluate the degree of mobility at the treated site. The opening of the angle between the two implant end plates, as shown in the flexion view in this patient, indicates that mobility is maintained. At the reevaluation 6 months later, the radiographic findings were unchanged.

study, except one in which the technique was improperly performed, showed improvement in the neurological status during the observation period. In the majority of dogs, the distraction was moderately lost, and mobility at the treated sites decreased or became undetectable over time (Figure 40.5). A subsequent study using a redesigned thinner disc (2nd-generation disc) with the internal convex surface replaced with polyether ether ketone (PEEK) and an additional tool (sizing probe) to probe/test the disc space during burring before final disc implantation showed similar results but with the advantages that the surgery was facilitated by less burring and less implant manipulation and the implant accommodated easier along the natural angle of the disc space [11]. A recent study evaluating 50 disc spaces in 33 dogs treated with CDA for DAWS showed that on the

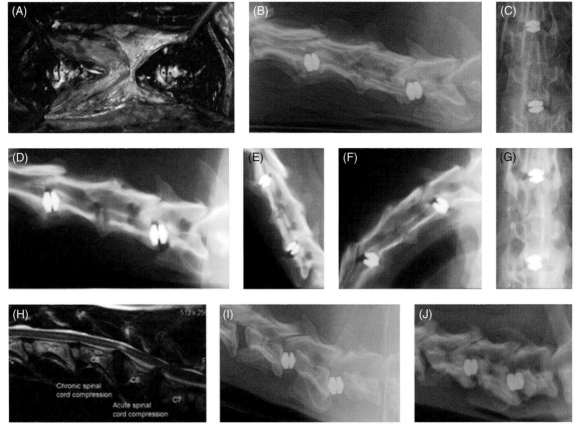

Figure 40.5 Two-level cervical disc replacement. Intraoperative photo (A) and immediate postoperative radiographs (B and C) of disc-associated wobbler syndrome (DAWS) at C3–C4 and C5–C6, with a suspected congenital vertebral fusion at C4–C5. Multiple cervical disc arthroplasty was recommended to avoid additional fusion at the affected spaces, which, in addition to the preexisting one, could have had predisposed the patient to a domino lesion at C6–C7. Nine-month postoperative radiographs with the neck in lateral (D), extension (E), flexion (F), and ventrolateral (G) positioning showed mild decrease of the original vertebral distraction, no heterotopic ossifications, and retention of mobility at both treated spaces. This dog had presented with a 4 month history of progressive ataxia/tetraparesis and regained full neurological function. MRI T2 weighted of 6-year-old Doberman with a 2-year history of ataxia/tetraparesis treated with NSAID who presented acutely tetraplegic; the MRI showed multilevel DAWS lesions at C5–C6 and C6–C7 (H). The dog was treated with double cervical disc replacement and the immediate postoperative radiograph showed adequate disc placement at both treated sites (I). At 7-month follow-up, recheck radiographs showed decreased vertebral distraction and heterotopic ossification at both treated spaces (J). Mobility was not detectable at C6–C7 and significantly decreased at C5–C6. However, this did not affect the clinical outcome. The dog became ambulatory 2 weeks postsurgery and neurologically normal 4 months later. He continued to maintain his normal neurological status without any adjuvant anti-inflammatory or analgesic medication.

immediate postoperative radiographs, 15 sites were overdistracted, 34 sites were adequately distracted, and only 1 site was underdistracted. Overdistraction was mostly observed with the 1st-generation (thicker) implant, while the adequate distraction was mostly observed with the 2nd-generation (thinner) implant. On serial radiographic evaluation, the distraction was gradually decreased compared to the immediate postoperative radiographs and subsidence (defined as reduction of the width of the disc space equivalent to or less than the width of the preoperative radiographs) was seen in 7/19 sites (37%) at 6 months postsurgery and progressed to all the five sites evaluated at 2 years postsurgery. Subsidence, except for one dog, was seen only when the disc spaces were overdistracted, and it was more pronounced with the 1st-generation (thicker) and narrower implants and less pronounced with the 2nd-generation (thinner) and wider implants (Adamo, personal observation). Mobility was not detectable in 8/36 treated sites (22%) 2 weeks after surgery in 24 dogs examined and was lost or not detectable in 17/22 sites (77%) at 6 months after surgery in 14 dogs examined. No implant migration or implant infections were observed on serial radiographs or on MRI when available. In this study, the mean and median follow up time was 16 and 12 months, respectively (range, 2 weeks to 42 months), and the outcome was considered good to excellent in 30 out of 33 dogs (91%). The three dogs with poor or unsatisfactory outcome were presented with over 2 months of nonambulatory tetraparesis and severe extensor rigidity in both thoracic limbs. Among these, one dog (12.4-year-old sheltie mix weighing 9 kg [19.5 lb]) was euthanized 2 weeks postsurgery because of a compressive fracture of C6 with ventral displacement of the implant, and another dog (13.5-year-old chow mix) was euthanized 8 months after surgery because of lack of significant improvement. Two dogs had recurrence of the neurological signs 18 months after surgery secondary to suspected osteophytes (noted on MRI) causing ventral spinal cord compression at the treated sites. Ventral osteophytes were seen at six treated sites, in four dogs on postoperative radiographs, causing bridging spondylarthrosis and ankylosis at three disc spaces in two dogs. No neurologic domino lesion adjacent to treated sites was seen in any of the dogs during the observation period. Median postoperative hospitalization time was 1 day (range 0–5 days), and 5 dogs

were discharged on the day of surgery. In this study, it was concluded that correct patient selection (dog's weight not less than 20 kg [44 lb]), neurological status at presentation, size of the implant, endplate preparation, and applied distraction during surgery were important factors that may influence the outcome (Adamo, personal observation).

These studies showed that cervical disc arthroplasty is well tolerated and might be a valuable method to treat DAWS [9–11]. Furthermore, these studies showed that the cervical cast used in the previous study was not needed.

Benefits of cervical disc arthroplasty

Cervical arthroplasty in people is still an area of active research, debate, and controversy, and a 5-year follow-up has been recommended to assess the long-term functionality of the prosthesis and its influence at adjacent levels [42]. A technology overview from the *American Academy of Orthopaedic Surgeons* analyzed the results of multiple clinical studies and concluded that artificial disc arthroplasty is more beneficial in the short term compared to ACDF, although its long-term benefit over standard ACDF remains unclear [43]. The impact of cervical disc replacement on adjacent segment degeneration and the degree of heterotopic ossifications (HOs) of the treated segments remain a subject of intensive investigation. HO is a pathologic condition that leads to the development of bone within nonosseous soft tissues [44]. The bone that forms is believed to develop through stimulation by cellular mediators and altered neurovascular signaling [44]. Although the precise cause of HO remains unclear, it is certain that it increases with time, it may occur at the four corners of the disc space (most commonly anterosuperior or posterosuperior), and it has been reported with an incidence as high as 60.3% [45].

A prospective, randomized, multicenter study comparing cervical arthroplasty with ACDF with a minimum of 2-year follow-up concluded that cervical arthroplasty was associated with significantly greater overall success rate than ACDF. Furthermore, there were significantly fewer patients in the cervical arthroplasty group showing severe adjacent-level radiographic changes at the 2-year follow-up [46]. Another study with an average follow-up of 49.4 months evaluated cervical disc replacement and its effects on adjacent segment discs and found satisfactory clinical and radiographic outcome. In this study, progression of adjacent segment degeneration was observed in 23% of patients, but this did not affect the clinical outcome [47]. A study of cervical arthroplasty with up to 2-year follow-up showed motion preservation at the treated site in 85% of patients, HOs in 4.5% of the treated levels, and radiological signs of adjacent-level degeneration in 9.1% patients. This study confirmed the efficacy and safety of the technique and concluded that the presence of HOs does not alter the clinical outcomes [48]. In another

study, HOs was detected in 27.7% of treated segments but did not affect the clinical outcomes, and no specific risk factors for HOs were identified [49]. Fitting of the implants to end plates has been identified as a factor to reduce the development of HO [45, 49]. Finally, multilevel cervical disc replacement with contiguous and noncontiguous implants has been reported to be a safe and effective alternative to fusion. However, the impact of multilevel arthroplasty, especially on the adjacent segments, remains to be evaluated [50–52].

In dogs, studies comparing long-term results of cervical disc arthroplasty with other surgical

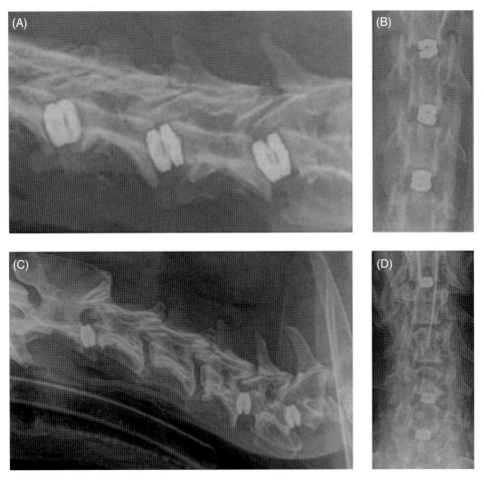

Figure 40.6 Three-level cervical disc replacement. Immediate postoperative radiographs of a 13-year-old dalmatian affected by disc-associated wobbler syndrome at C3–C4, C4–C5, and C5–C6. Correct positioning of the implant on the lateral (A) and ventrodorsal projection (B). The implant used is S1, which provides adequate distraction at all sites. Immediate postoperative radiographs of a 14-year-old chow–lab mixed affected by disc-associated wobbler syndrome at C2–C3, C5–C6, and C6–C7. Correct positioning of the implant on the lateral (C) and ventrodorsal projection (D). The implants used in this patient are M1 at C5–C6 and C6–C7 and S1 at C2–C3, which provide adequate distraction at all sites.

techniques are still lacking. However, there are several benefits of this technique including minimal invasiveness, quick recovery, spinal cord decompression, distraction with immediate relief of radicular pain and vascular compression at the intervertebral foramina, treatment of multilevel lesions at adjacent or nonadjacent sites (Figure 40.6), and ability to reassess the spine with MRI in the event of complications and for long-term assessment of domino lesions. Furthermore, because cervical disc arthroplasty is well tolerated and the neurological status does not worsen in the immediate postoperative phase, dogs that are ambulatory prior to surgery can be potentially treated as outpatients.

The advantage of cervical disc arthroplasty over a ventral slot procedure is that the prosthetic disc acts as a spacer preventing early collapse of the intervertebral disc space as may occur with a ventral slot alone. Collapse of the disc space can compress the nerve roots and vasculature at the intervertebral foramina, causing cervical hyperesthesia and focal spinal cord ischemia, which in turn may cause an immediate worsening from the preoperative neurological status. Ventral slot alone may also be ineffective in completely decompressing the spinal cord [53–56]. Clinical effectiveness of the ventral slot procedures is typically evident over time, and any instability may be alleviated because these disc spaces may eventually fuse [57–59].

An advantage of cervical disc arthroplasty over other distraction and stabilization techniques is that the prosthetic disc is retained in the slot without the use of additional fixation [8]. This eliminates complications associated with impingement on neurovascular structures, plate fractures, screws pulling out, and delayed graft incorporation [10, 57, 58, 60, 61]. An additional advantage is that cervical disc arthroplasty may prevent domino lesions [10]. However, long-term follow-up studies in a large number of dogs are needed to investigate this potential benefit.

Prophylactic treatment of mildly affected adjacent disc spaces has been suggested to reduce the incidence of domino lesions [57, 58]. Because the cervical prosthesis is relatively easy to implant, is cost-effective (its cost may be equivalent to the cost of the pins and PMMA), and does not require special instrumentation for plating, it could also be used at other mildly affected disc spaces in conjunction with disc replacement at the affected

space [10, 11]. This could be particularly indicated when at the suspected disc space there is a mild evidence of spinal cord signal hyperintensity on MRI T2-weighted images, which may be suggestive of "incipient lesions" (P.F. Adamo, personal communication).

Complications with cervical disc arthroplasty

In people, the most common complications include implant or end-plate subsidence (the penetration and collapse of the implant into the adjacent vertebral bone) [62, 63], splitting of the vertebral body during implantation [64], HOs and ankylosis at the treated site [65–67], adjacent disc degeneration including new formation or enlargement of osteophytes [65, 68], and device migration [69]. Less common complications include delayed hyperreactivity to metal ions and subsidence secondary to osteoporosis [62, 70].

In dogs, possible complications associated with this type of prosthesis may be similar to those reported in human patients. Among these, devices migrating out, infections, and subsidence would be the most serious. Although subsidence, HOs, and ankylosis have been observed, devices migrating out and infection have not been reported [9–11].

While canine disc arthroplasty may offer benefits over arthrodesis, it also requires that the surgeon acquire new operative techniques, and new complications might be introduced during this learning curve. Since the key to success in any surgical procedure is correct patient selection, treatment criteria also have to be determined in the future. Many patients may not be appropriate candidates for disc arthroplasty. Preoperative assessment should involve consideration of disc space width, although it is not clear at present whether there is a minimum width under which the device should not be used. Further, the effect of the artificial disc on angulation at the treated level and the overall spinal alignment may be important in long-term outcomes and rates of domino lesions. The angle of disc insertion is related to bone removal and end-plate preparation, and it is somewhat arbitrary, with no precise measure available to predict accurately the impact of the prosthesis on the vertebral alignment. However, the new generation of the thinner implants requires minimal end-plate bone removal, which allows the implant to follow the angle of the natural disc space [11].

Subsidence

Subsidence is defined as sinking of a body with a higher elasticity modulus (e.g., graft, cage, spacer) in a body characterized by a lower elasticity modulus (e.g., vertebral body), resulting in three-dimensional changes of the spinal geometry. Magnitude of subsidence is directly proportional to the load pressure and to the difference between the elasticity modules but inversely proportional to the area of the graft–bed interface. Both biological and mechanical qualities of the graft–bed interface are important for the subsidence process. End-plate preservation and a dynamic modification of cervical plates may enable surgeons to control subsidence and reduce the number of complications [71].

Possible factors for the decrease of distraction and subsidence over time may be a combination of overdistraction and bone resorption around the prosthesis [8]. In most dogs, distraction of 2–3 mm is enough to restore a normal disc width of 4–6 mm, and overdistraction should be avoided [10, 11, 58]. New disc designs of thinner prostheses are under investigation (P.F. Adamo, personal communication). Prevention of vertebral space collapse may be difficult because muscle and tensile forces that control postures in the horizontally oriented quadruped vertebral column cause an inherent axial compression of the spine [2]. Furthermore, a mild degree of collapse may be desirable to allow accommodation of the implant over time within the intervertebral space, and to decrease the biomechanical stress of distraction on adjacent vertebral motion unit. Selecting a prosthesis with a larger surface area would exert less force per unit area on the vertebral end plate and be less likely to cause subsequent subsidence [10]. Finally, to avoid bone resorption around the implant, bone–implant incorporation should be promoted [11].

Bone–implant interface incorporation

Generally, implant-induced osteolysis is a manifestation of an adverse cellular response to the phagocytosis of particulate wear and corrosion debris. This mechanism is also known as "particle-induced osteolysis" or "implant-related debris osteolysis." The effect of unintended debris resulting from wear and corrosion (e.g., micromotion between the interconnection mechanisms in spinal implants) remains a clinical concern [72].

Particulate debris should be expected any time an artificial disc implant is used. The generation of particulate debris can occur as a result of wear and corrosion. Titanium particulate debris has been shown to elicit a cytokine-mediated response with inflammatory infiltrates, increased intracellular tumor necrosis factor-α, increased osteoclastic activity and cellular apoptosis, and increased potential for aseptic osteolysis [72, 73]. Causes of implant failure in people have included failure of osseointegration, midsubstance elastomeric tears, and osteolysis, which may also result in heterotopic new bone equivalent to a fusion or pseudoarthrosis [74].

The presence of nonresorbable, osteoconductive hydroxyapatite (HA) particles could help maintain a denser and more functional peri-implant bone structure [75]. HA largely consists of calcium and phosphorous. This composition allows HA to function as a coating that promotes osseointegration between bone and various orthopedic implants. HA coating is wear-resistant and promotes osseointegration between bone and implant. The presence of HA seems to promote the maturation of collagen fibers surrounding the titanium implants and to support osteoconduction. Moreover, in an *in vivo* study, new formation of bone was faster in all samples where implants were inserted together with HA [76–79].

Coating with a modular bone growth factor "modular bone morphogenetic peptide (mBMP)" in orthopedic implants has also been recently investigated. The results of this study demonstrated that mBMP coated onto an HA–titanium implant stimulates new bone formation and may be useful to improve implant fixation in total joint arthroplasty applications [80].

However, excessive stimulation of bone formation at the intervertebral disc space with mBMP or other growth factors may be potentially deleterious, because it may induce excessive bone growth into the vertebral canal and subsequent compression of the spinal cord.

Improved bone–implant osseointegration may prevent subsidence, osteophytes, HOs, and ankylosis and therefore may reduce loss of mobility [81]. To promote bone–implant incorporation, the canine artificial disc presented in this book section has been upgraded with an external HA coating (third-generation disc) (Figure 40.7), and to decrease subsidence, additional wider and taller disc sizes have been made available. A clinical study using this third-generation disc implant is currently under investigation (Adamo, personal communication).

Decrease or loss of mobility over time

Decrease or loss of mobility over time could be secondary to the HO and ankylosis at the treated sites [10–12] and/or to fibrotic tissue ingrowth between the two articular faces of the implant. However, it has been postulated that the gradual decrease or loss of mobility at the treated sites

(when it occurs) allows the rest of the vertebral column to slowly and gradually accommodate to the new dynamic until a final dynamic stabilization occurs [10]. It is also possible that although some degree of mobility at the treated spaces persists, it is not detectable with the current method of investigation [10]. This could explain the excellent clinical outcome in dogs treated with cervical disc arthroplasty [10, 11]. New technical strategies to retain implant mobility at the treated disc spaces over time are currently under investigation [68]. Finally, packing the ventral edges of each vertebra facing the external surface of the implant with bone wax may prevent bone and fibrotic tissue ingrowth between the two articulated faces of the implant, as well as ventral bridging spondylarthrosis and ankylosis, which in turn may help in maintaining mobility at the treated site(s) (Adamo, personal communication).

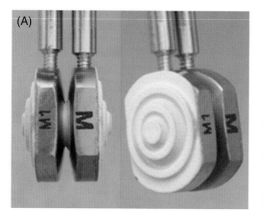
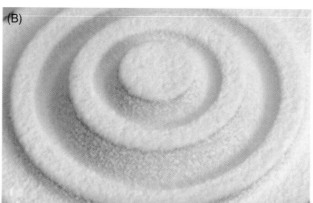

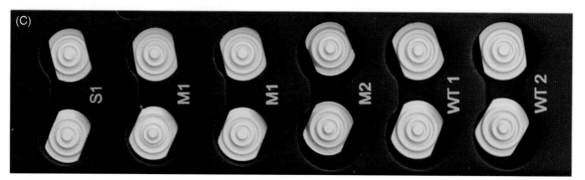

Figure 40.7 Third-generation Adamo spinal disc coated with hydroxyapatite (HA). The external surface of the implant is coated with HA to improve bone–implant osseointegration. Assembled disc (A); the micropores of the HA coating are visible in the external surface of the magnified picture of one shell of the disc (B). To allow adequate surface of contact between the implant and the vertebral end plates in larger-size dogs, additional wider and taller disc sizes labeled WT1 and WT2 are added to the original S1, M1, and M2 disc sizes (C).

Clinical concerns

An additional concern in humans is the longevity of the clinical outcomes. The average age of the patients considered appropriate candidates for disc arthroplasty is significantly younger than that of patients typically undergoing total appendicular joint replacement. This means that the longevity of the implants must be extended for decades compared with those of total hip or total knee replacements [71]. This problem might be less important in veterinary medicine because DAWS patients at presentation are usually at least 6 years old and have a shorter lifespan compared to people.

Conclusion

By preserving the motion segment, arthroplasty attempts to prevent adjacent segment degeneration while treating the underlying disease. Overall the results of the preliminary studies using cervical disc replacement in dogs affected by DAWS are encouraging. The minimal morbidity and the potential benefit of avoiding domino lesions, together with the other many advantages, may change the pet owner's perception of DAWS patients often having a guarded to a poor prognosis and may therefore increase their willingness to pursue this surgical treatment compared to other extant options.

Note

1. *Adamo spinal disc®*. Applied Veterinary Technology LLC, San Mateo, CA, 94403

References

1. DaCosta R. 2012. Comparison of cervical spondylomyelopathy in dogs and cervical spondylomyelopathy in people. In Proceedings of the Annual Meeting of the American College of Veterinary Internal Medicine Forum; New Orleans.
2. Smith TH. 2002. The use of quadruped as an in vivo model for the study of the spine—biomechanical consideration. Eur Spine J 11:137–144.
3. Hofstetter M, Gedet P, Doherr M, 2009. Biomechanical analysis of the three-dimensional motion pattern of the canine cervical spine segment C4–C5. Vet Surg 38:49–59.
4. Mummaneni P, Haid R. 2004. The future in the care of the cervical spine: interbody fusion and arthroplasty. J Neurosurg Spine 1:155–159.
5. DiAngelo D, Robertson J, Metcalf N, *et al.* 2003. Biomechanical testing of an artificial cervical joint and an anterior cervical plate. J Spinal Disord Tech 16: 314–323.
6. Wingfield C, Gill S, Nelson R, *et al.* 2002. Influence of an artificial cervical joint compared with fusion on adjacent-level motion in the treatment of degenerative cervical disc disease. J Neurosurg (Spine1) 96: 17–21.
7. Adamo PF, Kobayashi H, Markel M, *et al.* 2007. In vitro biomechanical comparison of cervical disk arthroplasty, ventral slot procedure, and smooth pins with polymethylmethacrylate fixation at treated and adjacent canine cervical motor units. Vet Surg 36(8):729–741.
8. Adamo PF, Burns G. 2009. Cervical arthroplasty in dogs with disc associated caudal cervical spondylomyelopathy and cervical disc herniation. Preliminary study in two cases. J Vet Int Med 23(3):71.
9. Adamo PF. 2011. Cervical arthroplasty in two dogs with disk-associated cervical spondylomyelopathy. J Am Vet Med Assoc 15;239(6):808–17.
10. Adamo PF, da Costa RC, Giovannella C, *et al.* 2012. Cervical disc arthroplasty in 12 dogs affected by disc associated Wobbler syndrome: preliminary results. In Proceeding of the Annual Meeting of the American College of Veterinary Internal Medicine Forum; New Orleans.
11. Adamo PF, da Costa RC, Kroll R, *et al.* 2013. Cervical disc arthroplasty using the adamo spinal disc in 18 dogs affected by disc-associated wobbler syndrome. In Proceedings of the Annual Meeting of the American College of Veterinary Internal Medicine Forum; Seattle.
12. Bolhman H, Emery S, Goodfellow D, *et al.* 1993. Anterior cervical discectomy and arthrodesis for cervical radiculopathy. Long term follow-up of one hundred and twenty-two patients. J Bone Joint Surg Am 75:1203–1232.
13. Goffin J, Geusens E, Vantomme N, *et al.* 2004. Long-term follow-up after interbody fusion of the cervical spine. J Spinal Disord Tech 17:79–85.
14. Hillbraund A, Carlson G, Palumbo M, *et al.* 1999. Radiculopathy and myelopathy at segments adjacent to the site of a previous anterior cervical arthrodesis. J Bone Joint Surg Am 81:519–528.
15. Eck J, Humphreys S, Lim T, *et al.* 2002. Biomechanical study on the effect of cervical spine fusion on adjacent-level intradiscal pressure and segment motion. Spine 27:2431–2434.
16. Matsunaga S, Kabyama S, Yamamoto T, *et al.* 1999. Strain of intervertebral discs after anterior cervical decompression and fusion. Spine 24:670–675.

17. Pospiech J, Stolke D, Wilke H, *et al.* 1999. Intradiscal pressure recording in the cervical spine. Neurosurgery 44:379–385.

18. Weinhoffer S, Guyer R, Herbert M, *et al.* 1995. Intradiscal pressure measurements above an instrumented fusion. A cadaveric study. Spine 20:526–531.

19. Urban JP, Holm S, Mardous A, *et al.* 1982: Nutrition of the intervertebral disc: effect of fluid flow on solute transport. Clin Orthop Relat Res 170:296–302.

20. Shoda E, Sumi M, Kataoka O, *et al.* 1999. Development and dynamic canal stenosis as radiologic factors affecting surgical results of anterior cervical fusion for myelopathy. Spine 24:1421–1424.

21. McGrory B, Klassen R. 1994. Arthrodesis of the cervical spine for fractures and dislocations in children and adolescents. A long term follow up study. J Bone Joint Surg Am 76:1606–1614 .

22. Chang UK, Kim DH, Lee MC, *et al.* 2007. Range of motion change after cervical arthroplasty with ProDisc-C and Prestige artificial discs compared with anterior cervical discectomy and fusion. J Neurosurg Spine 7:40–46.

23. Guilee J, Miller A, Bowen J, *et al.* 1995. The natural history of Klippel-Feil syndrome: clinical, roentgenographic, and magnetic resonance imaging findings at adulthood. J Pediatric Orthop 15:617–626.

24. Le H, Rhongtrangan I, Kim D. 2004. Historical review of cervical arthroplasty. Neurosurg Focus 17:1–9.

25. Mummaneni P, Haid R. 2004. The future in the care of the cervical spine: interbody fusion and arthroplasty. J Neurosurg Spine 1:155–159.

26. Wingfield C, Gill S, Nelson R, *et al.* 2002. Influence of an artificial cervical joint compared with fusion on adjacent-level motion in the treatment of degenerative cervical disc disease. J Neurosurg (Spine1) 96:17–21.

27. Goffin J, Casey A, Kehr P, *et al.* 2002. Preliminary clinical experience with the Bryan cervical disc prosthesis. Neurosurgery 51:840–847.

28. Baaj AA, Uribe JS, Vale FL, *et al.* 2009. History of cervical disc arthroplasty. Neurosurg Focus 27(3):E10.

29. Ferntrom U. 1966. Arthroplasty with incorporated endoprosthesis in herniated disc and painful disc. Acts Chir Scand Suppl 357:154–159.

30. Cummins B, Robertson J, Gill S. 1998. Surgical experience with an implanted artificial cervical joint. J Neurosurg 88:943–948.

31. Wigfield C, Gill S, Nelson R, *et al.* 2002. The new Frenchay artificial cervical joint: results from a two year pilot study. Spine 2446–2452.

32. DiAngelo D, Foley K, Morrow B, *et al.* 2004. In vitro biomechanics of cervical disc arthroplasty with Pro-Disc-C total disc implant. Neurosurg Focus 17:44–54.

33. Bryan VJ. 2002. Cervical motion segment replacement. Eur Spine J 11:S92–S97.

34. Du J, Li M, Liu H, *et al.* 2011. Early follow-up outcomes after treatment of degenerative disc disease with the discover cervical disc prosthesis. Spine J April 13;2(4):281–289.

35. Miao J, Yu f, Shen Ye, *et al.* 2014. Clinical and radiographic outcomes of cervical disc replacement with a new prosthesis. Spine J. Jun 1;14(6):878–83.

36. Mummaneni P, Haid R. 2004. The future in the care of the cervical spine: interbody fusion and arthroplasty. J Neurosurg Spine 1:155–159.

37. Jaramillo-de la Torre JJ, Grauer JN, Yue JJ. 2008. Update on cervical disc arthroplasty: where are we and where are we going? Curr Rev Musculoskeletal Med June;1(2):124–30.

38. Bao QB, Mc Cullen GM, Highham PA, *et al.* 1996. The artificial disc: theory, design and materials. Biomaterials 17:1157–1167.

39. Smolders LA, Bergknut N, Kingma I, *et al.* 2012. Biomechanical evaluation of a novel nucleus pulposus prosthesis in canine cadaveric spines. Vet J 192:199–205.

40. Klokkevoid PR, Johnson P, Dadgostari S, *et al.* 2001. Early endosseous integration enhanced by dual acid etching of titanium: a torque removal study in the rabbit. Clin Oral Implants Res Aug;12(4):350–7.

41. Le Guehennc L, Soueidan A, Layrolle P., *et al.* 2007 Surface treatments of titanium dental implants for rapid osseointegration. Den Mater Jul;23(7): 844–854.

42. Yi. S, Lee DY, Ahn PG, *et al.* 2009. Radiologically documented adjacent-segment degeneration after cervical arthroplasty: characteristics and review of cases. Surg Neurol 72:325–329.

43. Adopted by the American Academy of Orthopaedic Surgeons Board of Directors. 2010. March 8. http://www.aaos.org/research/overviews/overviewlist.asp. Accessed on August 4, 2014.

44. Zychowicz ME. 2013. Pathophysiology of heterotopic ossification. Orthop Nurs May–Jun;32(3):173–7.

45. Jin YJ, Park SB, Kim MJ, *et al.* 2013. An analysis of heterotopic ossification in cervical disc arthroplasty: a novel morphologic classification of an ossified mass. Spine J Apr;13(4):408–20.

46. Coric D, Nunley PD, Guyer RD, *et al.* 2011. Prospective, randomized, multicenter study of cervical arthroplasty: 269 patients from the Kineflex/C artificial disc investigational device exemption study with a minimum 2-year follow-up: clinical article. J Neurosurg Spine 15(4):348–354.

47. Ding C, Hong Y, Liu H, *et al.* 2012. Intermediate clinical outcome of Bryan cervical disc replacement for degenerative disk disease and its effects on adjacent segment disks. Orthopedics 1;35(6):e909–916. doi:10.3928/01477447-20120525-33.

48. Beaurain J, Bernard P, Dufour T, *et al.* 2009 Intermediate clinical and radiological results of cervical TDR (Mobi-C) with up to 2 years of follow-up. Eur Spine J 18(6):841–850.

49. Guerin P, Obeid I, Bourghli A, *et al.* 2012. Heterotopic ossification after cervical disc replacement: clinical significance and radiographic analysis. A prospective study. Acta Orthop Belg 78(1):80–86.

50. Phillips FM, Tzermiadianos MN, Voronov Li, et al. 2009. Effect of two-level total disc replacement on cervical spine kinematics. Spine 15;34(22):E794–9.

51. Cardoso MJ, Rosner MK. 2010. Multilevel cervical arthroplasty with artificial disc replacement. Neurosurg Focus 28(5):E19.

52. Huppert J. Beaurain J, Steib JP, et al. 2011. Comparison between single- and multi-level patients: clinical and radiological outcomes 2 years after cervical disc replacement. Eur Spine J 20(9):1417–1426.

53. Sharp N, Wheeler S. 2005. Cervical disc disease. In Sharp W, ed. Small Animal Spinal Disorders. 2nd ed. Edinburg, Elsevier Mosby, pp. 93–120.

54. Morio Y, Teshima R, Nagashima H, et al. 2001. Correlation between operative outcomes of cervical compression myelopathy and MRI of the spinal cord. Spine 26:1238–1245.

55. Sharp N. 2002. Neurosurgical disasters. In Proceedings of the 20th Annual Meeting of the American College of Veterinary Internal Medicine Forum; 338–340.

56. Lemarie RJ, Kervin S, Partington B, et al. 2000. Vertebral subluxation following ventral cervical decompression in the dog. J Am Anim Hosp Assoc 36:348–358.

57. Sharp N, Wheeler S. 2005. Cervical spondylomyelopathy. In Wheeler S, eds. Small Animal Spinal Disorders, Diagnosis and Surgery. 2nd ed. Edinburgh, Elsevier Mosby, pp. 211–246.

58. Trotter E. 2009. Cervical spine locking plate fixation for treatment of cervical spondylotic myelopathy in large breeds. Vet Surg 38:705–718.

59. Chambers J, Oliver J, Kornegay J, et al. 1982. Ventral decompression for caudal cervical disk herniation in large- and giant-breed dogs. J Am Vet Med Assoc 180:410–414.

60. Bergman R, Levine J, Coates J, et al. 2008. Cervical spine locking plate in combination with cortical ring allograft for a one level fusion in dogs with cervical spondylotic myelopathy. Vet Surg 37:530–536.

61. Swaim SF. 1974. Ventral decompression of the cervical spinal cord in the dog. J Am Vet Med Assoc 164(5):491–495.

62. Zhang X, Ordway NR, Tan R, et al. 2008. Correlation of ProDisc-C failure strength with cervical bone mineral content and endplate strength. J Spinal Disord Tech 21:400–405.

63. Lin CY, Kang H, Rouleau JP, et al. 2009. Stress analysis of the interface between cervical vertebrae and end plates and the Bryan, Prestige LP, and ProDisc-C cervical disc prostheses: an in vivo image-based finite element study. Spine (Phila Pa 1976) 34:1554–1560.

64. Datta JC, Janssen ME, Beckman R, et al. 2007. Sagittal spit fractures in multilevel cervical arthroplasty using a keeled prosthesis. J Spinal Disord Tech 20:89–92.

65. Beaurain J, Bernard P, Dufour T, et al. 2009. Intermediate clinical and radiological results of

cervical TDR (Mobi-C) with up to 2 years of follow-up. Eur Spine J 18:841–850.

66. Wang Y, Zhang X, Xiao S, et al. 2010. Clinical report of cervical arthroplasty in management of spondylotic myelopathy (in Chinese). J Orthop Surg [serial online] 2006;1:13. Available at: www.josr-online.com/content/1/1/13. Accessed on June 2010.

67. Denaro V, Papalia R, Denaro L, et al. 2009. Cervical spine disc replacement. J Bone Joint Surg Br 91: 713–719.

68. Hi S, Lee DY, Ahn PG, et al. 2009. Radiologically documented adjacent-segment degeneration after cervical arthroplasty: characteristics and review of cases. Surg Neurol 72:325–329.

69. Goffin J, Van Calenberg F, van Loon J, et al. 2002. Preliminary clinical experience with the Bryan cervical disc prosthesis. Neurosurgery 51:840–845.

70. Cavanaugh DA, Nunly PD, Kerr EJ III, et al. 2009. Delayed hyper-reactivity to metal ions after cervical disc arthroplasty: a case report and literature review. Spine (Phila Pa 1976) 1;34:E262–E265.

71. Hakato J, Wronski J, Ciupik L. 2003. Subsidence and its effect on the anterior plate stabilization in the course of cervical spondylodesis. Part I: definition and review of the literature. Neurol Neurochir Pol 37(4):903–915.

72. Hallab NJ, Cunningham BW, Jacobs JJ. 2003. Spinal Implant debris-induced osteolysis. Spine (Phila Pa 1976) Oct 15;28(20):S125–38.

73. Cunningham BW, Orbegoso CM, Dimitriev AE, et al. 2002. The effect of spinal instrumentation particulate wear debris: An in vivo rabbit model and applied clinical study of retrieved instrumentation cases. Spine J 2:69–70.

74. Meir AR, Freeman BJ, Fraser RD, et al. 2013. Ten-year survival and clinical outcome of the AcroFlex lumbar disc replacement for the treatment of symptomatic disc degeneration. Spine J Jan;13(1):13–21. doi:10.1016/j.spinee.2012.12.008.

75. Tami AE, Leitner MM, Baucke MG, et al. 2009. Hydroxyapatite particles maintain peri-implant bone mantle during osseointegration in osteoporotic bone. Bone 45(6):1117–24. doi:10.1016/j.bone.2009.07.090. [Epub 2009 Aug 11].

76. Allegrini S, Rumpel E, Kauschke E, et al. 2006. Hydroxyapatite grafting promotes new bone formation and osseointegration of smooth titanium implants. Ann Anat 188(2):143–51. doi:10.1016/j.aanat.2005.08.019.

77. Cecconi S, Mattioli-Belmonte M, Manzotti S, et al. 2014. Bone-derived titanium coating improves in vivo implant osseointegration in an experimental animal model. J Biomed Mater Res B: Appl Biomater. 102(2):303–310.

78. Lin A, Wang CJ, Kelly J, et al. 2009. The role of titanium implant surface modification with hydroxyapatite nanoparticles in progressive early bone-implant fixation in vivo. Int J Oral Maxillofac Implants Sept–Oct;24(5):808–16.

79. Jung UW, Kim S, Lee IK, *et al.* 2014. Secondary stability of microthickness hydroxyapatite-coated dental implants installed without primary stability in dogs. Clin Oral Implants Oct;25(10):1169–74.

80. Lu Y, Lee JS, Nemke B, Graf BK, Royalty K, *et al.* 2012. Coating with a modular bone morphogenetic peptide promotes healing of a bone-implant gap in an ovine model. PLoS ONE 7(11):e50378. doi:10.1371/journal.pone.0050378.

81. German JW, Foley KT. 2005. Disc arthroplasty in the management of painful lumbar motion segment. Spine 30:(16 Suppl):S60–S67.

Index

Note: Page numbers in *italics* refer to Figures; those in **bold** to Tables

Advances in Intervertebral Disc Disease in Dogs and Cats, First Edition. Edited by James M. Fingeroth and William B. Thomas.
© 2015 ACVS Foundation. Published 2015 by John Wiley & Sons, Inc.